Department
of
Economic
and
Social
Affairs

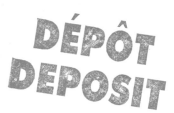

World YOUTH 2007 Report

**Young People's Transition to Adulthood:
Progress and Challenges**

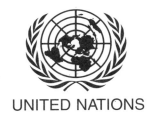

UNITED NATIONS

DESA

The Department of Economic and Social Affairs of the United Nations Secretariat is a vital interface between global policies in the economic, social and environmental spheres and national action. The Department works in three main interlinked areas: it compiles, generates and analyses a wide range of economic, social and environmental data and information on which States Members of the United Nations draw to review common problems and to take stock of policy options; it facilitates the negotiations of Member States in many intergovernmental bodies on joint courses of action to address ongoing or emerging global challenges; and it advises interested Governments on the ways and means of translating policy frameworks developed in United Nations conferences and summits into programmes at the country level and, through technical assistance, helps build national capacities.

Note:

The designations employed and the presentation of material in this publication do not imply the expression of any opinion whatsoever on the part of the Secretariat of the United Nations concerning the legal status of any country, territory, city or area or of its authorities, or concerning the delimitation of its frontiers or boundaries. The assignment of countries or areas to specific groupings is for analytical convenience and does not imply any assumption regarding political or other affiliation of countries or territories by the United Nations. The designations "developed" and "developing" are intended for statistical and analytical convenience and do not necessarily express a judgment about the stage reached by a particular country or area in the development process.

UN2
ST/ESA
2007W56

United Nations publication
Sales No. E.07.IV.1
ISBN 10: 92-1-130257-9
ISBN 13: 978-92-1-130257-8

Printed by the United Nations, New York

More than ten years after the adoption of the World Programme of Action for Youth to the Year 2000 and Beyond, it is clear that opportunities for young people have expanded in all world regions. However, major constraints persist. Youth around the world are presented with challenges and opportunities that are similar in many respects; however, the attendant dimensions and implications of these challenges and opportunities and the required policy interventions differ from one geographical and economic area to another.

In acknowledgement of these differences, the World Youth Report 2007 — Young People's Transition to Adulthood: Progress and Challenges *adopts a regional approach, highlighting the distinctive circumstances faced by young people living in each part of the world as they struggle to deal with issues of universal relevance. Each substantive chapter includes an overview of selected youth development challenges and constraints, focusing particularly on obstacles and opportunities relating to employment, education, poverty, and health (including HIV/AIDS), as well as area-specific socio-economic phenomena.*

The Report *highlights the unique aspects of youth development in various regions but emphasizes that young people the world over are ultimately constrained in their efforts to contribute to their own development and that of their communities by the absence of adequate opportunities to participate fully in the broader process of development. Priority must be given to enhancing the role of youth in all areas of social and economic development; this not only benefits young people themselves, but also fosters a sense of community and promotes national and international development.*

The theme of International Youth Day 2007 — Be Seen, Be Heard: Youth Participation for Development — resonates in the pages to come. In drawing attention to the obstacles and opportunities young people encounter in all regions of the world, this Report *effectively lays the groundwork for identifying and designing policy interventions that will offer youth the chance to be seen and heard.*

SHA ZUKANG
Under-Secretary-General for Economic and Social Affairs

Acknowledgements

This *Report* was produced through the collaboration of United Nations staff, experts and young people.

The World Youth Report 2007—Young People's Transition to Adulthood: Progress and Challenges represents a collaborative effort in which a number of experts, organizations and individuals—including young people—have participated.

The staff of the United Nations Programme on Youth, Department of Economic and Social Affairs, were responsible for the preparation of the report. Johan Schölvinck, Director of the Division for Social Policy and Development, and Sergei Zelenev, Chief of the Social Integration Branch, provided overall leadership and a review of the report as a whole.

Special gratitude goes to the consultants and specialists who provided textual and technical inputs for individual chapters. These individuals include Julio Carrion, University of Delaware, United States; Francis Chigunta, University of Zambia; Gaspar Fajth, UNICEF; David Gordon, Townsend Centre for International Policy Research, University of Bristol; Patricia Gordon, private consultant, London; Agnes Hars, KOPINT-DATORG Economic Research Institute, Budapest; S.T. Hettige, Social Policy Analysis and Research Center, University of Colombo, Sri Lanka; Graeme Hugo, National Center for Social Applications of GIS, University of Adelaide; Nader Kabbani, American University of Beirut; Om Mathur, National Institute of Public Finance and Policy, New Delhi; Mark J. Miller, University of Delaware, United States; Mansour Omeira, American University of Beirut; Ernesto Rodriguez, CELAJU-Latin American Center on Youth, Montevideo, Uruguay; Penelope Schoeffel, independent social development consultant, Sydney; Youfa Wang, Center for Human Nutrition, Department of International Health, Bloomberg School of Public Health, Johns Hopkins University, Maryland; and Jonathan J.H. Zhu, City University of Hong Kong. Although many of the submissions from the consultants have been revised or expanded to bring them in line with the theme of the report, the contributions of the consultants and specialists have been invaluable in shaping the final publication.

The report also builds upon background papers presented at various meetings organized by the Division for Social Policy and Development in 2006, including the Regional Expert Group Meeting on Development Challenges for Young People in Asia, hosted by the United Nations Economic and Social Commission for Asia and the Pacific in Bangkok from 28 to 30 March; and the Capacity-Building Workshop on Youth Development in Africa, hosted by United Nations Economic Commission for Africa in Addis Ababa from 27 to 29 June. Joop Theunissen played a key role in the conceptualization and organization of these meetings on youth and development.

Within the United Nations Secretariat, the core team charged with preparing the major inputs for the report included Fred Doulton, Anke Green, Charlotte van Hees, Peggy L. Kelly, Emily Krasnor, Julie Larsen, Jane Lowicki-Zucca, Girma Mulugetta, Eric Olson, Julie Pewitt, Patience Stephens, Makiko Tagashira and Sergei Zelenev. Inputs were also received from Samina Anwar, Irene Javakadze, Magdalena Krawczyk, and Dania Röpke. The United Nations Volunteers programme office in New York provided a number of examples of volunteerism in sub-Saharan Africa (see boxes 3.3–3.7). The staff of the United Nations Programme on Youth, led by Patience Stephens, the Focal Point for Youth, undertook the challenging task of arranging and integrating the voluminous and diverse pieces of information from various background papers, weaving them into a coherent story on the progress and challenges of young people around the world, and coordinating the production of the final report.

Emma Dumalag, Sylvie Pailler, Julie Pewitt and Dolores Vicente provided invaluable inputs and substantive editing of the report.

The World Youth Report 2007: Young People's Transition to Adulthood: Progress and Challenges also reflects the input of youth. The United Nations Secretariat is thankful to those young people and youth-led organizations that, through their contributions, have enabled us to see and reflect youth issues through the lenses, perspectives and experiences of young people themselves.

A special acknowledgement goes to the production team, including the editors, Ms. Terri Lore and Ms. Isabella Burns, and the design and layout by Ms. Diana de Filippi and Ms. Nancy Watt Rosenfeld, for their patience and dedication and for their assiduous work against tight deadlines to produce this report.

Deep gratitude also goes to all those who submitted designs, photographs and other contributions to be considered in the design of this volume.

**Unless otherwise indicated, the following country groupings
and subgroupings have been used in this report:**

Asia: China, Hong Kong Special Administrative Region of China, Macao Special Administrative Region of China, Democratic People's Republic of Korea, Japan, Mongolia, Republic of Korea, Afghanistan, Bangladesh, Bhutan, India, Islamic Republic of Iran, Maldives, Nepal, Pakistan, Sri Lanka, Brunei Darussalam, Cambodia, Indonesia, Lao People's Democratic Republic, Malaysia, Myanmar, Philippines, Singapore, Thailand, Timor-Leste, Viet Nam;

Sub-Saharan Africa: Angola, Benin, Botswana, Burkina Faso, Burundi, Cameroon, Cape Verde, Central African Republic, Chad, Comoros, Congo, Côte d'Ivoire, Democratic Republic of the Congo, Djibouti, Equatorial Guinea, Eritrea, Ethiopia, Gabon, Gambia, Ghana, Guinea, Guinea-Bissau, Kenya, Lesotho, Liberia, Madagascar, Malawi, Mali, Mauritania, Mauritius, Mayotte, Mozambique, Namibia, Niger, Nigeria, Réunion, Rwanda, Saint Helena, Sao Tome and Principe, Senegal, Seychelles, Sierra Leone, Somalia, South Africa, Swaziland, Togo, Uganda, United Republic of Tanzania, Zambia, Zimbabwe;

Latin America: Argentina, Belize, Bolivia, Brazil, Chile, Colombia, Costa Rica, Ecuador, El Salvador, Falkland Islands (Malvinas), French Guiana, Guatemala, Guyana, Honduras, Mexico, Nicaragua, Panama, Paraguay, Peru, Suriname, Uruguay, Venezuela;

Middle East and North Africa: Algeria, Bahrain, Djibouti, Egypt, Islamic Republic of Iran, Iraq, Israel, Jordan, Kuwait, Lebanon, Libyan Arab Jamahiriya, Malta, Morocco, Oman, Qatar, Saudi Arabia, Syrian Arab Republic, Tunisia, United Arab Emirates, Occupied Palestinian Territory, Yemen;

Eastern Europe and the Commonwealth of Independent States: Albania, Armenia, Azerbaijan, Belarus, Bosnia and Herzegovina, Bulgaria, Croatia, Czech Republic, Estonia, Georgia, Hungary, Kazakhstan, Kyrgyzstan, Latvia, Lithuania, Montenegro, Poland, Moldova, Romania, Russian Federation, Serbia, Slovakia, Slovenia, Tajikistan, Turkmenistan, Ukraine, Uzbekistan, former Yugoslav Republic of Macedonia;

Small island developing States: American Samoa, Anguilla, Antigua and Barbuda, Aruba, Bahamas, Barbados, Belize, British Virgin Islands, Cape Verde, Comoros, Cook Islands, Cuba, Dominica, Dominican Republic, Fiji, French Polynesia, Grenada, Guam, Guinea-Bissau, Guyana, Haiti, Jamaica, Kiribati, Maldives, Marshall Islands, Mauritius, Federated States of Micronesia, Montserrat, Nauru, Netherlands Antilles, New Caledonia, Niue, Northern Mariana Islands, Palau, Papua New Guinea, Puerto Rico, Samoa, Sao Tome and Principe, Seychelles, Singapore, Solomon Islands, Saint Kitts and Nevis, Saint Lucia, Saint Vincent and the Grenadines, Suriname, Timor-Leste, Tonga, Trinidad and Tobago;

Developed market economies: Australia, Austria, Belgium, Cyprus, Denmark, Finland, France, Germany, Greece, Iceland, Ireland, Italy, Japan, the Netherlands, New Zealand, Norway, Portugal, Spain, Sweden, Switzerland, United Kingdom of Great Britain and Northern Ireland, United States of America.

The following *abbreviations* have been used in the report:

ANSEJ	Algerian National Agency for the Support of Youth Employment
AUV	African Union Volunteers
CARICOM	Caribbean Community
CIS	Commonwealth of Independent States
ECOWAS	Economic Community of West African States
ESL	English as a second language
EU	European Union

GCC	Gulf Cooperation Council
GDP	gross domestic product
HDI	Human Development Index
HIV/AIDS	human immunodeficiency virus/acquired immunodeficiency syndrome
ICT	information and communication technologies
ILO	International Labour Organization
INJAZ	a Junior Achievement programme (Middle East/North Africa)
NAYOU	National Association of Youth Organizations in Uganda
NEET	not in employment, education or training
NEPAD	New Partnership for Africa's Development
OECD	Organization for Economic Cooperation and Development
PADEP	Peace and Development Programme (of ECOWAS)
PISA	Programme for International Student Assessment
PRSP	Poverty Reduction Strategy Paper
PSE	Poverty and Social Exclusion Survey of Britain
SADC	Southern African Development Community
SAR	Special Administrative Region (of China)
UNAIDS	Joint United Nations Programme on HIV/AIDS
UNDP	United Nations Development Programme
UNESCO	United Nations Educational, Scientific and Cultural Organization
UNICEF	United Nations Children's Fund
UNV	United Nations Volunteers
WAYN	West African Youth Network

Technical Note

In this publication, unless otherwise indicated, the term "youth" refers to all those between the ages of 15 and 24, as reflected in the World Programme of Action for Youth to the Year 2000 and Beyond. The term "young people" may be used interchangeably with the word "youth" in the text.

Photo credits:
Adam Rogers/UNCDF: cover and pages viii, xii, xiv, xlii, 5, 40, 78, 87, 113, 234.
Diego Goldberg/PixelPress/UNFPA, from the exhibition "Chasing the Dream, youth faces of the Millennium Development Goals" (www.chasingdream.org): pages 135, 139.
ShootExperience (UK):
  – Subira Mwanya: page xiii,
  – Simon Sewell: page 196,
  – Tanja Zenkovich: page 199
  – Laura Little: page 231
  – Ella Bryant: page 232
  – Joy Kim: page 247
TakingITGlobal: cover and page ix.
UN/DPI Photo Library: cover and pages x, xiii, xiv, 8, 10, 22, 41, 45, 46, 67, 72, 77, 82, 89, 114, 140, 154, 158, 165, 169, 170, 200, 227.
UN/DSPD staff: cover and pages i, vii, viii, xi, xiv.

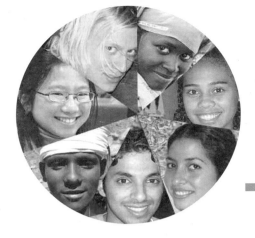

TABLE OF CONTENTS

Chapter 1
Asian Youth in the Context of Rapid Globilization   1

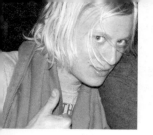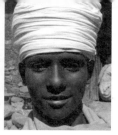

Chapter 2

Latin American Youth in an Era of Socio-Economic and Political Change 46

Chapter 3

Overcoming the Barriers of Poverty: Challenges for Youth Participation in Sub-Saharan Africa 78

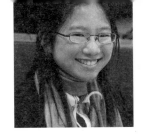

Chapter 4

Labour Market Participation among Youth in the Middle East and North Africa and the Special Challenges Faced by Young Women   114

Chapter 5

Tackling the Poverty of Opportunity in Small Island Developing States   140

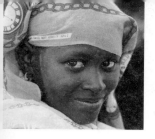

Chapter 6

Labour Market Challenges and New Vulnerabilities for Youth in Economies in Transition   170

Chapter 7

Opportunities for Youth Development in Developed Market Economies: an Unequal Playing Field   200

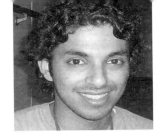

Chapter 8

Ensuring Youth Development around the World: the Way Forward 232

Statistical Annex

Introduction 249

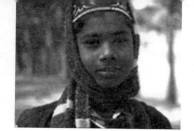

Tables

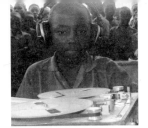
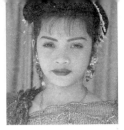

Figures

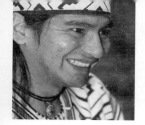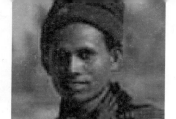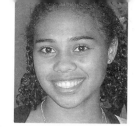

Figures (continued)

Boxes

The General Assembly, in paragraph 8(a) of the World Programme of Action for Youth, adopted by its resolution 50/81 of 14 December 1995, emphasized that "every State should provide its young people with opportunities for obtaining education, for acquiring skills and for participating fully in all aspects of society." Twelve years later, youth development in all world regions continues to be constrained by persistent obstacles at the community, national and international levels. For the purposes of this report, youth development entails actions and investments that enable youth to complete consistently and effectively the transition into adulthood and to take advantage of opportunities to develop and use their human capital in the process. Youth development requires that Governments and other stakeholders design and implement policies and programmes to protect young people from the negative social and environmental influences that can derail the transition into healthy adulthood.

The 1.2 billion people between the ages of 15 and 24 years in 2007—those the United Nations refers to as "youth" or "young people"—are the best educated youth generation in history. Constituting 18 per cent of the world's population, today's youth are a tremendous resource for national development. There is clear evidence of the determination of today's youth for self-improvement and their commitment to improving the social, political and economic fabric of society through individual and group action. For example, young people in all regions are actively exploiting the Internet to improve their education, upgrade their skills and find jobs; youth are contributing to the global debate on major development and policy issues through participation in social action groups and other volunteer activities, and they are migrating in large numbers, sometimes risking their own lives and losing connections to families and friends, to find better options outside their national borders.

However, the benefits that can be harnessed from the large and dynamic youth population do not accrue automatically. Since the period of youth is also one of transition from childhood dependency to independent adulthood, it can be tumultuous and prolonged. However, when societies provide adequate guidance and opportunities for youth to build their capacity to contribute to development by investing in their education, health, employment and sports and leisure activities, young people's abilities and capabilities can be unleashed early, and their contribution to development can be realized.

The *World Youth Report 2007—Young People's Transition to Adulthood: Progress and Challenges* argues that to benefit from young people's capabilities, societies must ensure that opportunities for youth to be engaged in development processes are nurtured and protected. Failure to do so can lead to the exclusion and marginalization of youth while depriving societies of their energy, dynamism and innovativeness. The report notes that the ability of youth to contribute to the development of their societies can be constrained not only by lack of capacity among youth, but also by the limited opportunities for participation in development as the global economy and social and political institutions undergo major change. For this reason, there is a pressing need for policies that not only build youth potential, but also open doors to youth participation in areas such as employment, civic engagement, political participation and volunteerism. An enabling environment must be created to provide youth with opportunities to be heard and seen as active players on the development stage.

In a review of key issues, opportunities and challenges for youth transitions in different world regions, the report finds that there are many unique aspects to the progress that youth have made and the challenges that they continue to face around the world. A common constraint everywhere, however, is the absence of an enabling environment for youth development and participation. Factors such as inadequate investments in education, high private costs of obtaining quality education and health care, and shrinking labour markets in which youth are often the last hired and first fired all present youth with real obstacles to meaningful participation in the development of their communities.

In some regions, large numbers of youth have not attained the levels of education that would enable them to compete effectively in the labour market. In other regions, youth have attained high levels of education but cannot find jobs because of a mismatch between the knowledge and skills they have acquired and those needed in a changing labour market. In all regions, globalization and changing labour markets have caused opportunities in the labour market for youth to shrink.

The focus of each of the core chapters of the World Youth Report 2007 on a different geographical or economic region allows more detailed examination of some of the specific factors that have fostered or constrained youth participation. Not all issues affecting youth transitions to adulthood are analysed in each regional chapter. Instead, aspects of a set of key interrelated issues that affect youth transition in the particular region are reviewed. Some issues, such as education, health, employment, and poverty, cut across all chapters as they crucially determine the nature and course of the transition of all youth. However, the findings and conclusions of each chapter lend unique insight into the factors that have enabled and constrained the transition of youth to adulthood around the world.

ASIA

Of the global youth labour force of 633 million in 2005, some 353 million (55.7 per cent) lived in Asia. Among the most important factors that will influence whether and how Asian economies continue to benefit from their sizeable youth population is how much of an opportunity youth have to develop their potential through education, decent employment opportunities and adequate health care.

Compared with other regions, globalization has arguably had the most impact on the rapidly growing Asian economies. In addressing the challenges and opportunities related to globalization and education in Asia, the report notes that the openness of these economies and the exposure to foreign goods, services and information has significantly changed the lives, values and culture of many young Asians. Globalization has, however, also fostered the coexistence of affluence and poverty and widened inequalities within and between countries. While many young people benefit from increased education options and from the new industries that moved to Asia, others continue to be restricted by inadequate schooling and poverty and are outside the reach of the basic information, goods and services that have become available with globalization.

Access to education has expanded in many parts of Asia, but the gains are most noticeable at the primary level. Girls are increasingly benefiting from primary education. In India, for example, the proportion of girls enrolled in primary education rose from 84 to 96 per cent between 1998 and 2002. Nevertheless, many countries in the region, particularly those in South Asia, still have a long way to go to achieve gender parity in education. The near-universality of primary education in Asia also comes too late for many of today's youth, who should have been in primary school some 10 to 20 years ago. In India, more than half of young women aged 15-19 years have no primary education.

Despite progress at the primary level, investment and enrolment rates at the secondary and higher levels lag. Though tertiary education has expanded rapidly in Asia in recent years, there continue to be shortfalls in availability and access, especially for marginalized groups of youth. This situation is worrisome in view of the fact that secondary education has increasingly become the lowest level of schooling required to participate in the global labour market.

Improvements have occurred in the quality of education in Asia, but progress has been uneven. This situation reflects a shortage of adequately trained teachers, large class sizes and high pupil-to-teacher ratios.

Youth living in poverty, youth living in rural areas, girls and young women, youth with disabilities, youth from ethnic minorities and youth who are refugees or who have been displaced by war or natural disasters have benefited less from progress in the region. As a result, these groups are likely to be excluded from household, community, and national decision-making processes.

Although many young people across Asia are now better prepared than ever before to enter the workforce, a large proportion are unable to secure employment. In South-East Asia and the Pacific, youth are five times more likely than older workers to be unemployed. In South Asia and East Asia, youth are almost three times as likely to be unemployed as adults. In all regions, the level of youth unemployment likely masks underemployment and poverty among working youth. Young women find it especially difficult to secure decent work and are more likely to be employed in the informal economy, where they are typically paid less than men and do a disproportionate share of unpaid domestic work.

Globalization has significantly changed the values and culture of youth, who more readily challenge traditional authority structures, but also experience disorientation and anomie caused by the day-to-day clashes between traditional and modern values and norms. Changing family structures have eroded many of the traditional constraints imposed on young people, but at a cost. The support systems on which they previously relied in times of difficulty have weakened. This has contributed to the emergence of lifestyles that place many young people at risk.

Interactions between injecting drug use and unprotected sex are driving serious HIV/AIDS epidemics. It is estimated that 2.2 million young people live with HIV/AIDS in Asia. Early pregnancy and its attendant risks of high maternal and child mortality also remain a problem in the region. Tobacco use, substance abuse and excessive consumption of alcohol, as well as poor dietary practices, all contribute to derailing the progress of young people towards independent and responsible adulthood. Young men are much more likely than young women to drink, smoke or use drugs and are more likely to start doing so at younger ages.

The challenges posed by unhealthy behaviour are compounded by difficulties in accessing health care. There is limited access to sexual education and inadequate access to youth-friendly health services. Family planning programmes, messages and information, for example, are often targeted at married people. Unmarried young people thus often have limited knowledge of contraception.

Asia is a major receiving and sending region for migrants. Job opportunities outside home communities and countries have encouraged millions of young Asians to become mobile on both a permanent and a non-permanent basis. Opportunities for migration to OECD countries have increased for highly skilled Asian youth, resulting in considerable outflows of the most qualified and brightest young people in many countries. Although women are underrepresented among international migrants living in Asia, they are dominant among migrant workers in several Asian sending countries. One dimension of migration that is of particular significance for Asian youth is student migration. East Asia and the Pacific are increasingly receiving international students. At the same time, these regions contribute the largest group of students studying abroad (29 per cent of the global total of mobile students worldwide). In absolute terms, China is the country with the largest share of internationally mobile migrants and accounts for 14 per cent of all mobile students.

In many cases, migration improves the status of youth within their families back home. Through the remittances they send home, young migrants may "earn the right" to participate in, and influence, family decision-making and the welfare of other family members.

The *World Youth Report 2007* addresses the transitions of Latin American youth to adulthood within the context of the profound political, economic and social changes that have occurred in the region over the past 30 years. A combination of low-quality education and lack of employment opportunities has contributed to poverty and fuelled widespread migration out of the region. The poor socio-economic situation has also negatively affected the political fervour once so characteristic of the region.

Latin American countries have made impressive progress in providing young people with educational opportunities. The net enrolment ratio for primary school is 95 per cent; this is higher than the developing world average of 85 per cent, and several countries in the region have achieved in universal primary enrolment. Gender disparity in literacy and educational attainment is also relatively small when compared with other regions in the world, with girls having higher enrolment rates than boys.

Despite educational gains, much more needs to be done to address large and persistent inequalities in access to education. Wide gaps persist between rich and poor, between those living in urban and in rural areas, and between indigenous and non-indigenous populations. A large proportion of the region's youth (almost one third of 20- to 24-year-olds in 2002) have not completed their primary education. The situation in terms of secondary education is even worse. Two out of three young people between the ages of 20 and 24 had not completed secondary school in 2002.

With respect to employment and income levels, Latin American youth are worse off today than they were 15 years ago. At a critical time in their lives, when they need to acquire skills and work experience, a significant proportion of youth is neither in school nor at work. In 2002, about 18 per cent of those between the ages of 15 and 19 were neither studying nor working, and about 27 per cent of those between 20 and 24 were in a similar situation. Although youth, as a whole, encounter severe difficulties in the labour market, those between the ages of 15 and 19 are most affected in terms of income and unemployment. If they abandon school at this age, as many do, it is very difficult for them to find a job. When young people do find jobs, they are often in family-owned businesses, small and low-productivity firms, domestic employment or the informal economy, all of which offer low incomes and little or no labour protection.

It appears that the educational attainment of young women in the region has not helped to improve their position in the labour market. Problems with unemployment and underemployment are particularly severe for young women, who face both higher unemployment rates and lower wages than their male peers.

Poverty and inequality continue to afflict Latin America. After children under 14 years (the poorest segment of society), young people aged 15-19 constitute the second highest proportion living in poverty. Non-monetary aspects of poverty, in particular the lack of a healthy living environment, impinge on many young people's successful transition to independent adulthood. Early pregnancy and early parenthood, as well as a large unmet need for reproductive health services, reduce young women's opportunities. Youth are also significantly affected by the spread of HIV/AIDS and by a high incidence of violence, in which young men tend to be both the main perpetrators and the main victims.

Migration has become one of the coping mechanisms with which young people seek to overcome the lack of opportunities at home. Migration is also a tacit acceptance of the status quo, which young people may view as unchangeable, or not worthy of the effort. Young people are more likely than adults to migrate within their own countries, but they also make up a sizeable share of international migrants. Better educational and work opportunities are the main drivers of both internal and international migration. However, the reality of migrants' lives is often not what youth had expected. Migrants are often concentrated in low-skill occupations, and potential questions about their legal status make many migrants reluctant to demand the observance of host country labour codes and to assert their human rights. Undocumented migrants can also be prey to exploitation, have little or no access to health care and face bleak educational prospects.

Despite recent evidence of youth engagement, a region-wide survey conducted in 2004 suggests that the political fervour that characterized many Latin American societies in the past may have receded. The survey results indicated that only slightly more than half of Latin American youth strongly preferred democracy to other types of Government, and only a third of young people claimed to be "very interested" or "somewhat interested" in politics. The relatively low levels of interest in politics among Latin American youth corresponded to relatively low levels of political activism, at least in the activities that were probed by the survey. Young people only outperformed older citizens in participation in illegal protests.

Many factors account for the transition in the political fervour in Latin America, including changing political structures, voter fatigue, a growing distrust of political parties and frequent political scandals. In addition to these political factors, however, the emergence and persistence of various social and economic constraints have impinged on the ability of young people to participate in political processes. Having to find means to survive may push youth out of the political landscape. A significant improvement in political engagement by young people cannot be achieved without addressing maladies that affect the citizenry at large and youth issues in particular. Evidence shows that education has a positive impact on political participation. Better educated youth are more likely to have greater knowledge of their rights and are more inclined to assert them by engaging in political activism. Education thus not only increases the potential for better earnings, but also the quality of participatory democracy by encouraging greater involvement in public affairs.

Youth are, and will remain, a significant share of sub-Saharan Africa's population for many years to come. The failure to provide opportunities for this large generation could have enormous economic, cultural, political and social consequences. Engaging youth fully in the region's development is thus not a matter of choice, but rather an imperative. The report addresses the role of poverty in constraining youth development in the region.

Between 1983 and 1992, when most of today's youth were born, the majority of sub-Saharan African countries suffered major social and economic setbacks. The measures taken to promote recovery, including structural adjustment and liberalization policies, resulted in major retrenchment and job losses and the withdrawal of State subsidies for social services. Many households experienced extreme difficulty in accessing basic goods and services, including those needed to support the education and health of their children, today's generation of youth.

The percentage of youth who live in poverty continues to be extremely high in sub-Saharan Africa. It is estimated, for example, that over 90 per cent of Nigerian and Zambian youth (almost 40 million) live on less than US $2 per day. Non-monetary dimensions of poverty, such as nutritional deprivation, as well as the lack of electricity and access to water, also affect large segments of the region's youth population. The importance of basic household facilities cannot be overemphasized. In the absence of water in the household, youth, especially girls, are often responsible for fetching water not only for their own households, but also for others. This detracts from self-development and involves risks of exploitation. Moreover, access to electricity is fundamental to benefiting from modern technologies such as computers, which not only facilitate communication but may also offer distance-learning opportunities for youth.

Compared with other areas of socio-economic development in sub-Saharan Africa, the greatest progress has been achieved in education. Net primary school enrolment increased from 57 per cent in 1999 to 70 per cent in 2005; however, on average, almost one in three children continue to be out of school. In comparison with other world regions, secondary school enrolment rates in sub-Saharan Africa also remain very low, with little change recorded in recent years. Similarly, young people's prospects of remaining in tertiary education for a substantial period of time are remote in most African countries.

Many factors account for the inability of youth to complete education in Africa. Foremost among these reasons is the cost of schooling, including non-tuition costs such as uniforms, books and transportation. The poor quality of the education system may also account for high repetition and low completion rates. In the mid-1990s, for example, more than 70 per cent of primary school teachers in Burkina Faso had no professional qualification. This has serious implications for the quality of education received by young people graduating from primary school.

For girls, low enrolment rates are due to persistent gender inequalities in access to schooling, especially at the tertiary level. Young women in Africa are therefore more likely to face a difficult transition into the workplace and into independent adulthood. This, in turn, contributes to their exclusion from decision-making, even about issues that affect their personal lives.

In recent years, there has been some improvement in access to education. Between 1991 and 2004, tertiary enrolment in the region nearly doubled, in part owing to increased investment and economic recovery in a number of countries. Nevertheless, one out of every 16 students from the region is pursuing tertiary education abroad because of the limited opportunities for quality education at home.

Young people's inability to continue their education and their need to earn an income to a large extent accounts for the many young people seeking work. The formal labour market in Africa is still small, however, and remains inaccessible to youth who lack adequate skills, experience and strong social networks. Because of the limited vacancies in the job market, the number of unemployed youth in all of Africa grew by about 34 per cent between 1995 and 2005. As the fastest growing labour force in the world, youth in sub-Saharan Africa will be increasingly difficult to accommodate in the labour market in the future if appropriate employment policies are not instituted in the next few years.

Many young people are forced to undertake jobs that are characterized by poor conditions. In addition to the informal sector, agriculture has been a refuge for many young people. In 2005, youth accounted for 65 per cent of agricultural employment. This sector is characterized by low and precarious incomes and the development of little, if any, useful work experience for youth. Consequently, many young people experience poverty despite the fact that they are working. Sub-Saharan Africa is the only region that has seen a sharp and continuous increase in the total number of working-poor youth.

In addition to lacking quality education and decent work opportunities, young people in sub-Saharan Africa also face serious health problems. The number of new HIV/AIDS cases in Africa continues to grow and is rising faster than treatment services are being scaled up. Estimates suggest that young women's HIV prevalence rates are twice as high as those for young men. HIV/AIDS has also had a major impact on other age groups, with repercussions for youth. For example, the high morbidity and mortality caused by the epidemic are also affecting the availability of teachers.

While HIV/AIDS has been devastating to Africa's youth, there are other causes for concern. Some of the leading causes of death for those aged 15 to 29 years of age in the region are tuberculosis, malaria, unsafe abortion and road traffic accidents, as well as war and violence.

The region has experienced many armed conflicts over the past decade, which has had both direct and indirect consequences for youth. Youth have not only been among the victims of violence; they have also frequently been recruited into the militias and armies that have perpetrated violence. In a culture where youth often have no voice and no opportunities to develop, recruitment into militias has been easy, especially when it comes with the promise of some meagre remuneration or power. There have also been indirect consequences resulting from armed conflict, including the displacement of populations, the breakdown of health and social services and the heightened risk of disease transmission. In combination with poverty, such conflict has deepened the alienation of young people from society and has hampered their ability to participate fully in development, even after the cessation of hostilities.

In view of the demographic and socio-economic realities in the region, African Governments are increasingly putting in place national youth policies aimed at supporting the well-being of young people. However, much remains to be done to advance a comprehensive approach to youth development. Intergenerational partnerships need to be strengthened and programmes undertaken that address the full range of priorities contained in the World Programme of Action for Youth. In addition to benefiting from Government policies, youth in sub-Saharan Africa are also increasingly taking their development into their own hands; the recent African Youth Charter is a testament to their effort. They are more and more involved in voluntary activities that promote both the development of their own potential and that of their communities.

MIDDLE EAST AND NORTH AFRICA

Shortages of decent jobs, low wages, a mismatch of skills and labour market needs, and socio-economic exclusion constrain the transition from school-to-work in the Middle East and North Africa countries. Young women, in particular, face numerous difficulties as the intersecting influences of gender and age limit the avenues for their economic participation. The report therefore examines progress and constraints in youth development in the countries of this region, with a focus on employment opportunities and related gender aspects.

Unemployment in the Middle East and North Africa is primarily a youth issue rather than a generalized population issue. Despite the fact that young people represent only about one third of the total working-age population, they account for almost half of all unemployed people in the region. The current labour market situation has evolved over many decades and is a result of a combination of demographic, social, economic, political and cultural factors.

The region's population more than tripled from 1960 to 2005, and between 1995 and 2005 the youth labour force grew by 30 per cent. The region is the only one in the world in which the share of youth who are employed has increased over the past decade. However, since not enough new jobs were created in either the public or private sectors to accommodate the entering young job seekers, unemployment rates soared and eventually led many young people to drop out of the labour force entirely. Consequently, the region now holds the distinction of having both the highest rate of youth unemployment in the world and the lowest rate of youth labour force participation (40 per cent), especially for young women (25 per cent). The region also has the lowest youth employment-to-population rate (29.7 per cent) in the world. This means that only one in three young people in the region has a job.

Since the 1970s, some countries in the region have spent more on public education as a share of GDP than any other developing region in the world. This investment has paid off in terms of higher levels of educational attainment. Literacy and average years of schooling have increased significantly across the region, and the gender gap in average years of schooling has been closing rapidly. Nevertheless, significant gender differences in illiteracy rates remain. In North Africa, illiteracy rates among young females are twice those of young males. The gender difference is, however, almost identical for youth and adults in the subregion, suggesting that illiteracy patterns may be persisting across generations.

In much of the Middle East and North Africa, increased education is not necessarily leading to more or better jobs for young people. The education that many young people in the region receive is not compatible with the needs and priorities of the labour market. In addition, the quality of education in some countries of the region has been considerably affected by armed conflict.

Apart from the labour market pressures caused by demographic factors and the mismatch between education and needed work skills, slow growth in many of the economies in the region has constrained opportunities for job creation. Job opportunities for youth in the private sector are also constrained by bureaucratic obstacles to the development and expansion of private enterprises.

The public sector in countries of the Middle East and North Africa has been the major source of employment since the 1960s, especially for those with high levels of education. In recent years, however, Governments have begun to implement rationalization programmes, to privatize State enterprises and to encourage youth to seek jobs in the private sector. As long as public sector wages and benefits remain high relative to those in the private sector, many young workers, especially women, will prefer to wait. Those who cannot afford to be unemployed are forced to accept work in the informal economy, often with lower wages, lack of benefits and poor working conditions.

Given the limited job opportunities at home, youth in the region have increasingly resorted to migrating internally and internationally in search of jobs. Trends towards increasing urbanization are prevalent throughout the region and are expected to continue. While 59 per cent of the Middle East and North Africa population lived in cities in 2003, this share is projected to increase to 70 per cent by 2030.

In all regions, certain groups of youth are excluded from accessing the full benefits of development. In the Middle East and North Africa, young women are among the most disadvantaged groups, particularly with respect to their employment situation. Although young women are increasingly participating in labour markets in the region, the rate of increase is slowing. The average labour force participation rate for female youth remained at 25.1 per cent in 2005, the lowest in the world and well below the rate of 54.3 per cent for young men in the region.

The economic participation of young women in the region is influenced by their roles in the family, worksite segregation, opportunities for advancement and inequality in incomes. Women are often restricted from commuting, travelling or migrating to take up a job. This can create barriers to women's entry into the labour force. Gender inequalities in social security regimes also hinder young women's transition to economic independence. In more than half of the States in the region, men and women are not equally entitled to non-wage benefits and young women are often dependent on their families for social and economic security.

Given the difficulties that youth in the region face in finding and securing decent employment opportunities and the restrictions that this places on their ability to participate fully in their societies, active policy interventions are indispensable in assisting youth to gain entry into the labour market. Early intervention is needed to avoid tracking girls into traditionally female specializations and to help open up new areas for them to fuel their confidence and ambitions. Labour demand, particularly in the private sector, must be further stimulated in order to absorb youth entering the labour market. For those who, for various reasons, continue to face difficulties finding decent employment, social protection systems that are available to both young men and women are crucial.

SMALL ISLAND DEVELOPING STATES

As in other regions, young people growing up in small island developing States have to cope with a lack of quality education and employment opportunities as well as with the resulting pressure to migrate. In contrast to other regions, the reasons behind these problems within the small island developing States tend to be related to the countries' small population sizes and relative geographical remoteness. Moreover, the fact that some of these States have only recently shifted from traditional societies to more modern lifestyles is creating not only opportunities, but also challenges for today's youth.

Youth make up a considerable portion of the populations living in small island developing States and are an important resource to be tapped. The share of youth in the total population ranges from about one eighth to almost one fourth, and the size of the youth population is expected to increase significantly by 2015.

To build the capacity of future generations of youth, the quality and reach of education must be improved. While education is expanding in the region, various challenges remain. Although most small island developing States have high primary enrolment rates, the survival rate to the last grade of primary school continues to vary widely. For example, whereas in Barbados 99.5 per cent of girls and 95.7 per cent of boys complete primary school, only 55.9 per cent of children in the Comoros stay in primary school until the last grade. Poverty hinders many young people from participating in education. Moreover, given their many isolated rural communities and outer-island populations, many small island developing States are struggling to provide education to children outside urban areas. Nevertheless, gross secondary enrolment rates have generally increased since the late 1990s, and the great majority of small island developing States have achieved gender parity in secondary education or have even more girls enrolled than boys.

Owing to their small population sizes and lack of suitably trained teaching staff, many small island developing States are also unable to establish national universities, forcing youth to pursue tertiary education abroad. To respond to this challenge, some of these States have set up joint universities through subregional partnerships.

Equipping those students who are able to attend school with skills to enable them to participate meaningfully in a volatile labour market is a major challenge for the education sector in most small island developing States. Governments are finding it difficult to keep pace with the rapid rate of change and technological development resulting from globalization and have stressed the need for curriculum reform. In addition, the quality of education provided by many schools in small island developing States is poor. Young people with secondary education frequently lack marketable skills, and vocational training opportunities continue to be limited. For example, vocational schools in Solomon Islands have only 1,200 places for a youth population of over 90,000.

Although it has slightly declined over the past decade, youth unemployment continues to be high in most small island developing States; one in five youth is unemployed in the Caribbean. Young women's higher attainments in education do not seem to translate into gains in their employment prospects, as they are still much more likely to be unemployed than young men. In Saint Lucia, almost half of all young women in the labour market are unemployed.

Small island developing States face a variety of structural problems that limit employment opportunities for all age groups. These include scarce resources, limited capital and a relatively undeveloped business sector. In addition, sustained population growth has led to annual labour force increases that greatly exceed the rate of job creation in the formal sector. Thus, job opportunities are frequently only available in informal or traditional sectors that do not meet young people's expectations and are not highly regarded by society.

The probability of youth migration in the region is among the highest in the world as rural youth seek job opportunities and a more exciting life in urban areas or overseas.

Remittances from international migrants have become an important supplement, not only to household incomes, but also to countries' GDPs. Of the 20 countries with the highest remittances as a percentage of GDP, seven are small island developing States. In Tonga, remittances make up 31 per cent of GDP, the highest percentage worldwide. Owing to the increased reliance on remittances in Pacific small island developing States, it is common for families to groom their youth for employment overseas. Many do not return.

Social change in small island developing States has had a profound effect on youth, particularly on young men. Traditionally, men and women have had ascribed social roles, particularly in the Pacific. Guided by these roles, youth were led into adulthood. Today, traditional male roles and activities have largely become obsolete, but for those without access to secondary education or employment, they have often not been replaced by alternative roles. In contrast, many young women continue to take on the traditional roles of wives, mothers and caregivers. Modernity has thus created far greater discontinuity between youth and adulthood for young men than for young women.

With traditional gender and other social norms persisting and large portions of the population remaining economically vulnerable, the health and safety of youth in small island developing States remains seriously at risk. Youth, young women in particular, continue to be at risk of contracting diseases such as HIV/AIDS, and of being abused and exploited in their homes and communities. The social alienation experienced by many young people expresses itself in a range of endemic social problems, ranging from violence to risky sexual behaviour to youth suicide.

Youth in small island developing States face a variety of health and related problems. Chief among them are teenage pregnancies and HIV/AIDS. Of all regions for which data are available, young people living in the Caribbean have sex at the earliest age. Early sexual activity and low rates of contraceptive use combine to produce high rates of teenage pregnancy, particularly for those with little education and those living in rural areas. Teenage pregnancies not only pose health risks, but given the limited support for child care, also reduce young women's life opportunities. In an effort to prevent premarital sex, adolescent girls are often denied the freedoms and choices allowed to adolescent boys, and families restrict their movements, including sometimes school attendance. While this certainly limits possibilities for girls' early sexual contacts, it also interferes with their chances of completing their schooling and thus the opportunities for their future lives.

Related to early sexuality and lack of sexual education in small island developing States is the increasing vulnerability of youth to HIV infection. The Caribbean as a whole has the second highest HIV prevalence rate in the world. In contrast, the overall picture of HIV/AIDS in the Pacific small island developing States is fairly positive, with relatively low youth prevalence rates.

Another health-related challenge in small island developing States is the high prevalence of non-communicable diseases, including the increase in the incidence of obesity over the past several decades. High rates of youth suicide are also a matter of serious concern and may be related to the lack of opportunities that young people face in some small island developing States.

A combination of social alienation, lack of opportunity, and high unemployment of large numbers of youth in unstable, poorly managed urban settings contributes to gang violence and civil unrest in the region. Evidence suggests that violent crime is usually concentrated in poor urban communities, and most offences are committed by young people. In Jamaica, for example, young people constitute almost two thirds of those found guilty of crimes, with men four times more likely to be found guilty than women.

COUNTRIES WITH ECONOMIES IN TRANSITION

Those who are now 15-24 years old in Eastern Europe and the Commonwealth of Independent States (CIS) were born in the last decade of the communist regimes. In the 1980s and 1990s, they experienced great change in their immediate social environments, which included a mix of difficulties and uncertainties, as well as new possibilities. In particular, the socio-economic transformation that has taken place in this region over the past two decades has given rise to significant changes in labour market prospects for youth. Many youth in the region are experiencing vulnerability, poverty and social exclusion that have in many cases encouraged risky behaviour, including substance abuse and unsafe sexual practices. This in turn has helped fuel the spread of HIV/AIDS. Numbers of new infections have increased twenty-fold in less than a decade, and 75 per cent of reported infections were in people younger than 30 years.

Under State socialism, work was provided by the State for all, and employment was not just an option but a duty. Efficiency considerations and market demands were not taken into account. When young people completed secondary school, they went through a regimented system of job placement. While choice was limited, the system provided young people a feeling of security, assured a largely predictable path from school to work and gave access to all benefits and social services provided by State-owned enterprises. The political and economic change brought on by democratization was accompanied by a diminished role of the State and carried with it new expectations for young people's self-sufficiency and initiative. Although new economic and social opportunities opened up, security and predictability were gone, creating new sources of vulnerability for societies at large, including the youth population.

With the demise of State socialism and the elimination of artificial labour hoarding, employment rates for youth, as well as for the general population, decreased rapidly in all countries of the region. Serious job losses accompanied economic restructuring. New jobs were created at a much slower rate and within different sectors, in information and communication technologies and other high-tech industries, or in services, trade and the banking sector. Those who could adjust to the new demands of labour markets were able to benefit from these new opportunities. New windows of opportunity are important, and quite often they are seized by young people, but such opportunities are limited and may not compensate for the risks associated with substantially decreased social protection.

Although the level of insecurity in the region has increased, young people as a rule remain more optimistic than the older generations. According to opinion polls conducted in the countries of the region, young people support political and economic change more strongly than older generations.

Faced with labour market difficulties, youth have resorted to self-employment, or temporary and part-time work. Others have withdrawn from the labour market altogether after having become discouraged with their prospects of finding formal employment. The percentage of youth who are not in school and not employed is a good indicator of the non-utilized potential of the young labour force. In Central and Eastern Europe, this percentage is 33.6, the highest in the world.

Education has also been affected by the demise of State socialism. Before the transition, primary and secondary school enrolment was very high. During the transition, both primary and secondary school enrolment decreased in some countries of the region. By contrast, higher education enrolment has continuously increased in most transition economies, slowly at the beginning of the transition and at a more rapid pace in recent years. The share of young women in tertiary education has grown in many countries of the region and now exceeds that of young men. This increase may reflect the fact that some youth, especially young women, tend to "hide" in the education system, and postpone the school-to-work transition in the hope that eventually the economy may improve to a point where decent jobs become widely available.

With a youth unemployment rate of more than double the overall unemployment rate, young people's social exclusion has increased in most transition economies. This exclusion undoubtedly underlies the growth of the HIV/AIDS pandemic in the region, as social exclusion, vulnerability and poverty among youth often lead to risky behaviours, including substance abuse and unsafe sex. These behaviours, in turn, have fuelled the rapid growth of HIV/AIDS in the region.

Eastern Europe and the CIS is the region with the fastest growing HIV/AIDS epidemic in the world, and young people account for over half of all new infections. Current statistics give a strong indication that the overwhelming majority of people living with HIV/AIDS in Eastern Europe and the CIS countries are under age 30. Injecting drug use, in particular the sharing of needles and syringes, accounts for more than 70 per cent of HIV cases in the region, and youth make up a significant number of injecting drug users.

Condom use is generally low among young people of the region, and unprotected sex with injecting drug users has led to increasing numbers of young women being infected with HIV. There is the risk that the disease will spread from mainly young injecting drug users to become generalized among the population. Fortunately, there is evidence of a growing political and civil society commitment to a strong AIDS response in the region.

Since youth are at the centre of the HIV/AIDS epidemic in the Eastern Europe and CIS region, specific policies directed towards youth must be designed and implemented. Central to the prevention of HIV/AIDS is information and education about the risks of HIV and how it is transmitted. Comprehensive and correct knowledge about HIV/AIDS is extremely low among youth in the region. School-based HIV prevention programmes exist in some countries but are not widespread enough. In addition, school-based HIV prevention programmes cannot reach youth who are not in school. Many youth who are injecting drugs may already have dropped out of or otherwise left school.

The region needs vital prevention and treatment strategies for youth to include access to condoms, treatment for sexually transmitted diseases, strategies to prevent mother-to-child transmission, and other specific programmes, including harm reduction programmes for injecting drug users to decrease the transmission of HIV among them.

DEVELOPED MARKET ECONOMIES

The opportunities available to youth living in developed market economies are unmatched in other parts of the world. Many youth benefit from a high standard of living, access to quality education and health care, and the ready availability of the Internet. Nevertheless, inequalities in youth development exist in all countries of the region for which data are available, often reflecting class, ethnicity, race, sex and migrant status. The report reviews the bases and consequences of these inequalities in youth development, with special attention to the impact of migration.

While enrolment and completion rates are high at all levels of education, major inter- and intra-country differentials are common. Differences in educational performance seem to reflect the socio-economic and ethnic background of youth. Whereas those from poorer backgrounds are more likely to drop out of school if they fail a grade or perform poorly, those from wealthier backgrounds are more likely to find the resources to take remedial action to ensure success. Tertiary education opportunities, in particular, are strongly linked to socio-economic status. The type of educational system, including the duration of degree programmes and the facilities available to different groups, also plays a role in determining educational opportunities and outcomes.

These educational inequalities result in an uneven playing field of opportunities. The disadvantaged face unemployment, underemployment, poverty, isolation from the rest of society, and the risk of being drawn into antisocial groups. Evidence that some of the education differentials across groups have diminished in the region give reason for hope, however.

Information and communication technologies play a major role in education systems and in the social and economic lives of youth in the developed market economies. Young people are increasingly using the Internet for job searches and training. In Europe, use of career resource sites jumped 21 per cent to involve 9.5 million youth between 2005 and 2006. In addition to using the new technology as an information source, youth have also made an impact on the landscape of the Internet and are prolific users of social networking sites. However, young people are also exposed to greater risk of exploitation, abuse and fraud as access to the Internet becomes easier and more widespread.

Youth in the developed market economies experience, overall, better labour market prospects than youth in developing regions. The total number of unemployed youth in these economies has declined over the past decade, and young men and women are almost equally likely to participate in the labour market. Even with the same qualifications, however, young women tend to earn less than young men.

Despite fairly good labour market conditions, many young people in developed economies have difficulty obtaining stable, decent and long-term employment corresponding to their skill levels. Although tertiary education is generally perceived as a guarantor of decent and well-paid jobs, even university graduates increasingly experience insecurity and uncertainty in their employment prospects. This is largely due to a lack of specific job training.

In developed countries, internships appear to have become a waiting stage for those who are unable to find suitable immediate employment or for those who seek to improve the chances of finding good jobs. This raises equity concerns for young people's opportunities to acquire work experience. Since internships are often poorly remunerated, those from mainly higher socio-economic groups can afford to position themselves for good future jobs. Greater corporate responsibility is required to ensure that internships are sufficiently remunerated, or to provide part-time options so that youth from all backgrounds are able to acquire work experience. Increased opportunities for apprenticeships and entry-level jobs that require little or no prior job experience are also needed. Finally, public or private stipends for volunteers and interns from disadvantaged backgrounds would ensure greater equality in entry-level labour markets.

The fact that labour market conditions have made it more difficult for young people to secure well-paid employment has been a major factor in slowing the transition of youth to independent adulthood in the developed market economies. Between 1985 and 2000, young adults' abilities to form independent households in the developed market economies declined. Employment has not only been a source of economic security and independence, but also an important avenue for youth to become integrated into society through contacts with colleagues and professional or labour organizations. Therefore, exclusion from employment can also mean exclusion from society.

Youth in developed countries generally experience the best health conditions in which to mature into healthy and independent adulthood. Nevertheless, there are pockets of youth in all developed countries that are excluded from quality and affordable health care, partly owing to parental background, residence, education, race or income. For example, death due to injury is two to three times higher for those coming from lower socio-economic groups compared with groups with higher socio-economic status.

In addition to inequalities in health, behavioural choices that young people make are compromising their well-being. The age at the onset of drinking and using illegal drugs is becoming progressively lower. Youth in the region are also choosing to have sex, frequently unprotected, at earlier ages than in the past. The resulting sexually transmitted diseases and early pregnancies seem to hit youth from disadvantaged backgrounds and youth with lower educational status the most. Barriers to prevention and treatment services for sexually transmitted diseases include lack of insurance, lack of transportation, and facilities or services that are designed for adults and may intimidate youth or compromise confidentiality. Although overall adolescent pregnancy rates have dropped significantly over the past 25 years, young women with low levels of education and income are more likely to become pregnant during their teenage years than their better-off peers.

To a large extent, unhealthy lifestyles reflect youth alienation from human development opportunities. Poverty, lack of access to education or employment, and limited opportunities for structured and constructive leisure activities may leave young people vulnerable to negative peer pressure. Policies to address the increasing lifestyle-related health challenges of youth in developed countries therefore require a more holistic approach. Reducing these risks involves changing personal behaviour, but it also requires changes in social and economic structures to foster the inclusion of youth, especially those of lower socio-economic backgrounds.

With the influx of young migrants, youth populations in developed countries are becoming increasingly diverse. Migrants now constitute 9.5 per cent of the developed countries' populations. Migrant youth are increasingly recruited to meet the demand for specific skills or the care-giving needs of an ageing population in the developed market economies. Schooling, particularly at the tertiary level, is also a major reason for immigration into these countries. Others migrate because of domestic, political and economic difficulties, or for family reunification.

The social inclusion of migrants remains a challenge, especially for undocumented migrants. Socially marginalized migrant youth are at risk of exploitation and might become involved in antisocial behaviour. In addition to improving the integration into the educational system, Governments must take steps to improve employment opportunities for youth with migrant backgrounds. Active labour market policies can be instrumental in this regard.

Inequalities in civic engagement can also be observed among youth in developed countries. Although youth involvement in formal political processes is often limited, many young people engage in community volunteer and development activities—new forms of expression and civic involvement that address their concerns and interests directly. Those with higher levels of socio-economic resources, however, are most likely to participate. Because participation in community volunteer activities is an important form of non-formal education, youth from lower socio-economic backgrounds are further disproportionately disadvantaged.

ENSURING GLOBAL YOUTH DEVELOPMENT: THE WAY FORWARD

This report's review of the progress and challenges in youth transitions to adulthood suggests clearly that although youth face a number of challenges as they try to make the transition into adulthood, many are determined to succeed and are using varied approaches to ensure their "survival." Some are staying in school longer; others are dropping out of school to work and earn an income. Some are joining the informal economy or setting up private businesses; others opt to migrate in search of greener pastures.

It is clear from these actions that youth are not a passive group waiting for resources and opportunities to be handed to them. In all regions, they want to make a better life for themselves. However, lack of adequate investments in youth, challenges related to globalization, and other changes in the world economy, as well as social and cultural constraints, have often combined to create unfavourable contexts for youth development and participation. An enabling environment for youth development and participation is urgently needed if youth are to attain their full potential and contribute to national development.

Although there are some variations in the challenges across regions, this report clearly suggests that, regardless of world region, there are a few common areas in which youth persistently experience difficulties that impinge on their transition to adulthood. Areas that are identified in this report as requiring priority attention include health, education, employment, poverty reduction, healthy leisure and volunteer programmes, and investment in protecting the rights and status of young women and girls. Marginalized youth in all countries require particular attention. Even in developed regions, many young people—especially those from poorer socio-economic backgrounds— suffer from the consequences of inadequate investment in these areas. The result is that young people's transition to adulthood can be compromised or stalled.

Given the large youth share of the global population, especially in less developed regions, the failure to ensure that young people have access to resources and opportunities for health maintenance, education, leisure and volunteer activities, poverty reduction, employment, and the protection of the rights of girls and young women will derail future national and global development. The similarities in the core challenges in youth development across regions suggest that there may be some common approaches to addressing these problems. However, it is important that interventions are properly tailored to the particular youth development issues of regions and communities, with special attention given to migrant communities.

An important challenge of youth policies and programmes in the coming decades is to make up for the major shortfall in investment in young people, especially women, in past decades. It is essential, in this regard, for all stakeholders to work towards eliminating discrimination against young women, to increase their access to education and literacy, including non-formal education and remedial programmes, and to develop gender-sensitive programmes, including sexual and reproductive health services. In addition, specific efforts should be made to provide skills training for young women and to increase their employment opportunities while ensuring their equal representation at decision-making levels.

Youth development is incomplete if young people are not given a chance to participate in society. Youth must also be engaged in all aspects of policy and programme development. The key to ensuring that today's young people's transitions are completed successfully and that they become responsible and productive adult members of their communities lies in enabling them to develop themselves while having opportunities to contribute to society on an equal basis. ▪▪▪▪▪

Introduction

The progress of civilization is largely determined by the extent to which each individual is given the opportunity to contribute to the development and advancement of society. The world's 1.2 billion young people aged 15-24 constitute 18 per cent of the global population and are an essential part of this process. Aside from their material and intellectual contributions, young people offer unique aptitudes and perspectives that must be assimilated into the broader development paradigm and translated into effective action on the ground. Unfortunately, negative perceptions of youth, the failure to help them develop to their full potential, the inability to recognize that investing in youth benefits national development, and the consequent unwillingness and incapacity of society to fully involve young people in a meaningful way have effectively deprived the world of a resource of inestimable value. Unless a sustained effort is made to ensure that youth are given the opportunity to contribute to the well-being of their societies, the goal of achieving of "a society for all," as called for at the World Summit for Social Development in Copenhagen in 1995, will never be achieved.

The vital role young people can play in the development of society was formally recognized by the United Nations for the first time in General Assembly resolution A/RES/2037 (XX) of 7 December 1965, comprising the Declaration on the Promotion among Youth of the Ideals of Peace, Mutual Respect and Understanding between Peoples. Noting that "young people must become conscious of their responsibilities in the world they will be called upon to manage," the resolution officially acknowledged the importance of youth engagement in addressing global development issues. Several decades later, the World Programme of Action for Youth to the Year 2000 and Beyond, adopted by the General Assembly in its resolution 50/81 of 14 December 1995, identified the "full and effective participation of youth in the life of society and in decision-making" as one of ten priority areas requiring action by Governments, the international community, civil society and the private sector. The Programme of Action (paragraph 107) recommended the following interventions to facilitate the achievement of this goal:

(a) Improving access to information in order to enable young people to make better use of opportunities to participate in decision-making;

(b) Developing and/or strengthening opportunities for young people to learn their rights and responsibilities, promoting their social, political, developmental and environmental participation, removing obstacles that affect their full contribution to society and respecting, inter alia, freedom of association;

(c)   Encouraging and promoting youth associations through financial, educational and technical support and promotion of their activities;

(d)   Taking into account the contribution of youth in designing, implementing and evaluating national policies and plans affecting their concerns;

(e)   Encouraging increased national, regional and international cooperation and exchange between youth organizations;

(f)   Inviting Governments to strengthen the involvement of young people in international forums, inter alia, by considering the inclusion of youth representatives in their national delegations to the General Assembly.

This call to action has not gone unanswered. Over the past decade, recognition of the importance of investing in young people has grown at the national and international levels, and numerous programmes and activities promoting youth development and participation in society have been implemented. The necessity of involving young people in both conceptualizing and implementing policies and programmes is widely acknowledged. The dialogue on youth development, which only a few years ago was characterized by a top-down, adult-to-youth approach, has broadened and now encompasses more planned consultations with youth organizations.

YOUTH DEVELOPMENT: PROGRESS AND CHALLENGES IN AN EVOLVING GLOBAL CONTEXT

The United Nations defines youth as those between the ages of 15 and 24; today, this group would include individuals born between 1983 and 1992. In its broadest sense, "youth" is not so easily circumscribed; it essentially represents the period of transition between childhood and adulthood, the nature and length of which vary from one individual or society to another. What is certain is that young people undergo a variety of new experiences; they take on new roles and responsibilities and make decisions that ultimately influence the course of their lives (Lloyd, 2006). When society provides adequate and appropriate guidance and opportunities for youth development in areas such as education, health, employment, and sports and recreation, young people are more likely to transition successfully into adulthood and contribute meaningfully to the development of their societies. Conversely, neglecting to support the development of young people and failing to provide them with the knowledge and resources they need to make informed choices and move forward can derail this transition process, with potentially disastrous consequences for society as a whole.

Youth development, as defined in this report, entails actions and investments that enable young people to build and utilize their human capital and become productive adults. It is essential that Governments and other stakeholders design and implement policies and programmes to protect young people from negative social and environmental influences that can interfere with their progress towards healthy adulthood. To benefit from youth capabilities, societies must ensure that opportunities for youth engagement in development processes are nurtured and protected. The failure to do so can lead to the exclusion and marginalization of young people, depriving society of their energy, dynamism and innovative spirit.

A number of historic events have occurred in recent decades that have helped shape the challenges and opportunities that young people now face. The toppling of dictatorships around the world, the collapse of communism, and the trend towards increased political and economic liberalization have brought about greater freedom of choice but have also produced a significant degree of uncertainty for the present generation of youth. Globalization has created tremendous potential for economic and social development, but it has contributed to heightened inequality and insecurity as well. The reverberations of the global economic recession in the 1980s and of the economic and financial crises of the late 1990s and the first part of the present decade are still being felt, undermining opportunities for youth development. Young people face harrowing difficulties entering and staying in the labour market; many cannot find jobs in the formal sector and may languish in the informal economy. Others are employed but remain poor because of inadequate remuneration; employers often discriminate against youth, especially young women. Labour market difficulties are related to issues, challenges, and policy and environmental factors specific to each region and are examined in some detail in the present report.

On a more promising note, the commitment of the international community to addressing the problems experienced by young people around the world is stronger than ever before. Global efforts in the area of youth development increasingly reflect explicit recognition of the importance of youth participation. Civil society groups active in this field, especially youth-led non-governmental organizations, are receiving growing international support. More is being done in direct collaboration with youth led-organizations to foster a broader understanding of the obstacles to youth participation and the benefits of involving young people in national development. Youth are frequently invited to join deliberations on major issues in global forums. Although many countries, particularly in the less developed regions, have yet to nominate youth representatives, youth delegate participation in United Nations meetings has grown considerably in recent years; past delegates, taking part in deliberations such as those on social development at sessions of the Commission for Social Development and within the General Assembly, have made significant contributions to the international debate on a range of issues. The international community as a whole has come to recognize the need for young people to be seen and heard in the development dialogue and has made a determined effort to involve them in global meetings and to support them in leading roles in such contexts.

At the country level, national youth councils are increasingly providing a common platform from which young people can work to influence decision-making. Young people, in particular those involved in youth organizations, have played a key role in establishing such councils in a number of countries, adopting a bottom-up approach in their formation and operation—even where they are institutions of State Governments. A national youth council promotes unity and provides the structure and focus needed for effective action and advocacy; it serves as an umbrella organization or national platform for youth associations, and its primary functions are to create linkages between youth organizations and the Government, particularly to ensure better communication and the implementation of youth programmes in the country; and to encourage youth participation less on an ad hoc, topic-specific consultation level and more on a coordinated and sustained basis (Kehler Siebert and Seel, 2006).

Youth organizations have been instrumental in bringing the perspectives of young people to the world's attention; they have fought to ensure that their members are included in the national and international dialogue, and that the needs and ideas of youth are considered in policy design, development and implementation.

As the needs of youth have become better recognized and understood, the collection and analysis of relevant data have expanded greatly, making it easier to monitor and evaluate the progress of young people over time. In spite of these gains, much of the discussion on youth participation continues to focus on strengthening youth involvement in political processes, neglecting the broader aspects of participation—in personal, educational, social and economic development—that are crucial for a successful transition to adulthood.

Although youth participation activities at the national and international levels are helping to facilitate the transition to adulthood, the potential for development in this area has not been fully realized. Approaches to fostering youth participation have remained rather narrow, with the benefits of inclusion sometimes regarded as accruing solely to youth rather than to society as a whole. Investments in youth have too often been viewed as a means of improving the welfare of young people rather than as part of an integrated national development strategy. Consequently, efforts to help youth understand their rights and responsibilities and to strengthen their social, economic, and political participation remain sporadic and diffuse. Government bodies responsible for youth development generally operate at the subministerial level or form part of underfunded joint ministries, such as those concerned with sports, culture or tourism, rather than being affiliated with the larger ministries in charge of labour affairs or economic development.

ORGANIZATION AND SCOPE OF THE REPORT

This report presents an overview of the challenges and constraints young people encounter during their transition to adulthood and assesses the progress made by Governments, youth and other stakeholders in facilitating this transition. The fundamental premise of the report and an analytical point of departure is that facilitating young people's transition to adulthood by improving their health prospects, expanding education and employment opportunities, and providing opportunities for participation in all aspects of development is an essential precondition for achieving the inclusive, equitable societies called for at the World Summit for Social Development in Copenhagen.

Youth are not a homogeneous group; the challenges and opportunities affecting their lives are broadly similar but are characterized by important differences deriving from unique contextual circumstances. To avoid addressing issues in a manner suggesting greater global uniformity than actually prevails, this report adopts a regional approach.

The seven geographic and/or economic groupings covered in the report include Asia, Latin America, sub-Saharan Africa, the Middle East and North Africa, small island developing States, Eastern Europe and the Commonwealth of Independent States (CIS), and developed market economies.[1] Because regions are defined in both geographic and economic terms, there is a certain degree of overlap, with countries sometimes identified as belonging to more than one region. For example, Japan belongs to the Asia group but is also listed among the developed market economies. Similarly, each of the small island developing States is part of a distinct geographic region. The trends examined in the report represent the conditions characteristic of a particular region or group and do not necessarily reflect the conditions prevailing in individual countries.

The succeeding chapters focus on various interrelated issues that have emerged as priorities based on recent economic and social developments in each region.

Chapter 1 highlights the challenges and opportunities related to globalization and education in Asia. Globalization has arguably had the greatest impact on the rapidly growing Asian economies. Large numbers of new industries have moved to Asia, attracted by low wages and production costs, and while many young people have benefited from this trend, others have not been able to find employment or are being exploited by those same industries in the absence of protective labour regulations. The progress made in the education sector has allowed some Asian youth to reap the benefits of globalization; however, inequalities in access and other significant challenges remain.

Chapter 2 addresses the transition from youth to adulthood in Latin America within a changing economic, social and political environment. The major economic transformations that have occurred in Latin American during the past couple of decades have dramatically affected the course of many young lives. Low-quality education and a lack of employment opportunities have contributed to increased poverty, fuelling widespread migration in many countries of the region. The socio-economic situation has also negatively affected the political fervor once so characteristic of the area.

The impact of poverty on the development of young people in sub-Saharan Africa is explored in chapter 3. There are presently large cohorts of youth in this region. With the consistent decline in population growth rates, a major demographic shift is occurring; however, the negative momentum created by past demographic growth is still being felt today in the form of intense pressure on limited government resources. For developing regions as a whole, the proportion of those living on less than US$ 1 a day fell from nearly one third of the population to about one fifth between 1990 and 2004, while in sub-Saharan Africa the corresponding decline was only from about 47 to 41 per cent (United Nations, 2007). The consequences for youth of various dimensions of poverty are addressed in the chapter.

Chapter 4 examines the progress and challenges in youth development in the Middle East and North Africa, with a special focus on employment and gender concerns. This region has the lowest rate of youth participation in the labour force. Young people account for only about one third of the total working-age population, but because they are seriously underrepresented in the workforce they constitute almost 50 per cent of the region's unemployed—one of the highest rates in the world (International Labour Office, 2006). Growing numbers of skilled young graduates are vying for a diminishing number of jobs in the public sector. Young women are becoming more actively involved in the region's labour markets, but the rate of increase is slowing, and labour force participation rates for females remain much lower than the corresponding rates for males (International Labour Office, 2006).

The unique situation of youth in small island developing States is featured in chapter 5. Young people growing up in these countries face many of the same challenges and constraints as their contemporaries in other parts of the world, but the educational, employment and other problems affecting them tend to be related to the small size, relative remoteness, and other special characteristics of the island States in which they live. In many of these countries (particularly the Pacific islands), new opportunities and challenges are also linked to the relatively recent transformation from traditional to more modern societies.

In chapter 6 the report reviews the major constraints to youth development in Eastern Europe and the Commonwealth of Independent States, focusing on labour market difficulties and the HIV/AIDS epidemic in the region. The socio-economic transformation that has occurred in this area over the past two decades has brought about significant changes in labour market prospects for young people. The vulnerability, poverty and social exclusion experienced by many youth in the region have been linked to a relatively high prevalence of risky behaviour, with substance abuse and unsafe sexual practices fuelling the spread of HIV/AIDS. The number of new infections has increased twenty-fold in less than a decade, and people under the age of 30 have accounted for 75 per cent of reported infections (Joint United Nations Programme on HIV/AIDS, 2006; Joint United Nations Programme on HIV/AIDS and World Health Organization, 2005).

Chapter 7 draws attention to inequalities in youth development in the developed market economies. Overall, young people in these countries have the best opportunities with respect to many of the priority areas of the World Programme of Action for Youth. However, access to these opportunities varies considerably. The chapter explores some of the more serious disparities, especially in the light of the demographic and socio-economic changes that are occurring within the context of increasing international migration into the region.

The final chapter summarizes the key issues and conclusions and offers a number of recommendations for future policy and programme development. A statistical annex reflecting the current situation of youth in a number of areas is provided at the end of the report. ▬▬▬▬▬▬▬▬▬

---

[1] A list of the countries included in each region is provided in the explanatory notes at the beginning of the present publication.

References

International Labour Office (2006). *Global Employment Trends for Youth 2006.* Geneva.

Joint United Nations Programme on HIV/AIDS (2006). *2006 Report on the Global AIDS Epidemic.* Geneva.

_____ and World Health Organization (2005). Eastern Europe and Central Asia. *AIDS Epidemic Update: December 2005.* Geneva.

Kehler Siebert, Clarisse, and Franziska Seel (2006). *National Youth Councils: Their Creation, Evolution, Purpose, and Governance.* Toronto: TakingITGlobal.

Lloyd, Cynthia B. (2006). *Growing Up Global: The Changing Transitions to Adulthood in Developing Countries.* National Research Council and Institute of Medicine of the National Academies. Washington, D.C.: National Academies Press.

United Nations (2004). *World Youth Report 2003: The Global Situation of Young People.* Sales No.E.03.IV.7.

_____ (2005). *World Youth Report 2005: Young People Today, and in 2015.* Sales No. E.05.IV.6.

_____ (2006). World population monitoring, focusing on international migration and development. Report of the Secretary-General (E/CN.9/2006/3).

_____ (2007). *The Millennium Development Goals Report 2007.* New York. Sales No. E.07.II5.

Chapter 1

ASIAN
YOUTH
in the context of rapid
GLOBALIZATION

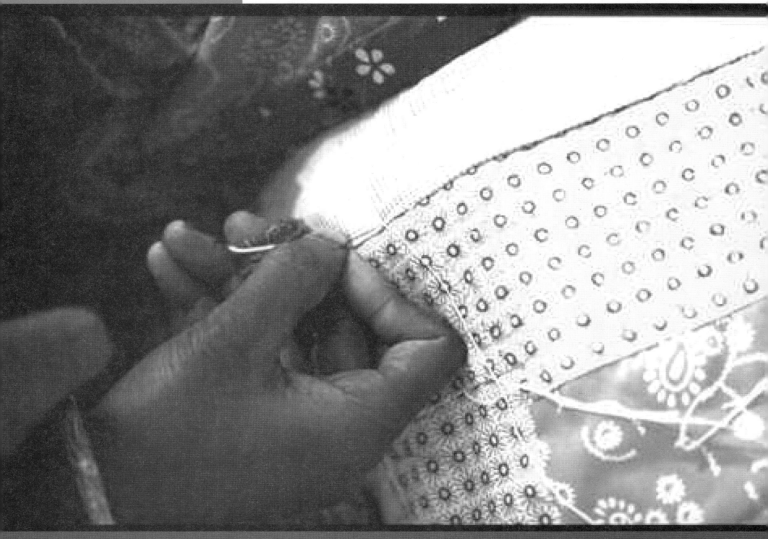

I n Asia as in other world regions, globalization has generated extraordinary opportunities. New avenues for education and employment have been created; improvements in technology have helped to raise the productivity of individuals as well as manufacturing and agricultural output; and many people, including youth, are reaping the benefits of major public health breakthroughs and interventions. The rapid processes of change and adjustment associated with globalization have, however, intensified poverty, unemployment and social disintegration in certain areas, especially among the most vulnerable populations. Factors such as the changing nature of work, a shrinking demand for young workers (who are more likely to be unskilled), and the emergence of new and less secure forms of employment are seriously undermining the ability of young people to contribute meaningfully to, and benefit fully from, the global economy. Young people often lack the financial resources necessary to access the opportunities and withstand the pressures created by globalization. Many are restricted by inadequate education and poverty, or are outside the reach of basic information and communication and of the goods and services that have become available with globalization.

Affluence and poverty have always coexisted, but globalization has had a polarizing effect, widening inequalities within and between countries and population groups. Perhaps nowhere has this change been as evident as in Asia, where, despite impressive achievements, substantial differences in social and economic development are apparent across subregions, and where globalization has contributed to increased marginalization and vulnerability for many groups. In Asia, as elsewhere, globalization is characterized by unprecedented economic interdependence driven by cross-border capital movement, rapid technology transfer, and information and communication flows. Non-governmental organizations and civic groups, which can complement and sometimes challenge State authority, have emerged as key players, as have global firms, production networks and financial markets. Governments are increasingly being pressured to conform to new international standards of governance, transparency and accountability and to ensure the fair and consistent application of the rule of law. In addition, a Western-leaning international culture has emerged, sparking concerns about the erosion of national identity and traditional values in Asian countries. This complex transformation process has produced dramatic economic, social and cultural changes in Asia during the past two to three decades. Young people in the region have benefited from the positive aspects of these developments, but many have been left vulnerable to the negative repercussions of modernization.

This chapter explores how young people in Asia have fared in the context of globalization, focusing particularly on whether they have the capacity and opportunity to participate more fully in their communities at the social and economic levels. It is argued that because Asian countries have been able to take advantage of a very large pool of young labour, youth in the region have been a strong, positive force in the development of their societies. Young people have, in turn, profited from a number of positive developments, including expanded educational opportunities, better health care, access to information and communication technologies, and enhanced leisure possibilities. Girls and young women have been given increased opportunities to contribute to development. The chapter acknowledges these important gains but also provides an assessment of the remaining obstacles and constraints and their consequences for youth development in the region.

It should be noted that many of the trends explored in this chapter reflect the inter-play of multiple forces and factors associated with globalization, not all of which are addressed in the present context.

THE DEMOGRAPHIC CONTEXT: NUMBERS MATTER

An estimated 738 million youth between the ages of 15 and 24 lived in Asia in 2007, accounting for more than 18 per cent of the region's population. The situation of Asian youth must be considered within the context of a substantial demographic shift that has both influenced and been affected by the social and economic transformation of the region (Hugo, 2005a). Changes in fertility and, to a lesser extent, mortality have had a profound impact on the age structure. During the second half of the twentieth century, high fertility dominated the demographic picture in the region, producing large cohorts of children that evolved into sizeable youth cohorts over the years. This trend peaked in 1985, when youth accounted for an all-time high of 22 per cent of the total population of Asia (see table 1.1).

Table 1.1
The youth population in Asia and its subregions, 1960-2050
(in thousands and as a proportion of the total population)

Year	Asia		West Asia		South-East Asia		East Asia		South-Central Asia	
1960	294 380	18.5	11 486	18.4	40 110	19.2	131 486	17.8	111 298	19.2
1965	325 702	18.4	12 781	17.8	43 086	18.2	149 465	18.4	120 370	18.5
1970	398 680	19.9	16 064	19.5	51 462	19.1	187 093	20.2	144 061	19.8
1975	460 113	20.4	19 520	20.4	63 082	20.8	206 080	20.0	171 431	20.9
1980	514 153	20.8	23 009	20.9	73 414	21.7	224 854	20.5	192 875	20.9
1985	591 992	22.1	26 591	21.1	82 478	22.1	268 174	23.3	214 748	20.8
1990	643 035	21.8	29 947	21.0	90 570	22.2	285 267	22.9	237 250	20.5
1995	645 844	20.1	33 577	20.9	96 683	21.6	251 609	19.2	263 977	20.4
2000	663 246	19.3	37 784	21.1	102 216	21.2	226 397	16.8	296 850	20.9
Change (1960-2000)	**368 866**	**0.8**	**26 298**	**2.8**	**62 107**	**1.9**	**94 911**	**-1.1**	**185 552**	**1.8**
2005	720 859	19.7	41 254	21.0	106 941	20.7	243 728	17.3	328 937	21.4
2010	749 527	19.2	43 944	20.4	108 953	19.7	243 697	16.4	352 933	21.3
2015	735 023	17.9	46 077	19.6	107 356	18.4	221 084	14.5	360 506	20.3
Change (2005-2015)	**14 164**	**-1.8**	**4 823**	**-1.4**	**416**	**-2.3**	**-22 644**	**-2.8**	**31 569**	**-1.1**
2020	714 618	16.6	47 184	18.6	106 659	17.4	201 051	13.0	359 724	19.1
2025	709 765	15.8	48 958	17.9	107 631	16.7	188 238	11.8	364 939	18.3
2030	718 880	15.4	51 296	17.6	106 209	15.8	189 567	11.7	371 809	17.7
2035	719 875	14.9	52 612	17.0	103 152	14.9	191 729	11.7	372 382	17.0
2040	706 101	14.2	52 878	16.3	100 330	14.0	188 789	11.5	364 104	

Source: United Nations, World Population Prospects: The 2006 Revision (New York: 2007a).

The proportion of youth in the total population of Asia has slowly begun to shift downward in all subregions. The attenuation of the "Asian youth bulge" is evident in figure 1.1, which projects a consistent decline in the share of the youth population after 2010. The actual number of young people in the region is expected to slowly decrease to around 706 million in 2040, with youth comprising 14 per cent of the total population.

Figure 1.1

Youth as a proportion of the total population in Asian subregions, 1950-2050

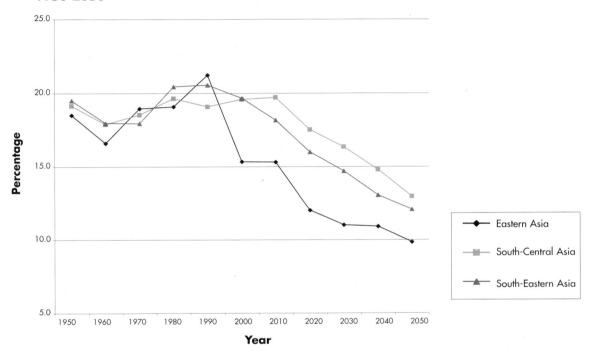

Source: *United Nations* (2007a), *World Population Prospects: The 2006 Revision* (New York).

The size of the youth population in Asia gives the region a major advantage in terms of development potential. Table 1.2 shows that of a global youth labour force of 633 million in 2005, some 353 million (55.7 per cent) lived in Asia. By 2015, the Asian youth workforce is expected to increase to 361 million. Countries in the region have been able to reap a "demographic dividend" from the production capacity of a labour force that is sizeable in relation to the dependent population; indeed, it is estimated that one third of East Asia's economic miracle (occurring between 1965 and 1990) can be attributed to this phenomenon (Bloom and Canning, 2003). The extent to which Asian economies will continue to benefit from this demographic picture will depend critically on how they develop and harness the potential of the youth population.

Table 1.2
Global and regional estimates and projections of the youth labour force, 2005 and 2015 (thousands)

Region	Youth labour force in 2005	Youth labour force in 2015	Change (2005-2015)
Developed economies	64 501	61 167	-3 334
Central and Eastern Europe (non-EU) and CIS	29 661	23 989	-5 672
East Asia	154 511	139 596	-14 915
South-East Asia and the Pacific	61 490	72 889	11 399
South Asia	136 616	148 293	11 677
Latin America and the Caribbean	57 149	56 649	-500
Middle East and North Africa	33 174	34 039	865
Sub-Saharan Africa	96 153	120 587	24 434
World	633 255	657 209	23 955

Source: *International Labour Office, Global Employment Trends for Youth 2006* (Geneva: International Labour Organization, August 2006).

One of the most important factors influencing whether and how Asian economies benefit from their sizeable youth population is how much of an opportunity young people have to participate in development, which includes strengthening their capacities through education, improved health care and productive employment. Maximizing the demographic dividend requires a favourable policy environment for human capital development (Bloom, Canning and Sevilla, 2003).

YOUTH PARTICIPATION IN EDUCATION

Developments in education represent perhaps the most important of the factors that have positioned Asian economies to take advantage of the demographic dynamic and globalization.

Access to quality education has expanded in many parts of Asia, making it possible for a much broader range of youth to contribute meaningfully to economic and social development. Improvements have occurred across the education system, though the gains are particularly noticeable at the primary level. Many countries in the region, including Bangladesh, Indonesia, Myanmar, the Republic of Korea, Sri Lanka, and Viet Nam, have implemented curricular reforms, while others, such as the Maldives and Thailand, are preparing for major curriculum changes (United Nations Educational, Scientific and Cultural Organization, 2006a). In line with the growing trend towards resource rationalization and cost recovery in the social sectors, many countries in the region have also begun to explore ways to make their education systems more efficient and effective.

Formal education

While youth are generally not enrolled in primary education, analysis of trends in this area is important from a youth development perspective. It is during the primary cycle that literacy, numeracy, and other fundamental skills and knowledge are obtained, providing the foundations for further education at the secondary and tertiary levels and ultimately for active participation in society.

Today, as a result of both demographic conditions and increased investment in education, more children than ever before are attending school in Asia. Gross primary enrolment ratios exceed 100 per cent in many countries, reflecting the participation of many children outside the official primary school age range (see table 1.3). Figure 1.2 indicates that between 2000 and 2004, net primary enrolment increased sharply in South Asia and West Asia and rose slightly in Central Asia; in East Asia and the Pacific, where this ratio has traditionally been high, a marginal decline (from 96 to 94 per cent) was registered.

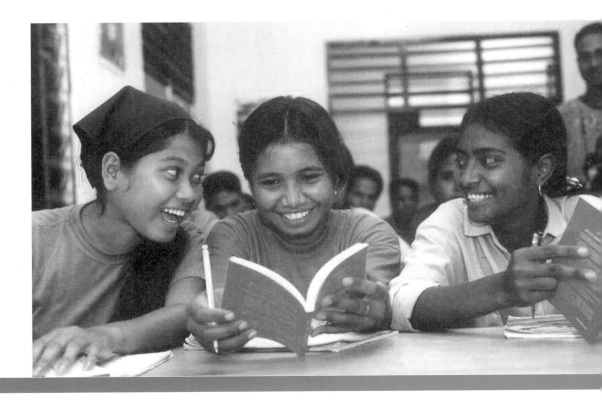

Table 1.3

Gross primary, secondary and tertiary enrolment ratios* in selected Asian countries, by sex, 2004

Region/Country	Primary			Secondary			Tertiary		
	Total	Male	Female	Total	Male	Female	Total	Male	Female
East Asia									
China	118	118	117	73	73	73	19	21	17
Hong Kong SAR**	108	111	105	85	86	83	32	33	32
Macao SAR**	106	110	101	96	94	98	69	84	54
Japan	100	100	101	102	102	102	54	57	51
Mongolia	104	104	105	90	84	95	39	29	48
Republic of Korea	105	105	105	91	91	91	89	109	67
South-East Asia									
Brunei Darussalam	109	109	109	94	91	96	15	10	20
Cambodia	137	109	109	29	35	24	3	4	2
Indonesia	116	117	115	62	62	61	16	18	14
Lao People's Democratic Republic	116	124	109	46	52	39	6	7	5
Malaysia	93	93	93	70	67	74	29	25	33
Myanmar	97	96	98	41	41	40	11	..	..
Philippines	113	113	112	84	80	88	29	26	33
Thailand	99	101	96	77	77	77	41	38	44
Viet Nam	98	101	94	73	75	72	10	11	9
South Asia									
Afghanistan	93	127	56	16	35	5	1	2	—
Bangladesh	109	107	111	51	49	54	7	9	4
India	107	111	104	52	58	46	11	14	9
Islamic Republic of Iran	103	98	108	82	84	79	22	21	24
Nepal	113	118	108	46	49	42	6	8	3
Pakistan	82	95	69	27	31	23	3	4	3
Sri Lanka	102	102	101	81	79	83	..	..	..

Source: *United Nations Educational, Scientific and Cultural Organization, Global Education Digest 2006: Comparing Education Statistics Across the World* (Montreal: UNESCO Institute for Statistics, 2006) (UIS/SD/06-01).

Notes: Two dots (..) signify that an item is not available. A dash (—) indicates that an amount is nil or negligible.

 *Gross enrolment ratios can exceed 100 per cent if a substantial number of pupils are not in the official age range, thus overstating the actual share of the school-age population participating in school.

**SAR: Special Administrative Region of China.

Figure 1.2
Trends in net primary enrolment

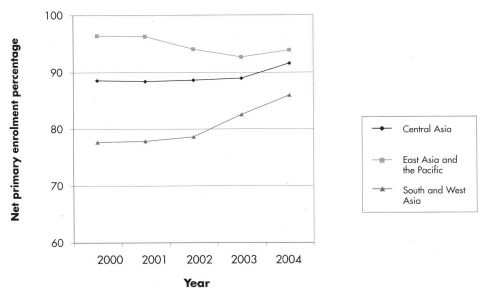

Source: United Nations Educational, Scientific and Cultural Organization, Institute for Statistics (data accessed from www.uis.unesco.org on 18 January 2007).

After decades of relative exclusion, girls are increasingly benefiting from the gains in primary education. India and Nepal have nearly achieved gender parity at this level; between 1998 and 2002, the proportion of girls enrolled in primary education rose from 84 to 96 per cent in the former and from 78 to 92 per cent in the latter. Parity had already been reached in Bangladesh, the Islamic Republic of Iran, the Maldives and Sri Lanka by 1998. A few countries have made less significant progress in this area. Afghanistan has the world's widest gap between boys and girls in primary education, and in Pakistan the primary enrolment rate for girls is only 73 per cent (United Nations Educational, Scientific and Cultural Organization, 2005b).

Improvements in primary enrolment in Asia are due to many factors, including State, private sector and international community commitments and investments in education. In most Asian countries, increases in government expenditure on primary education have meant that basic facilities and materials such as classrooms and textbooks are often provided free of charge, making school attendance possible for a broader segment of the target population. Countries such as Bangladesh, Brunei Darussalam, Indonesia, Sri Lanka and Thailand have adopted a free and universal system of basic education and literacy, which has allowed more children to transition into youth with the fundamental knowledge and skills required to participate effectively in society.

While statistics clearly indicate overall improvement in primary enrolment in the region, critical gaps remain. Bangladesh, India and Pakistan each have more than 1 million children not in school (United Nations Educational, Scientific and Cultural Organization, 2005a). In many parts of Asia, enrolment and retention in primary school are adversely affected by poor teaching and learning environments. Poverty often compels all fit members of a household to contribute to the family income, preventing many children from attending school. In half of the countries for which data are available, fewer than 78 per cent of pupils continue to the fifth grade. While grade repetition in Asia is low overall, in Nepal more than one fifth of all pupils are repeaters (United Nations Educational, Scientific and Cultural Organization, 2004). Quality and relevance remain key concerns; youth in Asia, as in other parts of the developing world, continue to be poorly prepared for work and life (World Bank, 2006).

Of even greater significance is the fact that the near-universality of primary education suggested in table 1.3 comes too late for many of today's youth, who should have been in primary school some 10 to 20 years ago. The educational situation of young people in Asia is illustrated by data from household demographic and health surveys conducted in various countries. Table 1.4 highlights the disparities in early educational attainment among young women in the region, indicating that while in Indonesia, the Philippines, Thailand, and Viet Nam fewer than 10 per cent of young women aged 15-19 years received no primary education, the same is true for over half of the young women in India and Nepal. More limited data suggest a somewhat better picture for males, with only Bangladesh showing more than 40 per cent of young men between the ages of 15 and 19 with no primary education. Reflecting improved participation rates in recent years, males aged 15-19 years have achieved a higher level of education than their counterparts in the 20-24 age group.

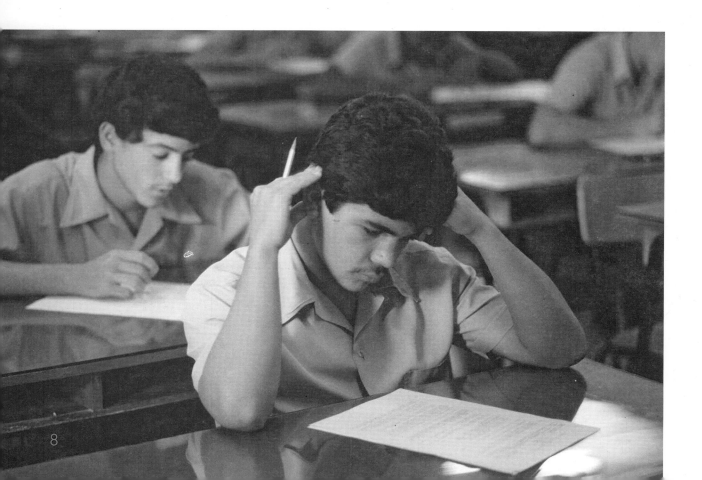

Table 1.4
Highest educational attainment of young females in selected Asian countries
(percentage)

Country	Year	Females aged 15-19 years			Females aged 20-24 years		
		No education	Primary education	Secondary or higher education	No education	Primary education	Secondary or higher education
Bangladesh	1993/94	48.7	33.0	18.3	53.3	28.1	18.6
	1996/97	40.8	34.3	24.8	49.8	26.9	23.3
	1999/2000	29.0	34.2	36.8	37.6	29.6	32.8
	2004	15.3	33.2	51.4	26.5	29.1	44.4
Cambodia	2000	18.8	56.6	24.6	27.4	51.8	20.8
India	1992/93	64.7	17.0	18.0	58.2	15.9	25.7
	1998/99	53.4	18.8	27.8	47.4	16.2	36.3
Indonesia	1987	8.1	76.2	15.7	12.5	67.4	20.1
	1991	5.3	77.1	17.7	7.6	66.1	26.2
	1994	3.9	73.3	22.8	5.5	62.2	32.3
	1997	2.8	72.0	25.3	3.3	60.5	36.1
	2002/03	1.5	51.6	46.9	1.7	49.4	48.9
Nepal	1996	69.0	19.1	12.0	68.1	15.7	16.2
	2001	52.2	26.1	21.7	59.2	18.2	22.6
Pakistan	1990/91	81.0	10.9	8.1	75.3	12.6	12.0
Philippines	1993	1.2	17.9	80.9	1.7	21.1	77.2
	1998	0.5	16.1	83.4	0.8	17.4	81.8
	2003	0.6	13.2	86.3	0.5	14.3	85.2
Sri Lanka	1987	15.8	24.1	60.1	11.4	29.9	58.5
Thailand	1987	7.5	83.3	9.2	5.9	79.8	14.3
Viet Nam	1997	7.3	41.6	51.1	6.5	25.3	68.2
	2002	6.6	40.6	52.8	8.8	31.0	60.2

Source: MEASURE DHS, STATcompiler (available from http://www.measuredhs.com; accessed 23 February 2007).

Children in Asia are better served by the educational establishment now than ever before. Primary enrolment figures are higher for those currently attending school than for the present youth cohort; however, there are indications that improvements were initiated early enough to benefit many of today's young people. In the countries in table 1.4 for which data exist for several points in time, the proportion of young women without any education has declined. The situation in the Philippines is particularly striking; by 2003, virtually all of the country's youth had been enrolled in primary school at some point, with males reportedly lagging slightly behind females in terms of early educational attainment.

Secondary education greatly improves employment prospects, providing an effective means for young people to acquire knowledge, skills and attitudes that will make it much easier for them to enter and remain in the labour market. In the context of globalization, secondary education has increasingly become the lowest level of schooling required for formal, productive employment. Asian countries have increased their investments in secondary education, and many have been successful in raising secondary enrolment rates. In just two generations, the Republic of Korea has made enormous strides and is now ranked among the world's top countries in terms of educational performance, as evidenced by its superior level of achievement within the framework of the OECD Programme for International Student Assessment (PISA) (Organization for Economic Cooperation and Development, 2006). Young women, who have typically had comparatively limited access to education in the region, have made considerable progress in obtaining secondary schooling. Table 1.4 indicates that secondary enrolment among young women rose dramatically over a relatively short period in virtually all of the countries for which multiple-year data were available; the Philippines, which registered the most modest increase, had already achieved a secondary school enrolment rate of 81 per cent for young women aged 15-19 years by 1993 but was able to raise the proportion further, to 86 per cent, by 2003.

In spite of these successes, there is much yet to be done. Table 1.3 reveals that secondary enrolment ratios are still low in a number of Asian countries, especially in the southern part of the region, and table 1.4 indicates that for many, educational attainment has not extended beyond primary schooling. There are countries in which a significant proportion of young women have not even had the benefit of a primary education. Educational coverage has improved considerably since the 1980s throughout much of the region, and differences in educational attainment among different age groups can be extreme. In Indonesia, for example, access to primary schooling is nearly universal today, but statistics for 2002/03 suggest that half of the country's young women aged 15-19 years had completed only primary schooling. As shown in figure 1.3, primary to secondary school transition rates vary greatly in Asia. In most countries boys are more likely than girls to move from primary to secondary education, though in Brunei Darussalam, Macao Special Administrative Region of China, Bangladesh, Sri Lanka and the Islamic Republic of Iran, transition rates are higher for girls.

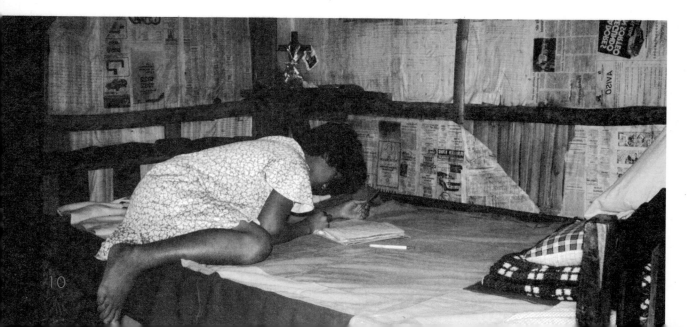

Figure 1.3
Rates of transition from primary to secondary education for selected countries, 2002-2004

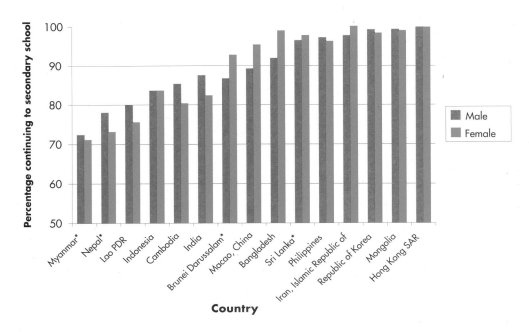

Source: United Nations Educational, Scientific and Cultural Organization, Institute for Statistics (data accessed from www.uis.unesco.org on 18 January 2007).
Note: * UNESCO Institute for Statistics estimate.

Even in countries with high primary to secondary school transition rates, participation in lower and upper secondary education is characterized by significant disparities. East Asian countries, in particular, have achieved high gross lower secondary enrolment ratios. These ratios are below 40 per cent in Afghanistan and Pakistan but are over 90 per cent in the Republic of Korea and Malaysia and as high as 98 per cent in Sri Lanka. Brunei Darussalam, China and Japan have gross lower secondary enrolment ratios exceeding 100 per cent. At the upper secondary level the figures decline sharply, with gross enrolment standing at 51 per cent for East Asia and the Pacific and only 40 per cent for South Asia and West Asia (United Nations Educational, Scientific and Cultural Organization, 2006b).

Besides the gains in primary enrolment, the most impressive development in educational attainment in Asia has been the dramatic upsurge in enrolment at the tertiary level. Globally, the number of students in tertiary education doubled between 1990 and 2004, reaching 132 million. East Asia and the Pacific led the trend with an increase of 25 million students during this period. In China alone, the number of students in tertiary education doubled between 1998 and 2002 and again between 2001 and 2004. By 2004, China had 19 million tertiary students, the largest number of any country and 15 per cent of the world total (United Nations Educational, Scientific and Cultural Organization, 2006b). The number of students enrolled at the tertiary level also doubled in South Asia and West Asia. India is mainly responsible for the increase in tertiary participation in South Asia, having registered annual growth rates averaging 13.4 per cent in the late 1990s. While tertiary expansion has proceeded at a more moderate pace in other countries, the overall picture reflects a tremendous numerical increase in post-secondary enrolment across Asia.

The substantial growth in Asian tertiary enrolment is largely a response to demographic exigencies, as countries have had to invest heavily in the education sector to meet the growing demand for schooling among members of the youth bulge. Larger numbers of students are choosing to continue their education, partly in response to high levels of unemployment and the need to gain a competitive edge through the acquisition of higher-level knowledge and marketable skills. Governments have also become more cognizant of the economic and social benefits of higher education. The OECD has estimated that among member countries the long-term effect on economic output of one additional year of education is between 3 and 6 per cent (Organization for Economic Cooperation and Development, 2006).

Increased private financing has also contributed to expanded access to tertiary education across the region. In countries such as India, most tertiary institutions are still financed by the public sector, but private provision of tertiary education is relatively widespread in East Asia. In Japan and the Republic of Korea about 80 per cent of post-secondary students are enrolled in independent private institutions, and in the Philippines, Indonesia, and Macao Special Administrative Region of China, the share is above 60 per cent. Access to private, often high-quality higher education is often the prerogative of the privileged elite, though in a few countries this is not the case; as suggested by the relatively high ratio of private tertiary enrolment, Japan and the Republic of Korea are among the exceptions (United Nations Educational, Scientific and Cultural Organization, 2006b).

Tertiary education in Asia has become increasingly attractive to foreign investors interested in providing various "transnational" study options; among the most popular are matriculation at an established facility or branch in the beneficiary's country, distance education, and Internet-based e-learning (Mohamedbhai, 2002). A benefit of these new configurations is increased access to tertiary education at no or low cost to Governments. Training young people in their home countries reduces the likelihood of brain drain. The Governments of countries such as China, India, Malaysia and Singapore have become increasingly aware of the advantages associated with these educational alternatives and are allowing prestigious foreign universities to set up local "branch campuses" or "subsidiaries"; indeed, many are actively seeking to establish such relationships (United Nations, 2006a). The downside of transnationally delivered private tertiary education is that profit—rather than the overall economic, social and cultural development of the host country—often constitutes the primary objective (Mohamedbhai, 2002). Quality control mechanisms must be established to ensure that the graduates of such systems are adequately prepared to compete in the job market. It is also necessary to provide equivalent opportunities for those in the public system who may not be able to afford options tailored to the privileged elite.

Vocational and technical education

In both developed and developing regions, vocational and technical education provides important job-related skills that are typically not acquired through academic studies. In Asia, such education is particularly critical in the less developed countries, where significant numbers of youth have had no access to formal education or have dropped out of primary or secondary school. These young people need alternatives to prepare them for the workforce and improve their opportunities in life.

There is limited information on the range of vocational and technical education opportunities across Asia. The Government of India, in collaboration with various non-governmental and intergovernmental organizations, runs the Swaranjayanti Gram Swarozgar Yojana for youth in both rural and urban areas. These schemes focus on self-employment through vocational training and entrepreneurship development. Industrial training institutes and upper secondary schools also provide vocational training courses both for youth who are in school and for those who have dropped out. The skills young people learn help them start and operate small businesses (Kingra, 2005). In some countries, education has become increasingly commercialized, with priority given to technical training for high-performing students. In China, vocational and technical education opportunities tend to be concentrated in cities; young people from rural and/or poor backgrounds are often at a clear disadvantage in terms of access (Xiaoying, 2005).

Successful vocational and technical education programmes focus on building practical skills but are also involved in employment promotion, ensuring that students learn job-search strategies and participate in internships. Graduates must possess broad competencies, transferable skills and relevant knowledge that will enable them to function effectively in today's flexible work environment (Alvarez, Gillies and Bradsher, 2003). Both the public and the private sector have a vital role to play in the development and provision of vocational training, with particular attention given to increased investment in internships, apprenticeships, and other opportunities for practical experience. When expanding the provision of vocational and technical education, Governments and policy makers should guard against investing in ad hoc crash-training courses aimed at addressing rising youth unemployment (Asian Development Bank, 2004). These often represent stopgap solutions and typically have no long-term impact. Finally, steps must be taken to ensure that disadvantaged youth have access to vocational and technical learning options.

Quality issues

According to a comparative study undertaken by the OECD, education systems in East Asia outperform those in other parts of the world. In 2003, the six East Asian countries participating in PISA, which measured the performance of 15-year-old students in mathematics, were ranked among the top ten in the final evaluation (Organization for Economic Cooperation and Development, 2006).

The quality of education tends to be high in East Asia but is somewhat uneven in other Asian subregions. Many countries that have achieved near-universal enrolment in basic education have substandard school, library and laboratory facilities, and learning environments are often less than optimal. Such conditions produce adults who are inadequately prepared to participate fully in society. The World Bank (2006) notes that in Nepal, for example, among the 30 per cent of 15- to 19-year-olds who never made it past the third grade, fewer than 60 per cent can read a sentence.

The lack of adequately trained teachers contributes to the poor quality of schooling in many parts of Asia. A considerable number of primary school teachers, particularly in rural areas, have only obtained a secondary education themselves. As illustrated in figure 1.4, the percentage of trained teachers at the secondary level varies widely from one country to another. In some countries, such as Bangladesh and Bhutan, the proportion of qualified teachers decreases at higher levels of education. The opposite is true in Myanmar, Nepal and Viet Nam, where the share of trained teachers increases with the level of education; this may be a reflection of the lower numbers of students at higher levels and the consequent need for fewer teachers. Priority must be given to strengthening teacher motivation and dedication. In many countries, teaching is one of the less economically rewarding jobs, so incentives might be needed to improve overall levels of commitment and performance. Governments could make teaching more attractive by raising salaries but also by introducing or strengthening opportunities for further training and career advancement. Better facilities and working conditions and improved access to teaching aids and materials would also enhance teacher performance.

Figure 1.4
Percentage of trained teachers in primary education and in lower and upper secondary education, selected countries in Asia

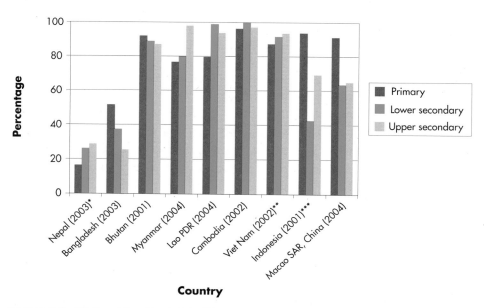

Source: United Nations Educational, Scientific and Cultural Organization, Institute for Statistics (data accessed from www.uis.unesco.org on 18 January 2007).
Notes: *Statistics for upper secondary education are based on 2002 data.
 **Data for upper secondary education are estimates from the UNESCO Institute for Statistics.
 ***Data for all types of education are estimates from the UNESCO Institute for Statistics.

Large class sizes and high student-teacher ratios are common in many Asian countries. Despite evidence suggesting that reducing class size does not necessarily influence student performance (World Bank, 2005), it is unlikely that the quality of education is completely unaffected by the ratio of pupils to teachers. As indicated in figure 1.5, Bangladesh, Cambodia and India have relatively high student-teacher ratios in primary education, ranging from an average of 40 to 55, whereas Brunei Darussalam, China and Malaysia report much lower ratios of between 15 and 21. Similar disparities are evident at the secondary level.

Figure 1.5
Student-teacher ratios in primary and secondary education in selected countries in Asia

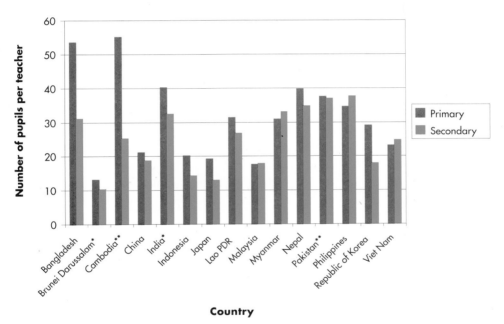

Country

Source: United Nations Educational, Scientific and Cultural Organization, Institute for Statistics (data accessed from www.uis.unesco.org on 18 January 2007).
Notes: *UNESCO Institute for Statistics estimate for primary education.
**UNESCO Institute for Statistics estimate for secondary education.

Content is a critical factor in determining the quality of education. The importance of a solid academic curriculum is undisputed, but there are other aspects of educational content that require consideration as well. It has been observed that rather than emphasizing pluralism and ensuring access and tolerance for all, education is at times excessively politicized and unduly influences young people's identity formation and political affiliations. This can contribute to the creation of segregated communities along ethno-linguistic and religious lines (Hettige, 2005).

Public expenditure on education is largely restricted to the primary level; as education at the higher levels has become increasingly privatized, public spending for tertiary and technical education has declined (Rizvi and others, 2005). While primary school enrolment has increased tremendously across the region, rates of investment and enrolment at the secondary and higher levels lag far behind. As a consequence, large numbers of young Asians are transitioning to adulthood lacking the knowledge and skills necessary to participate fully in their communities and in the global economy.

The impact of globalization

Globalization has improved the accessibility of a good education for many young people in Asia. Large numbers of previously unserved youth are benefiting from a wide range of innovative educational options, including opportunities originating outside their national borders; distance education is particularly important within this context. Many countries in the region are relying on information and communication technologies (ICT) to improve access to schooling. ICT-based distance education has been used to overcome time, space and geographic restrictions, allowing teachers and students to interact and share learning materials. In China, there are 2,735 radio and television universities at the national, provincial, prefecture and county levels offering more than 18,000 classes. In 2001, these universities produced 174,300 new graduates and enrolled 216,000 new students. According to incomplete statistics, at least 10 million students have successfully completed their studies through these university programmes (United Nations Development Programme, 2004). Young people pursuing their education through less traditional means are often better able to acquire knowledge and skills that will allow them to function effectively in a growing global economy driven by technology. Modern educational alternatives are generally positive for those who are able to benefit; however, they have also given rise to new inequalities, as youth from privileged families tend to be better placed to take advantage of the relevant opportunities.

The impact of globalization on the education sector is also evident in the increased demand for skills in science and engineering. Many Asian education systems have responded to this demand. In 2002, almost 650,000 science and engineering degrees were conferred in Asia, compared with approximately 357,000 in Europe and 100,000 in North America. The same year, Asian tertiary institutions granted twice as many degrees in the social and behavioural sciences as their European counterparts and about 160,000 more than North American institutions. Asian youth are also increasingly able to access higher education opportunities outside their national borders, competing successfully for places in science and engineering programmes abroad. Between 1983 and 2003, institutions of higher learning in the United States awarded 141,826 doctoral degrees to persons of Asian origin; of this number, 120,698 were in science and engineering (National Science Foundation, 2006). Asian youth able to take advantage of these opportunities are well prepared for entry into an international labour market in which science and engineering dominate as fields of specialization. Essentially, many young people in Asia are improving their ability to participate in the global economy by training in fields that currently have some of the lowest rates of unemployment.

Ultimately, the subjects studied and the qualifications obtained by students are a reflection of the socio-economic opportunities available to individuals or particular segments of society in each country. For example, poorer students cannot always afford programmes with higher unit costs. The divide frequently becomes apparent at the lower levels, where the quality of education may not be adequate to properly prepare students for tertiary studies. Schools in low-income countries, especially in rural areas, often have poorly equipped science facilities or no such facilities at all, limiting student choices with regard to fields of study. Rural-urban disparities persist, and poorer students in outlying areas are more likely than others in their age group to choose fields that have little relevance within the globalization framework.

New global production systems require a workforce that is skilled, flexible, and adaptable to rapid change in the business environment (United Nations, 2006b). Significant progress is being made in building such a workforce, but action must be taken to reach those who remain outside the education system, as they will be unable to transition successfully into gainful employment or to participate effectively in the global economy.

Aspects of inequity in access to education

In almost all Asian countries, regardless of development status, there are marked inequalities in access to education at all levels. Education is an indicator of social class and an avenue for upward social mobility and therefore plays a key role in determining social position. A university graduate is frequently perceived to have a higher social standing than a skilled worker (even one with vocational schooling), and a trained worker is ranked higher in the social hierarchy than someone without an education (Hettige, 1998). Easier access to schools and the ability to pay private tuition as well as after-school tutoring fees give well-to-do children a distinct advantage over their poorer peers. The result is considerable inequality in the level of preparedness among young adults to make the transition to productive adulthood characterized by active socio-economic, political and civic involvement.

Statistics showing wide income-based disparities in educational attainment confirm that poverty is a major barrier to schooling in Asia. Poor parents are often forced to involve their children in livelihood work and to choose which among them to educate. In the Philippines, more than 70 per cent of the shortfall in universal primary education consists of children from poor households. In India, the median number of years of schooling completed by 15- to 19-year-olds is 10 years higher among the richest 20 per cent than among the poorest 40 per cent (United Nations Population Fund, 2002).

Factors other than poverty also interfere with the educational participation of various socio-economic groups in Asia. Those living in rural areas, females of all ages, youth with disabilities, indigenous youth and ethnic minorities, and young people who are refugees or have been displaced by war or natural disasters often have limited access to education; because this places them at a social disadvantage, they tend to be excluded from household, community, and national decision-making processes.

Rural youth

In terms of educational opportunities, rural children and youth are particularly disadvantaged. Infrastructure and facilities are often substandard in rural areas, schools are fewer and farther away from the target population, and qualified teachers are reluctant to move to outlying districts. In developing countries, good schools tend to be scarce in remote locales. Access to well-equipped schools may depend on their affordability and on the availability of reliable transportation, neither of which is assured for most rural children in developing countries. Distance learning is rarely available outside the major cities. Educational disparities between rural and urban areas are far greater in less developed Asian countries such as Cambodia, India and Sri Lanka than in more developed countries such as Japan and the Republic of Korea.

Levels of academic performance tend to be considerably higher for urban students than for rural learners, particularly in science and mathematics, ICT education, and foreign language studies. Even in basic skills such as literacy, significant rural-urban disparities exist. In Pakistan, the adult literacy rate is 44 per cent in rural areas and 72 per cent in urban areas; however, the rural-urban ratio of 0.61 is nearly double the 1972 ratio of 0.34, suggesting that some progress is being made in bridging the rural-urban gap in literacy (United Nations Educational, Scientific and Cultural Organization, 2005a).

For many among the rural poor, personal circumstances preclude a sustained commitment to education. As rural incomes are often seasonal, poorer rural families may have to sacrifice their children's schooling for the family's sustenance. During harvest time, older children are sometimes needed to work in the fields or to care for younger siblings. In times of bad harvest or flooding, parents may be forced to pull their children out of school. Children who are poorly educated make the transition into youth and young adulthood with very limited job prospects; most inherit poor livelihoods, remaining unskilled and unprotected labourers for the rest of their lives. One of the dangers of such marginalization is radicalization.

Young Women

Gender disparities in access to education underlie the tendency for women to have fewer opportunities to contribute to decisions affecting them and their households. Long-standing cultural barriers, social customs and beliefs, and discriminatory practices place many girls and young women at a disadvantage in terms of educational access. Gender gaps tend to be greater at the secondary and tertiary levels; typically, fewer girls than boys remain in the education system once they have completed primary school. In some countries, however, girls are more likely than boys to continue their education. At the secondary level, female enrolment exceeds male enrolment in Bangladesh, Brunei Darussalam, Macao Special Administrative Region of China, Sri Lanka, and the Islamic Republic of Iran (see figure 1.3). In Brunei Darussalam, the Islamic Republic of Iran, Malaysia, Mongolia, the Philippines and Thailand, females outnumber males in tertiary education (see table 1.3).

Young men and young women are often steered into particular fields of study. Between 2 and 39 per cent of Asian university graduates in the countries highlighted in table 1.5 received degrees in science-and-technology-related fields, including traditional sciences, engineering, manufacturing and construction, with males constituting a clear majority in almost all cases. Asian females tended to pursue studies in disciplines such as health, humanities, education and social sciences; however, in Bangladesh, Cambodia and Lao People's Democratic Republic, males were also predominant in these fields of study. Mongolia is the only country in which females outnumbered males in science and technology (if only slightly), though this may derive from the fact that with 65 per cent of all graduates being women, young Mongolian females are significantly better represented than their male counterparts in tertiary education (United Nations Educational, Scientific and Cultural Organization, 2006b).

Table 1.5
Graduates by sex and field of education in selected Asian countries, 2004 or most recent data (percentage of the total)

Country	Science and technology fields	Percentage female	Other fields	Percentage female
Bangladesh	13	24	85	34
Brunei Darussalam	11	42	88	67
Cambodia	15	12	85	32
Hong Kong SAR[a]	28	26	47	68
Islamic Republic of Iran	37	30	60	56
Japan	22	15	73	59
Lao People's Democratic Republic	7	21	93	39
Macao SAR[a]	2	..	98	..
Mongolia	16	51	84	68
Philippines[b]	21	47	72	68
Republic of Korea	39	31	61	61
Viet Nam	18	14	77	52

Source: United Nations Educational, Scientific and Cultural Organization, *Global Education Digest 2006: Comparing Education Statistics Across the World* (Montreal: UNESCO Institute for Statistics, 2006) (UIS/SD/06-01).

Notes: Two dots (..) indicate that the item is not available.

[a] SAR: Special Administrative Region of China.

[b] Provisional data.

There appears to be no correlation between national per capita income and gender disparities in education, which supports the assertion that economic development alone does not translate into full access to education for females (Filmer, King and Pritchett, 1998). Where gender disparities have been reduced, policies and interventions have included provisions for economic investment but have focused primarily on eliminating cultural, social and ideological barriers to female education. The international community has placed the problem of gender disparities in education high on the development agenda, adopting international targets for improvement. The third Millennium Development Goal, for example, calls for the elimination of gender disparities in primary and secondary education, preferably by 2005, and at all levels by no later than 2015. The 2005 target has clearly been missed, and much greater effort is needed to achieve the objectives for 2015 in many parts of Asia.

Youth with disabilities

For youth with disabilities, inequalities in access to education are extreme. Reliable data on children and youth with disabilities are scarce, and many countries do not provide enrolment figures for this group. Estimates suggest that globally about 35 per cent of all out-of-school children have disabilities, and that less than 2 per cent of children with one or more disabilities are enrolled in school (United Nations Educational, Scientific and Cultural Organization, 2005b). Available statistics indicate that in the Asia-Pacific region less than 5 per cent of children with disabilities are enrolled in school (Jonsson and Wiman, 2001).

Some Asian countries are taking steps to improve educational access for children and youth with disabilities. In China, for example, children with physical disabilities are mainstreamed into regular schools, and 80 per cent of those between the ages of 7 and 16 who are blind or deaf or have intellectual disabilities are receiving a formal education. In the Republic of Korea, 83.6 per cent of children and youth with disabilities (aged 6-18 years) are enrolled in either special or regular school programmes at the primary or secondary level.

Although measures have been taken in some countries to facilitate the education and training of children and young people with disabilities, in many parts of Asia significant gaps remain. In the Philippines, for example, only 2 per cent of school-age children and youth with disabilities are enrolled in formal educational institutions (United Nations Economic and Social Commission for Asia and the Pacific, 2006a).

In December 2006, the United Nations adopted the Convention on the Rights of Persons with Disabilities and its Optional Protocol. Article 24 of the Convention recognizes the right of persons with disabilities to an inclusive education at all levels on an equal-opportunity basis. Inclusive education enables persons with disabilities to acquire the knowledge and skills needed to participate effectively in a free society while also allowing students without disabilities to experience diversity in various forms. The Convention requires States Parties to fulfil certain obligations. It is necessary to ensure that teachers receive adequate training and possess the requisite skills to provide quality education in inclusive settings. In addition, there must be "reasonable accommodation" of individual learners' needs, which means, inter alia, that the school environment must be characterized by full accessibility in all possible respects; this may involve, for example, providing both stair and ramp access to all physical learning sites, producing educational materials in accessible formats, and facilitating the learning of Braille and sign language. The Convention is currently in the process of signature and ratification, and several Asian countries have signaled their willingness to accept its terms.

Indigenous peoples and ethnic minorities

Many Asian countries have multi-ethnic populations. In fact, over 60 per cent of the world's indigenous peoples live in Asia. India alone is home to 90 million indigenous people distributed among approximately 400 tribal groups (United Nations Educational, Scientific and Cultural Organization, 2005b). Article 30 of the Convention on the Rights of the Child officially recognizes the right of children of ethnic, religious and linguistic minorities and persons of indigenous origin to use their respective languages, but the lack of bilingual and culturally sensitive formal learning opportunities prevents many young people from obtaining a decent education; children or youth who want to learn but are unable to understand or communicate well in the primary language of instruction are far less likely to succeed (United Nations Educational, Scientific and Cultural Organization, 1999). Because relatively little effort is made to accommodate their linguistic and cultural needs, indigenous children tend to complete fewer years of schooling than non-indigenous children, and their educational performance is frequently substandard. Many indigenous children live in remote areas with poor infrastructure, making access to schooling difficult or impossible. Dropout, repetition and failure rates are high in indigenous schools. Since education services in indigenous areas are generally underfunded, materials and facilities tend to be inadequate. In most cases, formal education systems are not well adapted to traditional ways of learning, and the curriculum does not address the histories, knowledge, technologies and value systems of indigenous peoples. This lack of adaptation and accommodation not only distances students from their own cultures but may also contribute to low self-esteem and the feeling of being unable to cope in a modern world (United Nations, 2007b).

Improved collection and appropriate disaggregation of data on indigenous peoples would make it easier to identify and address the obstacles faced by the younger members of this group in obtaining an education. Precise data on educational attainment among indigenous peoples are scarce, but the limited statistics that are available point to significant disparities between indigenous and non-indigenous populations. The results of the 1991 census in Bangladesh indicated that only 18 per cent of the country's indigenous peoples were literate, compared with a national figure of 40 per cent. Viet Nam has a national literacy rate of 87 per cent, though for some indigenous groups the corresponding rate is as low as 4 per cent (United Nations Educational, Scientific and Cultural Organization, 2005a). These data on literacy apply to entire populations, but one important implication is that indigenous youth often lack the basic skills they need to function effectively in their communities.

Because of cultural, social and economic barriers, young indigenous females are at a greater disadvantage than their male counterparts in terms of educational access. Statistics indicate that among indigenous communities in two Cambodian provinces the literacy rate is only 2 per cent for women but 20 per cent for men, and in Rajasthan, India, the corresponding rates are 8 and 39 per cent (United Nations Educational, Scientific and Cultural Organization, 2005a).

YOUTH PARTICIPATION IN THE LABOUR MARKET

Many countries in Asia have been able to take advantage of their large supply of young, cheap labour to develop vibrant export-oriented manufacturing sectors. Industrial development opportunities have expanded as foreign companies ranging from medium-sized enterprises to large transnationals, especially from OECD countries, have been forced by domestic production costs to move offshore in order to remain competitive. This is particularly the case for the production of goods such as shoes, clothes, toys and electronic appliances, for which low-skill, labour-intensive work is required (Oxfam, 2003). Industrial expansion has created millions of new job opportunities in Asia, initially in the vibrant economies of Hong Kong Special Administration Region of China, the Republic of Korea, Singapore, and Taiwan Province of China; later in China, Indonesia, Malaysia and Thailand; and more recently in Cambodia, Lao People's Democratic Republic, and Viet Nam. Young people are a major resource in these labour markets. They may be more flexible and industrious, more willing to relocate for work, and better attuned to modern technology. Because they must contend with competition from other youth as well as from older and more experienced members of the labour force, young workers are more likely than older workers to accept short-term contracts, low wages and minimal benefits.

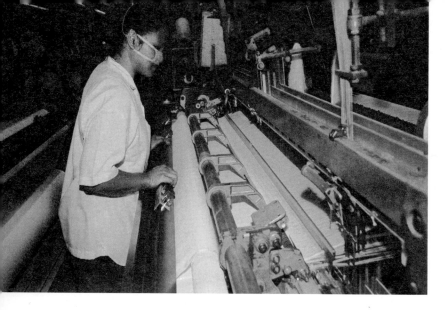

Younger workers constitute a ready supply of inexpensive labour and have played a key role in helping Asian economies meet the global demand for an ever-expanding array of goods. Many of the new job opportunities created by globalization, especially in manufacturing, have been in occupations dominated by women. Encouraged by improved prospects for employment, millions of young rural women have moved to urban areas, securing jobs in factories producing goods such as electronics, clothing and toys. Available data suggest that females represent an important part of rural-to-urban migration in Asia. Historical and cultural factors have combined with specific developments in the industrial and service sectors of cities to expand employment opportunities for women (Lim, 1993). At a broader level, young people in particular have helped the urban informal economy to diversify and become an integral part of the economy of Asian cities. More than half of Asian workers are employed in the urban informal economy (Hugo, 2003).

Unemployment, underemployment and the poor quality of work

Although large numbers of young Asians are better prepared than ever before to enter the labour force, many are unable to find a job. Unemployment is a major problem among youth, as opportunities for securing decent work remain limited. Employers may discriminate against young workers for various reasons, the most obvious being that youth are often at entry levels and lack the experience and knowledge needed in the workplace. In South-East Asia and the Pacific youth are five times more likely than older workers to be unemployed, and in South Asia and East Asia they are almost three times more likely to be without a job (International Labour Office, 2006). It should be noted that employment and unemployment figures mask problems of underemployment and poverty among working youth.

Since the dynamics of economic growth help determine a country's capacity to absorb new entrants to the labour market, employment prospects for young people are more sensitive to economic growth than are those for older workers (Morris, 2006). Figure 1.6 shows that the surge in unemployment in Thailand following the Asian economic crisis of 1997/98 was much higher for youth than for adults, and that while the post-crisis recovery saw a return to pre-crisis levels of unemployment for the population as a whole, youth unemployment declined only slightly, remaining five times higher than the adult level.

Figure 1.6
Youth, adult and total unemployment rates in Thailand, 1990-2004

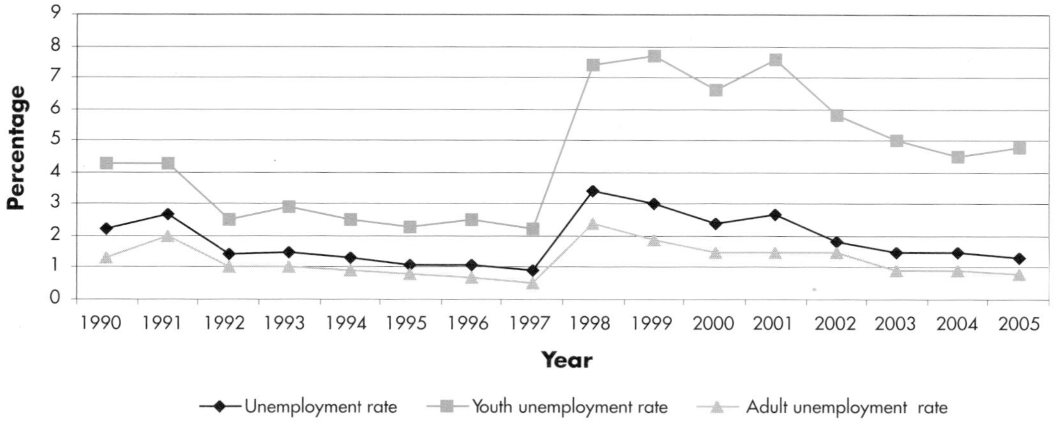

Source: Elizabeth Morris, "Globalization and its effects on youth employment trends in Asia", a paper presented at the Regional Expert Group Meeting on Development Challenges for Young People, Bangkok, 28-30 March 2006.

The Asian crisis had a similar impact on unemployment trends in other countries in the region. The most significant jump in youth unemployment between 1995 and 2005 occurred in South-East Asia and the Pacific, where the number of jobless young people rose by an astounding 85.5 per cent, compared with an increase of 14.8 per cent globally (International Labour Office, 2006).

Although it would appear that levels of educational attainment, employment and remuneration are positively correlated, this is not always the case in Asia. Unemployment levels in the region tend to be higher among those with a secondary or higher education than among those who have not made it past the primary level. Low levels of technology use translate into weak demand for better educated youth, resulting in unemployment in skilled categories (United Nations Economic and Social Commission for Asia and the Pacific, 2006b). This has certainly been true for Indonesia; in the years just before and after the Asian crisis, unemployment rates were highest among those with a senior high school or university education (see table 1.6). To some extent, this may reflect the willingness of better educated people to spend additional time looking for work commensurate with their expectations. Additionally, those who have obtained a higher-level education may find it easier to forego "employment at any cost" because they often come from better-off families (Ahmed, 1999). The unemployment of educated young people may also indicate a mismatch between their training and the types of jobs that are available.

Table 1.6
Unemployment trends in Indonesia by level of education, 1994-1998
(percentage)

Level of education	Unemployment rate			
	1994	1996	1997	1998
No schooling	0.4	0.5	0.3	0.4
Primary school not completed	0.9	1.0	1.0	1.3
Primary school	2.3	2.5	2.5	2.7
Junior high school (general)	6.3	6.8	6.0	7.5
Junior high school (vocational)	6.2	6.9	5.6	7.4
Senior high school (general)	16.9	14.9	14.1	15.3
Senior high school (vocational)	11.0	11.3	11.3	13.3
Diploma I/II	8.8	8.5	6.8	6.4
Diploma III	10.6	10.2	9.7	11.8
University	14.8	13.9	11.8	12.2

Source: Iftikhar Ahmed, "Additional insights on Indonesia's unemployment crisis", a paper presented at the Workshop on Food and Nutrition, Jakarta, 10-12 May 1999.

The figures in table 1.6 relate to open unemployment, but such data represent only the tip of the iceberg. Underemployment is also a major problem in Asia—one to which youth are particularly vulnerable. Unlike their more affluent peers, young people from poorer families cannot afford to be unemployed and are compelled to take whatever jobs are available. They often work part-time or intermittently and tend to become actively involved in the informal economy; their chances for upward mobility are generally limited. While short periods of job search are expected for new entrants to the labour force, extended periods of unemployment and economic non-participation can have serious consequences for national development in general and for young people in particular, resulting in a loss in production and an increase in poverty among youth (Morris, 2006). Many young people who are unable to find work become frustrated and discouraged and eventually give up and drop out of the labour force altogether. Others stay in the education system much longer than they intended. Providing young people with chances to obtain decent employment early in their working lives would help many avoid the vicious circle of chronic unemployment or underemployment, low income and poor working conditions, and social exclusion and despair.

Because of the demands of the labour market and intense competition, many young people who are able to obtain employment in the formal economy end up doing menial work, are vulnerable to abuse and job insecurity, and may face various workplace risks owing to the lack of occupational safety. In China, for example, 38 per cent of youth work without the protection of employment contracts and are therefore defenceless against job loss and exploitation (International Labour Office, 2006). Furthermore, foreign companies, which are often the primary source of the increased demand for labour, do not necessarily have long-term commitments to a particular country; as wages in the host country rise, many relocate to areas offering cheaper labour. In recent years a number of companies have moved from South-East Asian countries such as Malaysia to East Asian countries such as China and Viet Nam, where labour costs are lower.

In certain areas of the region, especially South Asia, young women are much less likely than young men to be part of the workforce. With labour force participation rates of 29.1 per cent for young women and 64.2 per cent for young men, South Asia has the largest gender differential in labour force participation in the world. This is largely a reflection of cultural constraints and the absence of opportunities for women to combine work and family roles.

Young women find it especially difficult to secure decent work (Morris, 2006). Those who do earn wages are likely to be employed in the informal economy. They are typically paid less than men and also do a disproportionate share of unpaid work at home. The labour market transformation brought on by globalization has exposed women to higher risks of exploitation in the workplace. Many new jobs are targeted at young women because they are perceived to be more amenable to control, more nimble-fingered, and cheaper to employ than their male counterparts. In many cases, young women work long hours in substandard conditions for subsistence wages, are subjected to sexual abuse, and are routinely discharged if they marry, become pregnant or grow "too old" (Hancock, 2000).

It is important to note that in response to youth employment challenges in the region, many Governments in Asia have encouraged the development of entrepreneurship and self-employment among young people. However, relatively few microfinancing initiatives specifically target this group. Those that do tend to be implemented by non-governmental organizations or private banks, and many initiatives are too small in scale and lacking in resources to make a noticeable dent in youth unemployment (United Nations Economic and Social Commission for Asia and the Pacific, 2006b). Consequently, even if youth are interested in establishing their own enterprises—an option that could help lift other youth out of poverty—relatively few will be able to obtain the resources necessary to do so.

Urbanization and related issues

Urban residents in Asia—more than 270 million of whom are youth—currently account for almost 50 per cent of the world's total urban population. By 2030, the number of youth living in urban areas in Asia is expected to climb to 533 million; the region's total urban population is projected to increase from 1,553 million to 2,663 million, with the proportion of urban residents rising from 40 to 55 per cent of the overall population (United Nations, 2005b). Many youth were born in cities, while others migrated there from rural areas either alone or as part of a family unit. East Asia is the most urbanized part of the region and South-Central Asia the least urbanized, with city-dwellers accounting for 41.6 and 29.8 per cent of the respective populations. At the subregional level, two in three residents in East Asia and almost one in two residents in South-Central and South-East Asia are expected to live in urban areas. Projections indicate even greater variations between individual countries (Hugo, 2003).

Although opportunities for education and employment are generally better in urban areas than in rural areas, inflexible labour markets and education systems have not always been able to adequately absorb urban youth, making the members of this group more vulnerable to poverty and social exclusion. In Asia, as in other regions, the process of urbanization has been accompanied by increased deprivation among certain groups. Poverty ranges between 12 and 40 per cent in urban areas, and in many Asian cities, 30 to 40 per cent of the population live in slums. In 2005, the slum populations of South Asia and East Asia were estimated at 276 million and 272 million respectively; with figures such as these, it is no surprise that the slum population in Asia far exceeds that in any other region of the world. In slums, residents of all ages commonly deal with challenges relating to inadequate shelter and the limited availability of public services such as water and sanitation; youth in such situations are at a particular disadvantage, given their insecurity of tenure, relatively poor job prospects, and often insufficient incomes. The anger and despair arising from these circumstances lead some youth to engage in crime, violence and other antisocial behaviour (Hugo, 2003). The emergence of various forms of delinquency, including the formation of youth gangs, is often a reaction to exclusion and marginalization in urban areas. According to the United Nations Centre for Human Settlements, developing countries have seen an overall increase in urban crime, and youth crime has risen exponentially. In crimes involving youth, young people are as likely to be the perpetrators as the victims. Young female migrants in urban areas are particularly at risk of sexual exploitation and abuse (Hugo, 2003).

The impact of globalization and urbanization on youth culture, values and social lives

Globalization, urbanization and the changes they have precipitated have brought about a profound transformation in the values, culture and everyday lives of young people. The openness of Asian economies and the exposure of youth to foreign goods, services and information have encouraged the development of an international youth culture and facilitated the spread of Western cultural practices, not all of which are positive. Rapidly developing communication technologies have enabled many young people from countries large and small to access information that may otherwise have been unavailable. Youth more readily challenge traditional authority structures that sometimes constrain or guide their development, but they also experience disorientation and anomie caused by the day-to-day experience of clashes between traditional and modern norms and values (Yap, 2004).

At the kinship level, the focus has shifted away from traditional extended families to more nuclear structures. This has been associated with a reduction in patriarchal power and control over younger family members. Young people in Asia today have greater autonomy than previous generations of youth, particularly with regard to choosing a partner. It has been asserted that no aspect of family life in Asia has changed more than matrimonial conventions (Jones and Ramdas, 2004). In the past, parents tended to play an active role in the selection of a spouse and the arrangement of the nuptials; today, however, the "love-marriage" paradigm is dominant. There have been significant increases in single-parent families and in single and two-person households. With rates of international migration on the rise, transnational families have also become more prevalent (Hugo, 2006). These changes in the family structure have contributed to the erosion of many of the traditional constraints imposed on young people, with mixed repercussions; young people have been given the opportunity to exercise their independence, but the support systems they were once able to rely upon in times of difficulty have weakened. As traditional norms are increasingly challenged and superseded by contemporary mores and values, new lifestyles are emerging that place many young people at risk in their personal and social lives.

The role of risky personal behaviour

Although information on sexual and reproductive health is readily available in most Asian countries, many young people engage in risky sexual practices and are therefore vulnerable to sexually transmitted diseases, unwanted pregnancies, and the dangers of unsafe abortions. A double standard prevails in the region whereby sexual promiscuity is accepted and even encouraged among men but strictly prohibited for women.

Early pregnancy, with its attendant high risks of maternal and child mortality, remains a problem in the region. In 2004, 33 per cent of the teenagers in Bangladesh and 21 per cent in Nepal were pregnant or had borne a child. The average age of first exposure to intercourse is low in Asia, contributing to early childbearing patterns; in some countries the vast majority of young people experience sexual intercourse before the age of 20. The results of a recent demographic and health survey indicate that more than 60 per cent of young women in Nepal have engaged in sexual intercourse by the time they are 18 years old, and almost 80 per cent have done so by the time they reach the age of 20 (see table 1.7).

Table 1.7
Age at first sexual experience for young women in selected
Asian countries

Country	Year	Percentage of youth experiencing first sexual intercourse by specified ages					Never had intercourse
		Age (years)					
		15	18	20	22	25	
Cambodia	2000	3.5	28.0	50.8	65.8	75.8	16.3
Indonesia	2002/03	6.7	27.8	45.9	60.9	75.4	13.9
Nepal	2001	16.7	61.3	78.6	86.8	91.8	4.5
Philippines	2003	2.8	14.8	33.6	49.3	68.2	18.3

Source: MEASURE DHS, STATcompiler (available from http://www.measuredhs.com; accessed on 28 March 2007).
Note: The women surveyed ranged from 25 to 29 years of age.

In several countries in the region, especially in South Asia, one third to one half of all childbearing occurs before the age of 25, and in rural areas the proportions are even higher. Early childbearing is associated with reduced participation in higher education and formal employment. Many engage in sexual intercourse and bear children at a relatively young age because of early marriage, but premarital sex is also increasing in the region despite strong cultural opposition (Gubhaju, 2002). Associated with this trend are heightened risks of sexual exploitation and disease transmission. In some countries, the sexual abuse of teenage girls and the increase in the proportion of sex workers under the age of 25 constitute serious problems (Haub and Huong, 2003); as shown in figure 1.7, young women in the latter group make up the majority of female sex workers in Asian cities.

Figure 1.7
Proportion of female sex workers who are teenagers or under the age of 25, selected sites in Asia

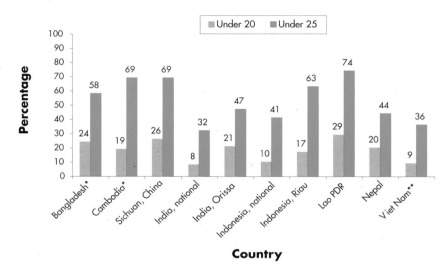

Source: National and regional behavioural surveillance survey data; see Cai Cai, "Globalization and its impact on youth health in Asia", a paper presented at the Regional Expert Group Meeting on Development Challenges for Young People in Asia, Bangkok, 28-30 March 2006.
Notes: * Data refer to brothel-based only.
** Data refer to street-based only.

The Joint United Nations Programme on HIV/AIDS (UNAIDS) reports that multiple forms of risky behaviour are driving serious AIDS epidemics in Asia, and the interplay between injecting drug use and unprotected sex, much of it commercial, is at the heart of the problem. Evidence of increased levels of sexual risk-taking among young Asians has raised concerns about the spread of HIV and other sexually transmitted infections (East-West Center, 2002). An estimated 2.2 million young people live with HIV/AIDS in Asia, and half of all new infections occur among youth (Cai, 2006). Statistics for the latter part of 2000 indicate that in Indonesia, HIV prevalence was highest for the age group 20-30, though the number of cases among 15- to 19-year-olds was also significant (see figure 1.8). Although data are limited, there is also evidence of an increase in sexually transmitted diseases among young people in Viet Nam, and youth are becoming an increasingly important group in the rapidly growing HIV-infected population (Haub and Huong, 2003).

Figure 1.8
HIV-infected population in Indonesia by age, November 2000

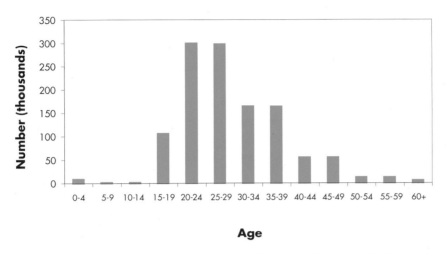

Age

Source: Indonesia, Directorate-General of Communicable Disease Control and EH Ministry of Health (2001).

Other negative lifestyle factors, including tobacco use, excessive alcohol consumption, substance abuse, and poor dietary practices, also undermine the ability of youth to move towards independent and responsible adulthood and full participation in society. Table 1.8 shows the prevalence of drinking, smoking and drug use among youth in selected Asian countries. Young men are far more likely than young women to engage in these practices and to start at a younger age (East-West Center, 2002).

Table 1.8
Percentage of males and females aged 15-19 years who drink, smoke or use drugs, selected countries in Asia

Country (year)	Drink		Smoke		Use drugs	
	Boys	Girls	Boys	Girls	Boys	Girls
China (2000)	37	9	36	1	..	..
India (1998/99)	2	1	14ª	2ª	..	..
Indonesia (1988)	2	—	38	1	1	—
Japan (2000)ᵇ	39	31	26	12	..	..
Nepal (2000)	21	11	12	4	..	..
Philippines (1994)	47	12	28	3	2	—
Republic of Korea (2000)	46	51	21	11	3	3
Thailand (1994)	43	16	33	2	6	1

Source: East-West Center Research Program, Population and Health Studies, The Future of Population in Asia (Honolulu: East-West Center, 2002).

Notes: Two dots (..) indicate that the information is not available. A dash (—) indicates that the amount is nil or negligible.
ª Includes chewing tobacco.
ᵇ For youth between the ages of 15 and 18 only.

The Centers for Disease Control and Prevention published data in 2006 showing that while the prevalence of cigarette use among young people in Asia is among the lowest in the world, the region ranks highest in terms of other tobacco use (this category includes but is not limited to chewing tobacco, snuff, dip and cigars). It is estimated that more than one third of the tobacco consumed in Asia is smokeless; some of the more traditional options include betel quid, tobacco with lime, and tobacco tooth powder. Tobacco use is prevalent not only among men and women, but also among children and teenagers (Gupta and Ray, 2003). In China and Indonesia more than 30 per cent of young men smoke, but only 1 per cent of young women do. In the Philippines, 14 per cent of children begin smoking before reaching age 10, and in some parts of China the corresponding proportion is over 20 per cent (Cai, 2006). Young women in Japan and the Republic of Korea are more likely to smoke than their female counterparts in other Asian countries.

The prevalence of precocious alcohol use varies considerably depending on the cultural and religious environment. Although alcohol consumption is very limited among young people aged 15-19 years in countries such as India and Indonesia, almost half of the young men in this age group drink alcohol in the Philippines, the Republic of Korea and Thailand. Among the countries surveyed in table 1.8, rates of alcohol consumption are generally lower among women, except in the Republic of Korea.

Asian countries report very low rates of drug use, but recent statistics point to a growing problem, especially in urban areas. One estimate indicates that in Indonesia drugs are used by around 2 per cent of the population, or around 4 million residents, 1.3 million of whom live in Jakarta (Utomo and others, 2000). Hospitals in the country's capital are reporting a surge in drug overdoses among young people. Survey data on 400 intravenous drug users in Jakarta indicated that 90 per cent were male and that 95 per cent were younger than 30 years of age. In China's Yunnan province, more than half of the registered drug users are under the age of 25, and more than half of the injecting drug users in India, Myanmar and Thailand are between 15 and 24 years old (Cai, 2006).

There is a clear link between globalization and the increased prevalence of obesity. Multinational fast-food companies in OECD countries are rapidly expanding into Asia, and the internationalization of the food industry is changing the diets of many young Asians, especially in the larger cities. Obesity exists alongside malnutrition in Asia and affects all age groups. One third of South Asians are dangerously overweight. In Chinese cities 12 per cent of adults and 8 per cent of children are obese, and in Thailand the prevalence of obesity among children aged 5-12 years increased from 12 per cent to between 15 and 16 per cent in two years (Cai, 2006). Obesity is often conceptualized as a problem of the affluent, but it actually occurs across the socio-economic spectrum. Overeating is certainly a factor, but obesity is also function of imbalanced nutrition and insufficient exercise. Unless action is taken to address the growing prevalence of obesity among young people in Asia, the youth of today will be more vulnerable than any previous generation to the early onset of degenerative and non-communicable diseases and to reduced longevity.

The challenges deriving from unhealthy behaviour are compounded by difficulties surrounding access to health education and health care. Though reproductive health information has been more widely disseminated in Asia in recent years, many young people have limited access to materials detailing contraceptive options and the risks of unprotected sexual activity, and youth-friendly health services are often unavailable. Substantial numbers of Asian youth simply cannot afford health care (Gubhaju, 2002). Demographic and health surveys indicate that young people in Cambodia frequently lack the knowledge, authority and financial resources to address their health needs.

The failure of the health-care establishment to address the needs of youth is particularly apparent in rural areas. Reproductive health is an urgent concern; though family planning programmes have been in place for some time, young people have limited knowledge of contraception. Throughout Asia, family planning information and programmes are almost exclusively targeted at married people, especially married women.

YOUTH MIGRATION: OPPORTUNITIES AND CHALLENGES

One of the most dramatic trends in Asia in recent decades has been the exponential increase in migration (Hugo, 2006). The region's population has become highly mobile, with growing numbers of residents resettling either permanently or temporarily in other Asian countries or abroad. Migration flows within, into, and out of the region are significant. In recent years there has been a substantial increase in migration from the less developed to the more developed countries in Asia and, to a much greater extent, to OECD countries. Statistics from the OECD Database on Immigrants and Expatriates indicate that relatively large numbers of Asians are relocating not only to traditional destinations such as Australia, Canada and the United States, but also to various European countries. In 2005, 28 per cent of all migrants worldwide lived in Asia, and Asians are increasingly moving abroad. Between 2000 and 2003 more than 2 million workers left Asian countries, compared with 1.4 million during the period 1990-1994 (United Nations, 2006a).

International migration takes many forms and directions; sizeable numbers of Asians relocate within the region or seek their fortunes in OECD countries or the Middle East, and there are "circular" as well as permanent flows, legal as well as undocumented migration, and both forced and voluntary movement. Although age-disaggregated data on migration are scarce, available evidence suggests that young adults make up a significant proportion of those leaving their countries for extended periods. As shown in table 1.9, for example, almost one third of Asian-born migrants arriving in Australia in the five years preceding the 2001 census were between the ages of 15 and 24. Other data suggest that levels of mobility are quite high among young adults; most Asian youth no longer have to limit themselves to the opportunities available in their local communities.

Table 1.9
Migrants from Asia arriving in Australia between 1996 and 2001

Birthplace	Number aged 15-24 years	Migrants aged 15-24 years as percentage of total	Total number of migrants (subregion and region)
South-East Asia	36 434	37.2	97 914
North-East Asia	28 452	29.2	97 526
South and Central Asia	12 069	21.9	55 163
Total Asia	76 955	30.7	250 603

Source: Australian Bureau of Statistics, *Census of Population and Housing* (2001) (data accessed at http://www.abs.gov.au on 10 May 2007).

Data on the age and sex composition of internal migrants are limited, but there are indications that youth constitute a major share of such migrants in various countries. In Indonesia, for example, internal migration rates for both sexes appear to rise progressively starting with the age group 10-14 years, peaking at various points between the ages of 20 and 35 for males and females (see figure 1.9). A distinctive feature of internal mobility in recent decades has been the increasing involvement of women. In Indonesia, where women comprise a relatively large proportion of the labour force, the migration rate is higher among females than among males (Chotib, 2003). Women migrate from rural to urban areas to work in factories but also seek employment in the informal economy; a great many are able to secure domestic service jobs. The rate of internal migration is highest for the age group 20-25, though the average ages of male and female migrant labourers are 21 and 17 years respectively (Chotib, 2003).

Figure 1.9
Recent Indonesian internal migrants as a proportion of the total population, by age and sex, 1990-1995

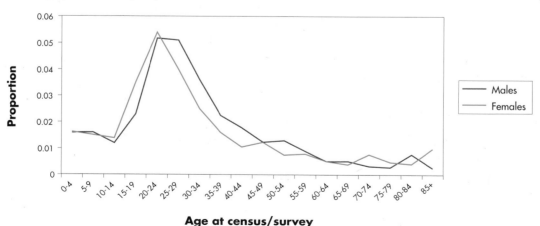

Source: Salahudin Muhidin, *The Population of Indonesia: Regional Demographic Scenarios Using a Multiregional Method and Multiple Data Sources* (Amsterdam: Rozenberg Publishers, 2002).

Opportunities for migration to OECD countries have increased for Asian youth with the requisite skills and qualifications but have decreased for those who are unskilled. As asserted previously, globalization has greatly expanded options for some while seriously limiting possibilities for others.

Women are underrepresented among international migrants living in Asia (United Nations, 2006a). However, in several of the region's labour-sending countries, females account for a sizeable proportion of the emigrant population (see table 1.10). Large numbers of young women from countries such as the Philippines and Sri Lanka are employed as domestic helpers in oil-rich Gulf States and some of the wealthier Asian countries. In many cases, this improves their status within their families back home. Because their remittances typically represent a significant proportion of the family income and may even be necessary for survival, these migrants often earn the right to participate in and influence family decision-making and assume responsibility for the welfare of other family members. However, their social status in their host countries is generally very low. They often work extremely long hours for little pay.

Table 1.10
Women as a proportion of international labour migrants, selected labour-sending Asian countries

Country of origin	Year	Number of workers sent	Women as a proportion of the workers sent
Philippines	2005	704 586	74.3*
Sri Lanka	2004	213 453	65.5
Thailand	2005	128 612	17.7
Indonesia	2004	382 514	78.0
Bangladesh	1999	268 182	0.1
Viet Nam	2000	30 000	15.0

Source: Graeme Hugo, "Globalization and Asian youth: a demographic perspective", a paper presented at the United Nations Regional Expert Group Meeting on Development for Young People in Asia, Bangkok, 28-30 March 2006.
Note: * New hires in 2004.

Globalization has been characterized by major changes in the loci of production and dramatic shifts in the number and spatial distribution of job opportunities. It has also made people more aware of possibilities outside of their immediate communities. The high mobility of Asian youth is a response to limited local opportunities coupled with the awareness, or at least the expectation, of better prospects elsewhere. This trend is fuelled by social and economic change that can provide new opportunities—but only for some.

Migration both within and outside of Asia is driven primarily by improved employment prospects, educational opportunities, marriage and/or family reunification, and escape from conflict situations or social unrest. All types of migration have been facilitated by the ICT revolution and reduced transportation costs. Social networks established by the growing Asian diaspora have allowed many new migrants to adjust more quickly and easily to their new surroundings (Massey and others, 1993). For young people, migration is often associated with increased social and economic independence, separation from traditional authority structures, exposure to new and different ideas and practices, and interaction with a wide range of people.

As the global demand for professionally and technically qualified youth increases, larger numbers of educated young people from poorer Asian countries are leaving home for well-paid jobs in wealthier countries. The resulting brain drain leaves developing countries unable to move from low-skill production to technologically advanced industrial production and service provision. Persistently low productivity levels in some developing Asian countries keep average incomes low, compelling even those with relatively limited skills to migrate to higher-income countries.

International student migration

Student migration is particularly significant among Asian youth. Global student mobility has increased exponentially in the past 30 years. In Afghanistan, Brunei Darussalam, Cambodia, Malaysia and Nepal, mobile students account for at least 5 per cent of domestic tertiary enrolment (United Nations Educational, Scientific and Cultural Organization, 2006b). Figure 1.10 indicates that East Asia and the Pacific has become an increasingly popular destination for international students, and figure 1.11 reveals that this subregion is the point of origin for the largest number of individuals migrating for educational purposes, accounting for around 700,000 students, or 29 per cent of the global total. Approximately 40 per cent of these students remain in the Asia-Pacific area (Australia and Japan each account for 15 per cent), 34 per cent travel to North America, and 25 per cent study in Western Europe. In absolute terms, China is the country with the largest share of student migrants, accounting for 14 per cent of the world total. India, Japan and the Republic of Korea each have more than 60,000 students in educational institutions abroad.

Figure 1.10
International students by region of study, 1975-2004

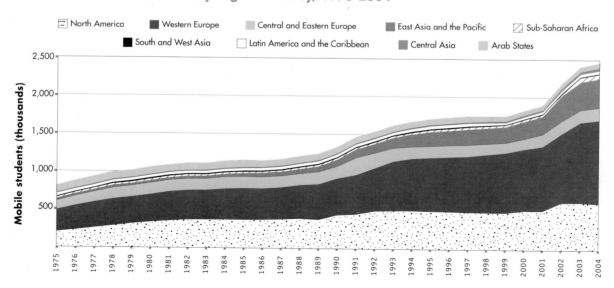

Source: United Nations Educational, Scientific and Cultural Organization, *Global Education Digest 2006: Comparing Education Statistics Across the World* (Montreal: UNESCO Institute for Statistics, 2006) (UIS/SD/06-01).

Figure 1.11
Mobile students by region of origin, 1999 and 2004

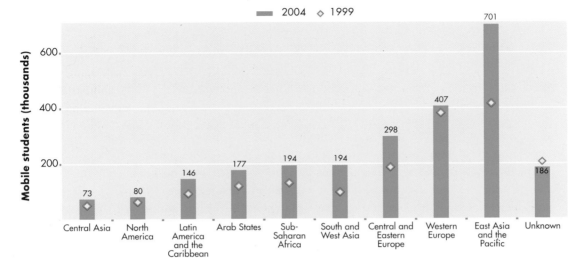

Source: United Nations Educational, Scientific and Cultural Organization, *Global Education Digest 2006: Comparing Education Statistics Across the World* (Montreal: UNESCO Institute for Statistics, 2006) (UIS/SD/06-01).

Many international students decide to stay and seek employment in their host countries, contributing to the massive brain drain from the poorer Asian nations. In 2004/05, 16,485 people on student visas in Australia successfully applied for permanent residence, and the majority of these were young Asians (Australia, Department of Immigration and Multicultural and Indigenous Affairs, 2006).

Consequences of migration

As international migration from and within Asia has increased, so have transnational marriages. Various factors are associated with this trend. Increased global travel and the emergence of commercial enterprises that facilitate marriage raise the likelihood of partnering with a foreign person. As a result of long-standing reproductive trends favouring males, eligible young women are in short supply in some countries, especially in rural areas. According to a report by the Chinese State Population and Family Planning Commission, around 118 boys are born for every 100 girls in China (Wang, 2007). In India in 2001, there were 93 girls aged 0-6 years for every 100 boys (Dasvarma, 2006). It has been estimated that by 2020 the male "surplus" could number more than 20 million in India and 30 million in China (Dasvarma, 2006; Wang, 2007). Even now, there are unprecedented numbers of young adult males who are unlikely to find marriage partners in the future. The report by the Chinese State Population and Family Planning Commission warns that the growing difficulties men face in finding wives may lead to social instability (Wang, 2007). Hudson and den Boer (2004) observe that those males who cannot find spouses generally have low socio-economic status, tend to be unemployed or underemployed, have relatively few ties to the community, and are otherwise marginalized in Chinese society. A marriage migration industry has emerged in which brides are recruited for males in other countries. In Taiwan Province of China, the practice has spread to such an extent that currently 32.2 per cent of marriages are to foreigners, and 13.4 per cent of births are to foreign women (Tsay, 2004).

International migration has opened up a vast range of new possibilities for Asian youth, particularly in terms of job and learning opportunities. Spending time abroad, away from the family, gives young people a chance to gain independence and develop their own opinions and ideas. Evidence shows that in many cases international migration has a positive impact on young Asians, allowing them to obtain work and personal experience, build self-confidence, and acquire skills and attitudes beneficial to themselves and their countries. Migration can lift barriers to participation in employment, particularly for the well-educated, and allow young people to earn decent wages and send remittances back home. This can facilitate young people's engagement with their families and communities in their countries of origin. Migrants who return bring back experience, expertise, and access to strategic contacts in their host countries. The "diaspora effect" has stimulated the growth of high-technology and other industries in several East Asian countries and India (International Labour Office, 2004).

International migration has created not only opportunities but also serious challenges for Asian youth and their home countries. There is ample evidence of expatriate contract workers being exploited. Levels of protection are often inadequate, especially for the large numbers of undocumented labour migrants (Battistella and Asis, 2003). The Philippines has put a number of protections in place for its contract workers living abroad, but few other countries in Asia have done the same.

Although women are still underrepresented in international migrant flows, their share is increasing. Growing numbers of females are entering the job market, many as breadwinners, and those who travel abroad for work are particularly vulnerable to exploitation and degradation. Among these are several million who provide domestic and care-giving services and work in the sex and entertainment industries (Yeoh and Huang, 1999; Lim, 1998; Jones, 1996; 2000). Criminal groups are becoming increasingly involved in human trafficking and other forms of undocumented migration and mainly target young people—in particular girls and young women, who are often forced into the sex and entertainment trades (Skrobanek, Boonpakdi and Janthakeero, 1997; Jones, 1996; 2000). The victims of the thriving Asian sex industry are predominantly poor youth. The exploitation and deprivation of human rights in this area is extreme.

Some Asian countries are experiencing substantial outflows of their brightest and most qualified young people. Aside from the implications of this exodus for national development, there are social costs associated with the separation of family members. Psychological stress is experienced by everyone involved, in part because young migrants and those they leave behind are often unable to fulfil the implicit terms of the "intergenerational contract". Ageing members of labour-sending families suffer because they are not able to rely on their children for day-to-day support and assistance, and the young migrants lose opportunities to benefit from the experience and guidance of their family elders.

Young people who migrate may be less able to benefit from their family's physical and emotional support and to provide such support to their families. However, remittances can have a significant impact on the well-being of household members back home; along with covering basic needs, these funds can provide young people in the family who have not migrated with the opportunity to obtain an education. Figure 1.12 shows that remittances account for a substantial proportion of both foreign exchange earnings and gross domestic product (GDP) in many Asian countries. India and China, with their large cohorts of young people, are the top two recipients of remittances in the world in absolute value (United Nations, 2006a). If channelled effectively, these resources can be used to enhance the educational and professional prospects of young people who are less able to take advantage of cross-border opportunities.

Figure 1.12
Remittances to selected Asian countries, 2004

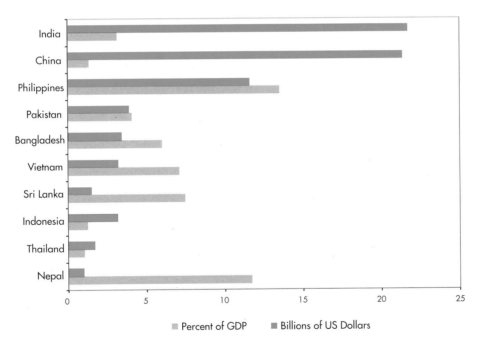

Source: Graeme Hugo, "Globalization and Asian youth: a demographic perspective", a paper presented at the United Nations Regional Expert Group Meeting on Development for Young People in Asia, Bangkok, 28-30 March 2006.

SUMMARY AND CONCLUSIONS

Globalization and major improvements in access to education have allowed many Asian youth to both benefit from and contribute to the development of their countries. Asian culture, values and ways of life have changed considerably as a result of increased economic openness and exposure to foreign goods, services and information. The new perspectives and modes of behaviour adopted by the region's young people sometimes place them at risk but have also allowed them to become a strong, positive force in the development of their societies. Younger workers constitute a ready pool of human capital and are industrious, competitive, adaptable and technologically savvy, but they are often underutilized or exploited in the labour market.

Factors such as the changing nature of work, diminishing demand for unskilled labour, and the emergence of new and less secure forms of employment effectively prevent young people from participating fully in the global economy. Although large numbers of Asian youth are better prepared now than ever before to enter the workforce, many are unable to secure decent employment. The relatively high rate of joblessness among educated youth is believed to derive at least partly from the misalignment or lack of correspondence between their training and the skill requirements for the types of jobs created by globalization. Young people unable to find work may become frustrated and discouraged and eventually give up and drop out of the labour force altogether. Others stay in the education system much longer than they intended.

Females may face additional obstacles. Although more women have found jobs in the era of globalization, the gender gap in employment remains significant; young women in many countries are often less qualified than their male counterparts and are not given an equal opportunity to acquire skills and participate in the labour market.

The population of Asia has become highly mobile in recent decades; temporary and permanent migration within and from the region have increased dramatically as millions of young Asians have left their homes to pursue educational and employment opportunities abroad. Many are taking advantage of the vast range of learning options now available in other countries. International demand for youth with professional and technical skills is growing, and highly qualified young people in poorer countries are drawn to well-paid jobs in wealthier parts of the world. Some Asian countries are experiencing substantial outflows of their brightest and most competent young people. Spending time abroad, away from the family, can provide youth with an important opportunity to gain independence. However, young migrants often experience poverty, deprivation and marginalization as they struggle to become part of their new communities.

Large numbers of Asian youth are highly educated, but strong academic qualifications do not appear to be sufficient to ensure their effective participation in society and the global economy. In the context of rapid globalization, it does not take long for the knowledge and skills of educated youth to be rendered redundant, and securing employment is often just as difficult for this group as for those with little education and training. It is imperative that Governments invest the time and resources necessary to ensure that the education young people receive, especially at the secondary and tertiary levels, prepares them for meaningful participation in the labour market. Private sector educational provision is growing rapidly but is often available only in urban areas. Governments must work to improve the content, quality and accessibility of education in rural areas in order to prevent the education gap from widening in the coming years. Making sure schools in remote locations have the facilities and resources to teach science, mathematics and technical subjects can expand career options for rural youth. Education policies and programmes must also address the special needs of vulnerable and marginalized groups such as girls and young women, youth with disabilities, those living in poverty, ethnic minorities, migrants, refugees, internally displaced persons, and other young people in areas affected by conflict. Given the economic and cultural diversity of Asia, it is important for Governments to ensure that the educational establishment does not contribute to the further marginalization of these groups. Multilingual and multicultural education should be encouraged to increase inter-ethnic and intercultural understanding and communication. Ideally, education should be used not only to enhance prospects for gainful employment and a sustainable livelihood, but also to combat crime and violence and to promote pluralistic, democratic values and peace.

Investment in education must be scaled up, particularly at the higher levels, as Asia has a large youth cohort that in many areas constitutes a significant share of the total population. Traditional secondary and tertiary education should be expanded, but there is also an urgent need to provide non-formal education, literacy programmes, accelerated and distance learning options, vocational training, and other "catch-up" opportunities to the millions of young Asians (especially women) who have never completed primary school.

To ensure that today's children and underserved youth ultimately have the opportunity to contribute meaningfully to community and national development, sustained interventions are needed to achieve universal primary education and higher rates of secondary enrolment. Incentives such as compensating poorer households for keeping their younger members in school, providing free education and materials, and giving a subsistence allowance to children and youth from poor backgrounds who attend school should be introduced or expanded in order to reach those who are not receiving an education.

Schools have a vital role to play in preparing young people for employment. Keeping up with an ever-changing job market is challenging even for the most advanced educational systems, and the majority of developing countries struggle to maintain complementarity between school curricula and workplace requirements. Even in the best situations, however, producing qualified professional and technical personnel does not necessarily translate into guaranteed employment, and graduates are not automatically equipped with the social, moral and attitudinal skills needed to find and keep a decent job. As education in Asia becomes increasingly commercialized and profit oriented, regulation is needed to ensure the availability of a broad range of disciplines and fields of study for young people in both urban and rural areas. Policy makers must ensure that educational curricula prepare young people for the job market, providing them with professional, entrepreneurial and job-search skills.

Today, education is incomplete without ICT integration, which entails both ICT training and the use of ICT as an educational tool. Within Asia, ICT exposure and access and overall e-readiness vary considerably. The Internet and other ICT applications are widely used in most of the higher-income East Asian countries, while in the region's less developed countries ICT penetration is extremely limited. Young people without foreign language skills and those in rural areas are at a particular disadvantage. Without access to ICT, young people are effectively isolated from the global market and unable to take advantage of an immense network of informational and educational resources. The digital divide is expected to narrow over time as the public and private sectors work to ensure universal ICT access, but the existing gap is having an enormous impact on the present cohort of Asian youth.

Governments, international organizations, the commercial private sector, and civil society all have roles to play in enhancing ICT-led education. Both individually and collaboratively, these actors must work to develop the telecommunications infrastructure, provide ICT facilities in schools, and strengthen e-literacy. They can also help to provide wider access to schooling through investments in non-formal education and distance learning with a view to reaching youth in rural and remote areas.

It is essential that young people be given the opportunity to develop in a balanced manner and to make a positive contribution to society. The pursuit of excellence in education (or the lack of opportunity to pursue an education), combined with the evolving challenges associated with rapid globalization, can place young people under extreme stress and interfere with their healthy transition to adulthood. A concerted effort must be made to provide youth with social, economic, personal and other forms of support both within and outside the education system as well as structured opportunities for healthy leisure activity. Active citizenship, intercultural understanding and social solidarity among young people are necessary to ensure equitable development, social justice, peace and social cohesion.

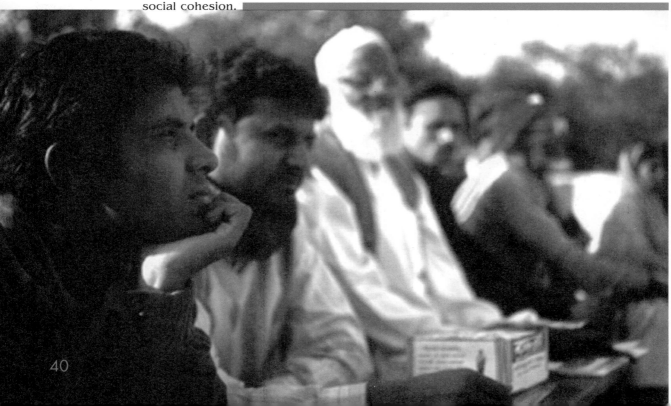

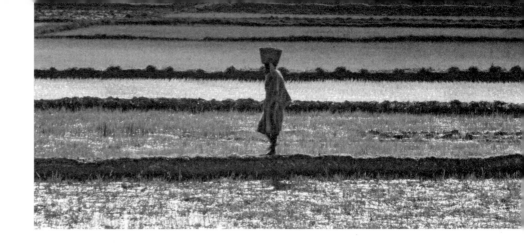

References

Ahmed, Iftikhar (1999). Additional insights on Indonesia's unemployment crisis. Paper presented at the Workshop on Food and Nutrition, Jakarta, 10-12 May 1999.

Alvarez, Benjamin, John Gillies and Monica Bradsher (2003). *Beyond Basic Education: Secondary Education in the Developing World*. Washington, D.C.: World Bank.

Amnesty International (2007). People's Republic of China. Internal migrants: discrimination and abuse—the human cost of an economic "miracle" (ASA 17/008/2007). Available from http://web.amnesty.org/library/index/engasa/70082007 (accessed on 1 March 2007).

Arnove, Robert F. (1973). Education and political participation in rural areas of Latin America. *Comparative Education Review*, vol. 17, No. 2 (June), pp. 198-215.

Asian Development Bank (2003). *Asian Development Outlook 2003*. New York: Oxford University Press.

_____ (2004). *Improving Technical Education and Vocational Training: Strategies for Asia*. Manila.

Australian Department of Immigration and Multicultural and Indigenous Affairs (2006). Population Flows: *Immigration Aspects, 2004-05 Edition*. Available from http://www.immi.gov.au/about/reports/annual/2004-05/contents.htm (accessed on 15 January 2007).

Australian Bureau of Statistics (2001). *Census of Population and Housing*. Data available from http://www.abs.gov.au (accessed on 3 April 2007).

Battistella, Graziano, and Maruja M.B. Asis, editors (2003). Unauthorized Migration in Southeast Asia. Quezon City: Scalabrini Migration Center.

Bloom, David E., and David Canning (2003). The health and poverty of nations: from theory to practice. *Journal of Human Development*, vol. 4, No. 1 (March), pp. 47-71.

_____ and Jaypee Sevilla (2003). *The Demographic Dividend: A New Perspective on the Economic Consequences of Population Change*. Santa Monica, California: Rand. Published under the auspices of Population Matters, a RAND programme of policy-relevant research communication.

Cai, Cai (2006). Globalization and its impact on youth health in Asia. Presentation to the Regional Expert Group Meeting on Development Challenges for Young People in Asia, Bangkok, 28-30 March 2006.

Caritas (2006). Nepal: Bhutanese refugee education programme needs emergency funds. Press release (30 January). Available from http://www.reliefweb.int/rw/rwb.nsf/db900sid/dpas6ljfxd?opendocument&rc=3&cc=npl (accessed on 17 November 2006).

Centers for Disease Control and Prevention (2006). Use of cigarettes and other tobacco products among students aged 13-15 years: worldwide, 1999-2005. *Morbidity and Mortality Weekly Reports*, vol. 55, No. 20 (26 May), pp. 553-556. Available from http://www.cdc.gov/MMWR/preview/mmwrhtml/mm5520a2.htm#tab (accessed on 27 March 2007).

Chotib (2003). Age pattern of migration from and into DKI Jakarta, Indonesia: an analysis of the 1995 Intercensal Population Survey. In *Asians on the Move: Spouses, Dependants and Households*, a collection of papers by Chotib and others. Asian MetaCentre Research Paper Series, No. 8. Asian MetaCentre for Population and Sustainable Development Analysis at the Asian Research Institute, University of Singapore.

Dasvarma, Gouranga (2006). Vulnerable females: the case of declining femininity ratio in India's population. Paper presented at the International Geographical Union Conference, Brisbane, Australia, 3-7 July 2006.

East-West Center Research Program, Population and Health Studies (2002). *The Future of Population in Asia*. Honolulu: East-West Center.

Filmer, Deon, Elizabeth M. King and Lant Pritchett (1998). Gender disparity in South Asia: comparisons between and within countries. Policy Research Working Paper 1867. Washington, D.C.: World Bank Development Research Group, January.

Gubhaju, Bhakta B. (2002). Adolescent reproductive health in Asia. *Asia-Pacific Population Journal*, vol. 17, No. 4, pp. 97-119.

Gupta, Prakash C., and Cecily S. Ray (2003). Smokeless tobacco and health in India and South Asia. *Respirology*, vol. 8, No. 4, pp. 419-431.

Hancock, P. (2000). The lived experience of female factory workers in rural West Java. *Labour and Management in Development Journal*, vol. 1, No. 1, pp. 2-19. Canberra: Asia Pacific Press, Australian National University.

Haub, Carl, and Phuong Thi Thu Huong (2003). *Adolescents and Youth in Viet Nam*. Hanoi: Center for Population Studies and Information.

Hettige, S.T. (1998). Pseudo-modernization and the formation of youth identities in Sri Lanka. In *Globalization, Social Change and Youth*, S.T. Hettige, editor. Colombo: German Cultural Institute.

_____ (2005). A concept paper on counselling and guidance within the school system in Sri Lanka. Paper submitted to the Sri Lanka Ministry of Education.

Hettige, S.T., Markus Mayer and Maleeka Salih, editors (2004). School-to-work transition of youth in Sri Lanka. Employment Strategy Papers, No. 2004/19. Colombo: International Labour Office, Sri Lanka.

Hudson, Valerie M., and Andrea M. den Boer (2004). *Bare Branches: The Security Implications of Asia's Surplus Male Population*. Cambridge, Massachusetts: MIT Press.

Hugo, Graeme (1998). The demographic underpinnings of current and future international migration in Asia. *Asian and Pacific Migration Journal*, vol. 7, No. 1, pp. 1-25.

_____ (2003). *Migration and Development: A Perspective from Asia*. IOM Migration Research Series, No. 14.

_____ (2005a). A demographic view of changing youth in Asia. In *Youth in Transition: The Challenges of Generational Change in Asia*, Fay Gayle and Stephanie Fahey, editors. Bangkok: UNESCO Publishing, Regional Unit for Social and Human Sciences in Asia and the Pacific.

_____ (2005b). Migration in the Asia-Pacific region. Paper prepared for the Policy Analysis and Research Programme of the Global Commission on International Migration. September.

_____ (2006). Migration and development in Asia. Keynote presentation to the International Conference on Population and Development in Asia: Critical Issues for a Sustainable Future, Phuket, Thailand, 20-22 March 2006.

Indonesia (2001). Directorate-General, Communicable Disease Control; and EH Ministry of Health.

International Labour Office (2004). *A Fair Globalization: Creating Opportunities for All*. Report of the World Commission on the Social Dimension of Globalization. Geneva.

_____ (2006). *Global Employment Trends for Youth 2006*. Geneva: International Labour Organization, August.

Jones, G.W. (1997). Population dynamics and their impact on adolescents in the ESCAP region. *Asia Pacific Population Journal*, vol. 12, No. 3 (September), pp. 3-30.

Jones, Gavin, and Kamalini Ramdas, editors (2004). *(Un)tying the Knot: Ideal and Reality in Asian Marriage*. Singapore: NUS Publishing.

Jones, Sidney (1996). Women feed Malaysian boom. *Inside Indonesia*, vol. 47, Nos. 16-18 (July September).

_____ (2000). *Making Money off Migrants: The Indonesian Exodus to Malaysia*. Amsterdam: CLARA Publications.

Jonsson, Ture, and Ronald Wiman (2001). Education, poverty and disability in developing countries. Technical note prepared for the Poverty Reduction Sourcebook. 21 June. Available from http://siteresources.worldbank.org/DISABILITY/Resources/Education/Education_Poverty_and _Disability.pdf (accessed on 19 January 2007).

Kingra, Hardip Singh (2005). Government policies and programs for youth development in India. In *Youth in Transition: The Challenges of Generational Change in Asia*, Fay Gayle and Stephanie Fahey, editors. Bangkok: UNESCO Publishing, Regional Unit for Social and Human Sciences in Asia and the Pacific.

Lim, Lin Lean (1993). Growing economic interdependence and its implications for international migration. Paper presented at the Expert Group Meeting on Population Distribution and Migration, Santa Cruz, Bolivia, 18-22 January 1993.

_____, editor (1998). *The Sex Sector: The Economic and Social Bases of Prostitution in Southeast Asia*. Geneva: International Labour Office.

Massey, Douglas S., and others (1993). Theories of international migration: a review and appraisal. *Population and Development Review*, vol. 19, No. 3, pp. 431-466.

MEASURE DHS (2007a). Demographic and health surveys, various years. STATcompiler. Available from http://www.measuredhs.com (data accessed in March 2007).

_____ (2007b). HIV/AIDS Survey Indicators Database. Data tables available from www.measuredhs.com/hivdata/data (accessed on 23 February 2007).

Mohamedbhai, Goolam (2002). Globalization and its implications on universities in developing countries. Paper presented at the conference Globalisation: What Issues Are at Stake for Universities?, Université Laval, Québec, 19 September 2002.

Morris, Elizabeth (2006). Globalization and its effects on youth employment trends in Asia. Paper presented at the Regional Expert Group Meeting on Development Challenges for Young People, Bangkok, 28-30 March 2006.

Muhidin, Salahudin (2002). *The Population of Indonesia: Regional Demographic Scenarios Using a Multiregional Method and Multiple Data Sources*. Amsterdam: Rozenberg Publishers.

National Science Foundation (2006). Science and Engineering Indicators for 2006. Available from http://www.nsf.gov/statistics/seind06/tt02-04.htm (accessed on 2 March 2007).

Organization for Economic Cooperation and Development (2006). *Education at a Glance: OECD Indicators—2006 Edition*. Paris.

Oxfam (2003). Export oriented manufacturing industries and young workers. In *Highly Affected, Rarely Considered—Youth Commission Report into Globalisation*. Available from http://iyp.oxfam.org/documents/Chapter%203%20Young%20Workers.pdf.

Philippine Overseas Employment Administration (2005). *Annual Report 2004*. Mandaluyong City.

Rizvi, Fazal, and others (2005). Globalization and recent shifts in educational policy in the Asia Pacific: an overview of some critical issues. APEID/UNESCO Bangkok Occasional Paper Series, No. 4. Available from http://www.unescobkk.org/index.php?id=1271 (accessed on 5 March 2007).

Siddiqui, Tasneem (2003). Migration as a livelihood strategy of the poor: the Bangladesh case. Paper presented at the Regional Conference on Migration, Development and Pro-Poor Policy Choices in Asia, Dhaka, 22-24 June 2003.

Sjőholm, Frekrik (2002). Educational reforms and challenges in Southeast Asia. European Institute of Japanese Studies Working Paper, No. 152. Stockholm. Available from http://web.hhs.se/eijswp/152.pdf (accessed on 12 January 2007).

Skrobanek, Siriporn, Nataya Boonpakdi and Chutima Janthakeero (1997). *The Traffic in Women: Human Realities of the International Sex Trade*. London and New York: Zed Books.

Sri Lanka. Department of Census and Statistics (2002). Some key statistics on education—2002. Available from http://www.statistics.gov.lk/education/edustat-2002.pdf (accessed on 20 January 2007).

Tsay, Ching Lung (2004). Marriage migration of women from China and Southeast Asia to Taiwan. In *(Un)tying the Knot: Ideal and Reality in Asian Marriage*, Gavin Jones and Kamalini Ramdas, editors. Singapore: NUS Publishing.

United Nations (2005a). *The Inequality Predicament: Report on the World Social Situation 2005*. Sales No. E.05.IV.5.

_____ (2005b). *World Population Prospects: The 2004 Revision*. New York.

_____ (2006a). International migration and development. Report of the Secretary-General (A/60/871).

_____ (2006b). Promoting full employment and decent work for all. Report of the Secretary General to the Commission for Social Development at its forty-fifth session (E/CN.5/2007/2).

_____ (2007a). *World Population Prospects: The 2006 Revision*. New York.

_____ (2007b). *Report on the World Social Situation 2007*. New York.

United Nations Children's Fund (2004). *The State of the World's Children 2005: Childhood under Threat*. Sales No. E.05.XX.1.

United Nations Development Programme, India (2004). *Promoting ICT for Human Development in Asia 2004: Realising the Millennium Development Goals*. Regional Human Development Report. New Delhi.

United Nations Economic and Social Commission for Asia and the Pacific (2006a). *Disability at a Glance: A Profile of 28 Countries and Areas in Asia and the Pacific*. Bangkok: October. Sales No. E.06.II.F.24.

_____ (2006b). *Economic and Social Survey of Asia and the Pacific 2006: Energizing the Global Economy*. Bangkok. Sales No. E.06.II.F.10.

United Nations Educational, Scientific and Cultural Organization (1999). *Manual on Functional Literacy for Indigenous Peoples. Bangkok: UNESCO Principal Regional Office for Asia and the Pacific*. Available from http://www2.unescobkk.org/elib/publications/functional/manual_functional.pdf (accessed on 22 August 2007).

_____ (2004). *Education for All Global Monitoring Report 2005: The Quality Imperative*. Paris: UNESCO Publishing.

_____ (2005a). *Education for All Global Monitoring Report 2006—Literacy for Life*. Paris: UNESCO Publishing.

_____ (2005b). *Global Education Digest 2005—Comparing Education Statistics Across the World* (UIS/SD/05-01). Montreal: UNESCO Institute for Statistics.

_____ (2006a). *Education for All Global Monitoring Report 2007—Strong Foundations: Early Childhood Care and Education*. Paris: UNESCO Publishing. Available from http://portal.unesco.org/education/en/ev.php-URL_ID=24242&URL_DO=DO_TOPIC&URL_SECTION=201.html (accessed on 5 March 2007).

_____ (2006b). *Global Education Digest 2006: Comparing Education Statistics Across the World* (UIS/SD/06-01). Montreal: UNESCO Institute for Statistics.

_____ Institute for Statistics (2004). Data on regional youth and adult literacy rates and the illiterate population by gender for 1990 and 2000-2004. July 2004. Data available from uis.unesco.org (accessed on 19 January 2007).

_____ Institute for Statistics (2007). Data available from www.uis.unesco.org (accessed on 18 January 2007).

United Nations Population Fund (2002). *State of World Population 2002—People, Poverty and Possibilities: Making Development Work for the Poor*. Sales No. E.02.III.H.1.

Utomo, B., and others (2000). *Behavioural Surveillance Survey among Injecting Drug Users in Jakarta 2000*. Survey carried out by the Center for Health Research, University of Indonesia, through the HIV/AIDS Prevention Project at the Ministry of Health, with technical assistance from Family Health International and funding from the United States Agency for International Development.

Wang, Shanshan (2007). 30m men face bleak future as singles. *China Daily* (12 January).

World Bank (2005). *World Development Report 2006: Equity and Development.* Washington, D.C.

_____ (2006). *World Development Report 2007: Development and the Next Generation.* Washington, D.C.

Yap Kioe Sheng (2004). Youth and urban conflict in Southeast Asian cities. In *Youth, Poverty, and Conflict in Southeast Asian Cities*, Lisa M. Hanley, Blair A. Ruble and Joseph S. Tulchin, editors. Comparative Urban Studies Project. Washington, D.C.: Woodrow Wilson International Center for Scholars.

Yeoh, B.S.A., and S. Huang (1999). Spaces at the margin: migrant domestic workers and the development of civil society in Singapore. *Environment and Planning A*, vol. 31, No. 7, pp. 1149-1167.

Xiaoying, W. (2005). The only-child generation: Chinese youth in a transformative era. In *Youth in Transition: The Challenges of Generational Change in Asia*, Fay Gale and Stephanie Fahey, editors. Bangkok: UNESCO Publishing.

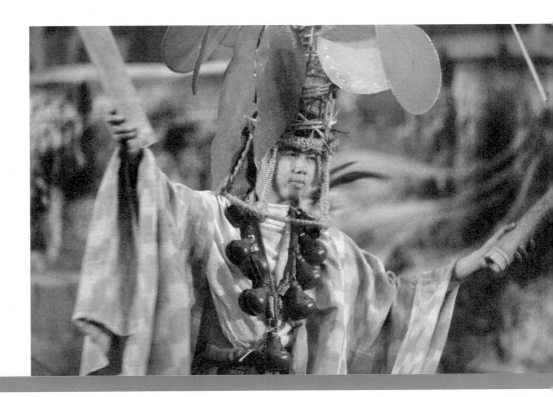

Chapter 2

Latin American YOUTH

in an era of socio-economic and political change

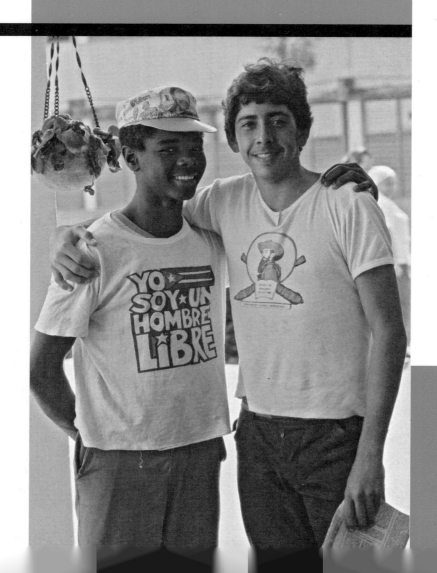

atin America has undergone significant changes in the past 30 years. Most countries in the region adopted democratic forms of government in the early 1980s. The accompanying economic reforms and new approaches to development brought about important social transformations (Agüero and Stark, 1998; Garretón and Newman, 2001; Teichman, 2001). The region has also experienced major demographic shifts. These factors, taken together, have affected young lives in both positive and negative ways. They also appear to have played an important role in determining how young people perceive the political sphere and their role in shaping it. The present chapter reviews recent demographic, social and related trends affecting youth in Latin America and assesses their impact on young people's political and socio-economic participation. The chapter emphasizes that the apparent political apathy among young Latin Americans is not the result of conscious choice, but rather a product of the circumstances in which they live; youth who find it difficult to meet their essential needs in the areas of education, employment, health and social integration tend to attach less priority to political involvement.

CHANGING ECONOMIC AND DEMOGRAPHIC CONTEXT
The repercussions of economic change

The combination of economic recession and rampant inflation following years of both fiscal and external disequilibrium provided the impetus for the adoption of a new economic model in the region. One by one, most of the countries in Latin America abandoned the old import-substitution industrialization model, which aimed at achieving economic independence through the local manufacture of goods previously imported from abroad, and introduced market-oriented economic policies that significantly reduced State participation in the economy (Haggard and Kaufman, 1995). The repercussions of this shift were dramatic. Protected industries collapsed in the face of increased competition from abroad as tariffs were lowered and commercial barriers were lifted. State enterprises were privatized, and many of their workers were dismissed. Old labour codes were replaced with new ones that offered workers less protection. To fight inflation and narrow the fiscal gap, Governments reduced or eliminated State subsidies for various goods and services, including foodstuffs.

Although the new economic policies produced some of the desired results, including reduced fiscal deficits and lower inflation, they also gave rise to serious social dislocations that have been particularly detrimental to youth. Increases in income poverty, unemployment, and overall inequality have had a tremendous impact on young people's schooling, health, and social and economic welfare. Few among the poor have had the benefit of a full, high-quality education that might allow them to improve their socio-economic situation (Sáinz, 2007). Many youth have been unable to secure domestic employment and have sought relief through migration.

Changing population dynamics

The political transition and socio-economic crisis in Latin America coincided with important demographic changes. Higher levels of educational attainment, improved health coverage, and important medical advances contributed to a precipitous decline in fertility, morbidity and infant mortality and an increase in life expectancy. These trends had an impact on the age structure of the region. The proportion of youth in the total population peaked in the 1970s and began to decline thereafter; their share is expected to diminish further over the next several decades as people live longer and have fewer children (Economic Commission for Latin America and the Caribbean, 2004a).

Despite this decline, youth remain a significant demographic and social group in Latin America. Young people between the ages of 15 and 24 currently number close to 100 million and constitute 18.5 per cent of the region's total population. This proportion is almost identical to that recorded in 1950 (see table 2.1). Although their demographic share is projected to decline in the coming decades, young people will continue to represent a major socio-economic group requiring adequate health, education, and other social services.

Table 2.1
Estimated and projected youth population in Latin America, 1950-2015

Region/Country	1950		2005		2015	
	Youth population (thousands)	Percentage of the total population	Youth population (thousands)	Percentage of the total population	Youth population (thousands)	Percentage of the total population
Central America	7 199.5	19.2	26 946.5	18.5	29 675.9	17.9
Belize	13.2	19.2	56.7	20.4	67.1	19.8
Costa Rica	165.4	17.1	856.4	19.5	850.9	16.8
El Salvador	379.6	19.5	1 260.4	18.7	1 411.6	18.3
Guatemala	630.3	20.0	2 559.8	20.0	3 337.8	20.4
Honduras	277.4	18.7	1 445.1	21.0	1 740.4	20.8
Mexico	5 330.3	19.2	19 004.8	18.0	20 336.7	17.3
Nicaragua	250.9	19.4	1 184.4	21.5	1 293.8	20.4
Panama	152.3	17.7	578.7	17.7	637.5	16.6
South America	21 307.9	18.9	69 894.5	18.5	70 431.6	16.5
Argentina	3 146.7	18.3	6 603.4	16.7	6 886.5	15.7
Bolivia	523.8	19.3	1 779.4	19.3	2 159.8	19.7
Brazil	10 420.4	19.3	35 348.3	18.7	33 595.6	15.7
Chile	1 104.3	18.2	2 785.3	16.8	2 817.1	15.3
Colombia	2 326.2	18.5	8 395.1	18.5	8 999.3	17.5
Ecuador	601.9	17.8	2 513.7	19.0	2 697.7	18.2
French Guiana	4.2	16.5	32.7	16.9	44.7	18.4
Guyana	75.6	17.9	128.6	17.2	134.9	18.6
Paraguay	282.0	19.1	1 224.5	20.6	1 363.5	19.2
Peru	1 432.9	18.8	5 320.1	19.3	5 653.7	18.1
Suriname	39.0	18.1	88.8	19.5	79.0	16.4
Uruguay	394.8	17.6	497.1	14.5	519.3	14.5
Venezuela	955.8	18.8	5 177.1	19.2	5 479.9	17.3
Latin America	28 507.5	18.9	96 840.9	18.5	100 107.4	16.9

Source: United Nations, *World Population Prospects: The 2006 Revision*, Extended Dataset, CD-ROM edition (New York: 2007).

The young people of Latin America constitute a tremendously important but largely underserved segment of the population. While many countries have become more responsive to the development needs of youth, young people continue to encounter serious obstacles in a number of areas, giving rise to marginalization, frustration, political dissent and, for some, the active pursuit of better opportunities elsewhere.

Education: continued exclusion despite major gains

Overall, Latin America has made impressive progress in providing young people with educational opportunities; it has been observed that the constituent countries are showing "some signs of breaking with the political and social history of education-based mechanisms for exclusion" (De Ferranti and others, 2004, p. 179). The region's net primary enrolment ratio of 95 per cent is much higher than the developing world average of 85 per cent, and several countries have achieved universal primary enrolment or are close to doing so. Participation in secondary and tertiary education is also growing, though access to the latter remains limited (United Nations Educational, Scientific and Cultural Organization, 2006).

Progress in education has varied from one country and socio-economic group to another. Since the early 1990s, educational gains have been made among urban youth in virtually all of the Latin American countries listed in table 2.2. In some countries, including Argentina, Brazil, Guatemala and Peru, the average period of education increased by 1.5 years or more. In other countries, such as Chile, Ecuador, El Salvador, Honduras, Nicaragua and Panama, the educational gains were more modest (one year or less). In Costa Rica the average number of years of education fell slightly, declining from the relatively high level of 9.1 to 9.0. Though disparities still exist, the decline in the standard deviation (the difference between the average number of years of education for each country and the regional mean) suggests that the region's youth are becoming more educationally homogeneous.

Table 2.2
Average number of years of education completed by different age groups in urban areas, selected Latin American countries

Country (census years)	Earlier census Age group (years)		More recent census Age group (years)	
	15-24	25-59	15-24	25-59
Argentina[a] (1990, 2004)	9.0	8.8	10.5	10.5
Bolivia (1994, 2002)	10.0	9.3	10.1	9.2
Brazil (1990, 2003)	6.6	6.2	8.4	7.5
Chile (1990, 2003)	10.1	9.7	10.9	11.1
Colombia (1990, 2002)	8.5	8.2	9.8	9.3
Costa Rica (1990, 2002)	9.1	9.6	9.0	9.4
Dominican Republic (2000, 2003)	9.4	8.9	9.6	9.1
Ecuador (1990, 2002)	9.4	8.9	9.7	10.1
El Salvador (1997, 2003)	8.8	7.9	9.2	8.6
Guatemala (1989, 2002)	6.7	5.6	8.2	7.4
Honduras (1990, 2003)	7.0	6.4	7.9	7.5
Mexico (1989, 2004)	8.7	7.5	10.0	9.4
Nicaragua (1993, 2001)	7.0	6.4	7.9	6.9
Panama (1991, 2002)	9.6	9.6	10.2	10.8
Paraguay[b] (1990, 2001)	9.3	9.0	9.6	9.6
Peru (1997, 2003)	9.0	10.1	10.6	10.6
Uruguay (1990, 2002)	9.2	8.3	9.6	9.7
Venezuela (1990, 2003)	8.4	8.2	9.0	8.6
Regional average	8.65	8.25	9.45	9.18
Standard deviation	1.10	1.34	0.91	1.24

Source: Economic Commission for Latin America and the Caribbean, *Panorama Social de América Latina 2005* (LC/G.2288-P/E); adapted from tables 33 and 34 of the statistical appendix.

Note: Population census years are shown in parentheses next to the name of each country. All averages are simple averages.

[a]Greater Buenos Aires.
[b]Asunción.

Gender disparities in literacy and educational attainment are relatively small in Latin America. The literacy gap is less than two percentage points for most countries. In Argentina, Brazil, Chile, Colombia, Costa Rica, Ecuador, Honduras, Mexico, and Venezuela, literacy rates are higher for young females than for young males. A similar situation prevails with regard to gross tertiary enrolment in both Central America and South America. Argentina has the highest gross tertiary enrolment ratio in the region, with more than three quarters of its young women and slightly over half of its young men pursuing higher studies (UNESCO Institute for Statistics, 2007). At the country and regional levels there appears to be little gender discrimination in terms of educational opportunities; however, national statistics often mask high illiteracy and low school participation rates among females from indigenous groups. In Bolivia, for example, more girls than boys are in school, but more than half of the indigenous girls drop out before the age of 14 (United Nations Educational, Scientific and Cultural Organization, 2006).

While educational gains have been impressive, much remains to be done to address substantial and enduring inequalities in access. Statistics for 2002 indicate that only 68 per cent of Latin Americans between the ages of 20 and 24 had completed the primary cycle, and that roughly a third (32.7 per cent of young men and 36.6 per cent of young women) had obtained a secondary education (Economic Commission for Latin America and the Caribbean and Organización Iberoamericana de Juventud, 2004).

Serious educational deficiencies persist even in urban areas. In 1990, urban youth between the ages of 15 and 24 had completed an average of 8.7 years of formal education; by 2002 that figure had climbed to 9.5 years (see table 2.2). This represents a respectable gain, but the fact remains that the majority of Latin American youth are not even close to finishing secondary school.

School attendance is strongly influenced by household income (see table 2.3). Across Latin America, urban youth from the poorest households are consistently less likely than their wealthier counterparts to attend school. The difference is especially pronounced among those aged 20-24 years, and poor young women seem to be particularly disadvantaged. In all the countries featured in table 2.3, with the exception of El Salvador and Mexico, attendance rates for 13- to 19-year-old females from the richest quintile are higher than the corresponding rates for males in the same age group and income quintile. In 10 of the countries, however, teenage women from the poorest households are less likely than young men from similar households to attend school. Statistics suggest that educational opportunities remain inadequate for a large proportion of urban youth; young people in rural areas tend to have even less access to formal schooling and are often effectively excluded from secondary and tertiary education.

Table 2.3
School attendance among urban youth in Latin America by sex, age group and per capita household income quintile, 2005*

Country		Percentage in school Quintile 1[a] (lowest income)		Percentage in school Quintile 5[a] (highest income)	
		Age group (years)		Age group (years)	
		13-19	20-24	13-19	20-24
Argentina	Both sexes[b]	75.1	22.4	90.0	62.7
	Men[b]	75.6	22.2	87.9	59.5
	Women[b]	74.7	22.6	91.7	65.7
Bolivia	Both sexes	83.5	28.2	90.6	64.8
	Men	82.3	33.6	89.9	61.4
	Women	84.6	23.3	91.2	68.5
Brazil	Both sexes	73.6	17.4	89.8	53.9
	Men	74.1	17.4	88.7	53.7
	Women	73.2	17.4	90.9	54.1
Chile	Both sexes	81.4	18.9	94.1	67.8
	Men	82.9	16.8	93.7	69.1
	Women	79.7	20.5	94.5	66.3
Colombia	Both sexes	70.1	11.6	89.2	56.6
	Men[c]	70.7	13.5	88.7	58.7
	Women[c]	69.5	10.1	89.6	54.4
Costa Rica	Both sexes[s]	78.4	26.4	93.4	67.5
	Men	79.9	33.3	92.0	63.5
	Women	76.7	21.5	95.1	72.0
Ecuador	Both sexes	70.2	21.4	88.9	52.0
El Salvador	Both sexes	67.5	14.5	90.2	43.6
	Men	72.7	19.7	90.8	43.7
	Women	62.6	10.3	89.6	43.6
Guatemala	Both sexes	63.3	11.1	78.3	43.9
	Men	70.2	15.4	76.7	44.9
	Women	58.1	8.1	80.0	42.9
Honduras	Both sexes	55.8	13.3	83.6	53.0
	Men	54.0	10.6	82.9	53.1
	Women	57.4	15.5	84.2	53.0

Country		Percentage in school Quintile 1[a] (lowest income)		Percentage in school Quintile 5[a] (highest income)	
		Age group (years)		Age group (years)	
		13-19	20-24	13-19	20-24
Mexico	Both sexes	60.5	14.4	87.1	48.7
	Men	61.9	14.5	88.1	49.7
	Women	59.4	14.3	86.0	47.9
Nicaragua	Both sexes	61.5	15.4	79.2	52.1
	Men	58.3	14.6	74.2	47.5
	Women	65.1	16.2	83.2	56.8
Panama	Both sexes	76.4	20.8	94.4	52.5
	Men	74.0	17.6	93.6	50.4
	Women	79.1	23.3	95.1	55.0
Paraguay	Both sexes	70.7	10.4	88.2	57.2
	Men	68.9	13.0	87.3	55.5
	Women	72.2	8.1	88.9	59.2
Peru	Both sexes	74.3	24.4	77.0	61.0
	Men	76.9	23.6	73.8	72.6
	Women	72.0	25.0	81.9	49.6
Uruguay	Both sexes	66.4	14.1	96.2	72.5
	Men	63.9	10.8	95.9	68.6
	Women	69.0	16.8	96.7	77.2
Venezuela	Both sexes[d]	74.4	34.3	80.6	60.4
	Men[d]	72.3	30.4	78.1	55.9
	Women[d]	76.3	37.3	83.3	65.2

Source: Economic Commission for Latin America and the Caribbean, *Statistical Yearbook for Latin America and the Caribbean 2006* (United Nations publication, Sales No. E/S.07.II.G.1).

Notes: *Data are for the years closest to 2005.

[a] Household income is classified by quintile, based on per capita income; quintile 1 is composed of the poorest 20 per cent of households, while quintile 5 corresponds to the richest 20 per cent.

[b] Twenty-eight urban agglomerations.

[c] Municipality capitals.

[d] National statistics.

Table 2.4 highlights different aspects and indicators of educational performance in Central America and the Dominican Republic, but the assessment is in many ways representative of the challenges faced by the region as a whole. Nine basic areas are evaluated on a scale ranging from "very poor" to "excellent". Arrows indicate whether progress, deterioration, or no visible change occurred between 2000 and 2005, as assessed by the Task Force on Education Reform in Central America. The "very poor" rating on equity issues is significant, given the considerable progress achieved by the region in educational provision.

Table 2.4
Educational "report card" for Central America and the Dominican Republic, 2007

Subject	Grade	Tendency	Comments
Test scores	Poor	⟷	Student scores on national tests remain low. Very few students have adequate reading comprehension and problem-solving skills.
Enrolment	Good	↑	Although enrolment continues to increase, fewer than half of boys and girls attend pre-school, and only four in ten attend secondary school.
Staying in school	Poor	⟷	Repetition is still high, especially in the first grade, and many students drop out prematurely. Average years of schooling remain low, and the situation has not improved in recent years.
Equity	Very poor	⟷	Wide gaps persist between rich and poor, between those living in urban and rural areas, and between indigenous and non-indigenous populations. Girls repeat grades and drop out less often than boys.
Authority and accountability at the school level	Average	⟷	Several countries have been pioneers in increasing school autonomy and community involvement, but only in certain areas. Little progress has been made in recent years, and there are signs of reversal in some countries.
Investment in primary and secondary education	Poor	⟷	Few countries in the region have increased public spending to the recommended 5 per cent of GDP. Public spending per pupil remains very low, and resources are not used efficiently.
Teaching profession	Poor	↑	Although some progress has been made, only three quarters of teachers have the minimum training required by their countries. Little social value is given to the profession, and wages are unrelated to performance.
Standards	Average	⟷	Several countries have drawn up standards establishing what students should learn. These standards, however, are neither broadly disseminated nor broadly applied, and they are not yet linked to assessment, teacher training, textbooks, and other classroom resources.
Assessment systems	Average	↑	Most countries have continued to test what students learn, but most systems are still not fully consolidated. Test results are not widely disseminated and are seldom used.

Grading scale	Excellent Good Average Poor Very poor	Tendency	↑ Improving ⟷ No change

Source: Partnership for Educational Revitalization in the Americas, *A Lot to Do: A Report Card on Education in Central America and the Dominican Republic* (Task Force on Education Reform in Central America, 2007).

Rising unemployment and declining wages

For young people, the employment and income situation is worse today than it was 15 years ago. In the early 1990s, Rodríguez and Dabezies (1991) described the labour situation of Latin American youth as being characterized by instability, inadequate remuneration, and limited access to social security. Although isolated gains have been achieved in some areas, the overall situation has deteriorated since then. During this critical period in their lives, when they need to be acquiring skills and job experience, a significant proportion of Latin American youth are neither in school nor at work; in 2002, about 18 per cent of young people between the ages of 15 and 19 found themselves in such circumstances, and the same was true for around 27 per cent of 20- to 24-year-olds (Economic Commission for Latin America and the Caribbean, 2004b).

Recent data indicate that youth unemployment was higher in 2002 than in 1990. Rates of joblessness rose for all three age groups highlighted in table 2.5, but the increase was less pronounced for adults than for young people. In 2002, unemployment among 15- to 19-year-olds was roughly twice that for 25- to 29-year-olds. In urban areas, rates of unemployment were higher for youth than for the labour force as a whole (Economic Commission for Latin America and the Caribbean, 2005).

Table 2.5
Gender-disaggregated unemployment rates for selected age groups in Latin America

Age group (years)	Males		Females	
	1990	2002	1990	2002
15-19	15.6	19.8	22.1	27.0
20-24	11.2	14.5	16.7	21.5
25-29	7.3	9.0	11.7	14.8

Source: Adapted from Economic Commission for Latin America and the Caribbean, *Panorama Social de América Latina 2004* (United Nations publication, Sales No. S.04.II.G.148), graph III.14, p. 169.

Young people who are employed often work in family-owned businesses, small companies with low productivity, the domestic service industry, or the informal economy. Such employment offers very little in the way of wages or benefits. Table 2.6 shows the proportions of Latin Americans from different age groups engaged in low-productivity activities; this category includes self-employed workers, unpaid workers with no technical or professional training, employees of companies with fewer than five workers, and domestic workers. The figures indicate that more young people were employed in low-productivity occupations in 2002 than in 1990.

Table 2.6
Proportions of workers engaged in low-productivity occupations in Latin America, by age and sex

Age group (years)	Sex	Year		Difference
		1990	2002	
15-19	Both sexes	63.3	69.1	9.2
	Males	59.7	67.3	12.8
	Females	68.6	72.0	5.1
20-24	Both sexes	46.8	49.4	5.5
	Males	45.3	48.5	6.9
	Females	48.6	50.5	4.0
25-29	Both sexes	42.7	45.1	5.7
	Males	41.2	43.7	5.9
	Females	44.1	46.9	6.2
30-64	Both sexes	48.9	51.7	5.7
	Males	45.2	48.2	6.7
	Females	54.9	56.6	3.2

Source: Taken from Economic Commission for Latin America and the Caribbean and Organización Iberoamericana de Juventud, "La juventud en Iberoamérica: tendencias y urgencias" (LC/L.2180) (Santiago, October 2004), p. 222.

More than two thirds of young people between the ages of 15 and 19 begin their working lives in environments that offer few or none of the labour protections or benefits typically available to other workers. Low-productivity employment declines after this entry phase, but the proportions remain high for all groups, hovering around 50 per cent. It is evident from table 2.6 that, throughout their lives, women are more likely than men to be engaged in this type of work.

The employment situation in Latin America is particularly problematic for young women, who have a harder time finding work, are paid lower wages, and are less likely than their male counterparts to participate in the job market. In 2004, about 62 per cent of young men and 42 per cent of young women were part of the labour force (Economic Commission for Latin America and the Caribbean, 2005). Some argue that the rise in unemployment among young women is the product of intermittent increases in their labour force participation; more females are competing for a limited number of jobs, and the share of those who are unable to secure employment is growing (Duryea, Jaramillo and Pagés, 2003).

The educational gains achieved by females in Latin America have not translated into an improved labour market position. The widening gender gap in employment at the regional level derives largely from the dramatic deterioration in the job situation for young urban women in several countries as a result of the 2001 economic crisis. In Argentina, unemployment among female youth in urban areas doubled between 1990 and 2004, and in Uruguay, the increase in unemployment was linked to the severe crisis in neighbouring

Argentina. In Venezuela, high inflation and economic recession seriously affected job prospects for young urban women. The substantial increases in unemployment among young women in Brazil and Colombia were related to the higher rates of female labour force participation in those countries (Economic Commission for Latin America and the Caribbean, 2005).

There are a number of important factors to consider in connection with unemployment among female youth in Latin America. Reproductive responsibilities and other family obligations interfere with labour market entry for many young women. The relatively high probability of unemployment may compel some young women to continue their education. Unemployed female youth with little education are more vulnerable to poverty, social exclusion, personal frustration, substance abuse, and the threat of HIV/AIDS.

This section has highlighted the challenges faced by Latin American youth in their pursuit of gainful employment. As a group, young people are at a relative disadvantage in the labour market, but those between the ages of 15 and 19 are especially vulnerable. Teenagers (especially females) who abandon their studies often find it extremely difficult to secure employment, and those who do are likely to be paid very little for their efforts.

The prevalence and severity of poverty

Poverty and inequality remain key issues in Latin America, and they have a profound impact on young people's education, employment opportunities, access to essential services, and overall well-being. Among the Latin American countries for which relevant data are available, Bolivia, Guatemala, Nicaragua and Peru have the highest proportions of youth living in absolute poverty. In 15 of the region's countries at least one in four residents live below the poverty line, and in seven of these more than half of the population is poor (United Nations Development Programme, 2004a). Almost a quarter of those living in Latin America subsist on less than US$ 2 a day (United Nations Millennium Project, 2005).

Poverty levels vary from one age group to another. Children under the age of 14 represent the poorest segment of society, followed by young people between the ages of 15 and 19. In 2002, about 45 per cent of 15- to 19-year-olds were considered "poor" (with incomes of less than twice the cost of a basic food basket), and 17 per cent were considered "indigent" (living on incomes lower than the cost of one basic food basket); the corresponding figures for those aged 30 years and above were 33 and 12.5 per cent respectively (see table 2.7). Youth aged 20-24 years fared slightly better than their younger counterparts; poverty rates were significant for this group but were closer to the figures recorded for adults. Gender-based income disparities were greatest among older youth and young adults; only in their twenties were females more likely than their male peers to experience poverty, reflecting the precariousness of the labour situation for young women.

Table 2.7

Poverty and indigence among selected age groups in Latin America, by sex (percentage)

Age (years)	Percentage poor		Percentage non-indigent poor		Percentage indigent	
	Males	Females	Males	Females	Males	Females
0-14	56.8	56.9	30.7	30.9	26.1	26.1
15-19	45.0	45.3	27.3	27.6	17.7	17.7
20-24	35.4	39.6	23.2	25.3	12.2	14.3
25-29	35.6	39.8	23.0	24.9	12.6	14.9
30 and above	33.5	33.5	21.0	20.9	12.5	12.6

Source: Adapted from Economic Commission for Latin America and the Caribbean and Organización Iberoamericana de Juventud, "La juventud en Iberoamérica: tendencias y urgencias" (LC/L.2180) (Santiago: October 2004), table III.7, p. 118.

Note: Statistics are based on the most recent available data.

Aggregate poverty estimates often hide significant disparities between groups and may also mask pockets of extreme poverty. In Latin America, poverty averages tend to obscure the dire situations of slum-dwelling youth, rural youth, and youth of African descent, many of whom are not reached by social services. Indigenous youth and their families are more likely than non-indigenous groups to experience poverty. In Mexico, for example, 81 per cent of indigenous residents live below the poverty line, compared with 18 per cent of the general population (United Nations Development Programme, 2004b).

Non-monetary dimensions of poverty

Poverty is linked to income insufficiency but is also manifested in the inaccessibility of basic necessities such as clean water, sanitation, and health and other social services. It is believed that many households in Latin America face serious water deprivation; statistics indicate that more than 10 per cent of the young people living in Bolivia, Colombia, Guatemala, Guyana, Nicaragua, Paraguay, Peru and Venezuela do not have access to clean water.

For many young women, early pregnancy and parenthood and the scarcity of reproductive health services seriously interfere with the transition to independent adulthood. Early motherhood contributes to intergenerational poverty, largely because young mothers tend to complete fewer years of schooling than other women their age. High rates of maternal mortality persist in some parts of the region. In Brazil, Colombia, Nicaragua, Panama and Venezuela, adolescent fertility rates exceed 17 per cent. In Chile and Uruguay, more than 5 per cent of 15-year-old girls have given birth (Economic Commission for Latin America and the Caribbean, 2004b). Early pregnancy and motherhood are strongly correlated with socio-economic and geographic factors. A rural 17-year-old female living in relative poverty is 4 to 10 times more likely to have a child than a young urban woman at the other end of the socio-economic spectrum (Economic Commission for Latin America and the Caribbean, 2004b).

According to UNAIDS, an estimated 1.6 million individuals (or 0.5 per cent of the population) between the ages of 15 and 49 were living with HIV in Latin America in 2005; the corresponding rates for male and female youth were 0.5 and 0.3 per cent respectively (Joint United Nations Programme on HIV/AIDS, 2006b). Belize, Guatemala, and Honduras have the highest rates of HIV prevalence in the region, but Brazil has the largest number of cases in absolute terms; a national prevalence rate consistent with the regional average obscures the fact that one in three people living with HIV in Latin America resides in Brazil. Because one third of Brazilian youth are sexually active before the age of 15, there are serious concerns about the rapid spread of HIV among young people (Joint United Nations Programme on HIV/AIDS, 2006a). The country's efforts in the provision of treatment have greatly reduced rates of death from HIV/AIDS. Youth in high-risk groups such as injecting drug users, sex workers and men who have sex with men require urgent attention, with interventions tailored to their specific needs.

The transmission of HIV between female sex workers and their clients contributes significantly to the spread of the disease in Latin America. In Honduras, which has a prevalence rate of 1.5 per cent and is one of the worst-affected countries in the region, one in twelve female sex workers in the capital city tested positive for HIV; though the data do not indicate the ages of the sex workers, most are believed to be relatively young. Similar trends are observed in Guatemala, where the prevalence rate is 0.9 per cent. In Guatemala City, HIV prevalence was found to be 15 per cent for street-based sex workers and 12 per cent for men having sex with men (Joint United Nations Programme on HIV/AIDS, 2006a).

There is a high incidence of violence among young people in Latin America, often in connection with youth gangs (pandillas). It is contended that much of this violence derives from the intense resentment and frustration bred by inequities in society and by the failure of adults to address youth concerns. In an era of weakening family and community ties, many young people find the companionship and support they crave and are able to establish peer relationships based on loyalty and trust through membership in antisocial and often criminal groups (Merkle, 2003). The violence perpetrated by young gang members represents a serious threat to society and to the youth themselves. In Colombia, 62.5 per cent of males who die between the ages of 15 and 24 are murder victims, and homicide is the leading cause of death for young males in Brazil (42 per cent), El Salvador (46.1 per cent), and Venezuela (38.3 per cent) (Economic Commission for Latin America and the Caribbean, 2004b).

In many areas, urban violence has become so widespread that it is rightly considered a major impediment to development, weakening the social fabric and jeopardizing the health and well-being of the population. Levels of violence vary considerably according to age and gender. In most settings, males are far more likely than females to be both the main perpetrators and the main victims. In Brazil, for example, the homicide rate among young men 15 to 24 years of age was 86.7 per 100,000 in 1999, compared with only 6.5 per 100,000 among young women in the same age group. Even in countries with much lower levels, the incidence and intensity of violence among juvenile males is increasing (Moser, 2005).

ON THE MOVE: MIGRATION AS A COPING STRATEGY

Migration has allowed large numbers of young people with limited opportunities to explore other alternatives. An upward trend has been observed in recent years as traditional rural-urban migration has been supplemented by increased migration to other Latin American countries and to Europe and the United States.

Internal migration

Young people are more likely than adults to relocate within their own countries (Rodríguez Vignoli, 2004). Figure 2.1 shows the proportions of Latin Americans in different age groups living in a state, province, department or other major administrative unit different from the one they were living in five years before the census was taken. The figure indicates that youth between the ages of 20 and 24 are most likely to migrate from one administrative unit to another, followed by youth aged 15-19 years. Progressively fewer residents migrate within their countries after the age of 25.

Figure 2.1
Rates of internal migration for different age groups in selected Latin American countries

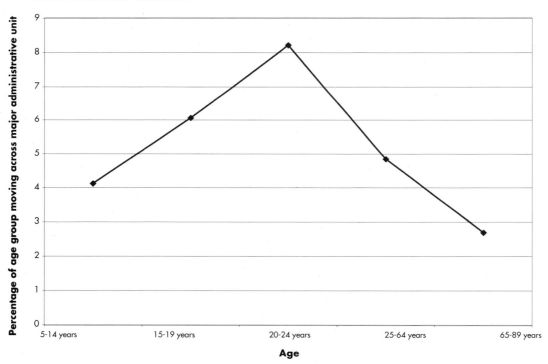

Source: Based on data from the Latin American and Caribbean Demographic Center, Database on Internal Migration in Latin America and the Caribbean (CELADE/MIALC) (available from http://www.eclac.cl).
Note: Statistics are based on the most recent available data.

Table 2.8 indicates that among the 12 Latin American countries for which recent data are available, five (Bolivia, Chile, Ecuador, Panama and Paraguay) have recorded internal migration rates of at least 9 per cent for young people aged 20-24 years. Rural-urban migration gained considerable momentum in the 1950s and 1960s and has continued to expand in many parts of the region. Youth have always represented a significant share of internal migrants and are now underrepresented in rural areas and overrepresented in the cities (Economic Commission for Latin America and the Caribbean, 2002); the dramatic shift in the demographic balance has played a critical role in the transformations occurring in countries such as Bolivia, Panama and Paraguay.

Table 2.8
Age distribution of internal migrants in selected Latin American countries (percentage)

Country	5-14 years	15-19 years	20-24 years	25-64 years	65-89 years
Argentina	2.6	3.0	5.5	3.5	1.8
Bolivia	4.2	8.1	10.3	3.2	2.6
Brazil	3.3	3.7	5.2	3.2	0.7
Chile	5.0	6.4	10.3	5.8	2.7
Costa Rica	5.3	5.6	7.6	5.6	3.0
Dominican Republic	3.5	5.0	6.5	4.0	2.5
Ecuador	4.1	7.2	9.0	4.9	2.8
Honduras	3.2	5.9	7.0	4.0	3.5
Mexico	4.0	5.1	6.5	4.4	1.9
Panama	4.0	7.6	10.7	6.7	3.5
Paraguay	5.8	9.2	12.7	7.6	4.4
Venezuela	4.4	5.9	7.3	5.0	2.8
Mean	4.1	6.1	8.2	4.8	2.7

Source: Based on data from the Latin American and Caribbean Demographic Center, Database on Internal Migration in Latin America and the Caribbean (CELADE/MIALC) (available from http://www.eclac.cl).
Note: Statistics are based on the most recent available data.

There are a number of reasons for these trends. As might be expected, employment and education are the main drivers of internal migration, especially among the young. In Paraguay, more than 68 per cent of recent migrants cited work, education and undefined "family circumstances" as the three most important reasons for migration (Molinas Vega, 1999).

In some countries, internal migration is also triggered by humanitarian crises caused by internal strife or natural disasters. Forced displacement was once a significant problem in many parts of the region but today is largely limited to Colombia. By the end of 2002, an estimated 2.2 million Colombian residents had been forced to leave their homes as a result of political violence (International Organization for Migration, 2005); many of the displaced were of indigenous origin, and around half were under the age of 18 (Human Rights Watch, 2005).

Internal migration rates for youth tend to be lower in Central America than in South America, perhaps because young people in the former are geographically better situated to take advantage of international migration opportunities. Many Central American youth migrate to the United States, but a significant number move to countries such as Mexico and Costa Rica, which have solid economies and attractive educational opportunities.

Panama has one of the highest rates of internal migration in Central America, which may have something to do with the fact that it is geographically most distant from the United States but is probably more directly related to the domestic construction boom and the growing demand for service jobs in the cities.

Young women in rural areas are often compelled to move to the cities because they have fewer opportunities than their male counterparts in their places of origin. Combined statistics for 12 Latin American countries indicate that young women between the ages of 15 and 24 constitute an average of 52-54 per cent of all internal migrants (see figure 2.2) Some female youth relocate to take advantage of secondary or tertiary educational opportunities, but a substantial number of young rural women travel to the cities in search of employment, especially domestic work (Rodríguez Vignoli, 2004).

Figure 2.2
The proportion of female internal migrants in 12 Latin American countries, by age group

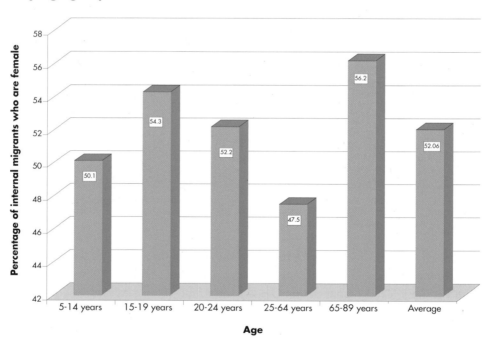

Source: Based on data from the Latin American and Caribbean Demographic Center, Database on Internal Migration in Latin America and the Caribbean (CELADE/MIALC) (available from http://www.eclac.cl).
Note: Statistics are based on the most recent available data.

International migration

Internal migration may be undertaken in search of better educational or employment opportunities or in response to serious humanitarian crises. International migration occurs for the same reasons, though the costs and benefits are potentially much greater. Those who move to other countries within or outside the region may be vulnerable to exploitation, especially if they lack the proper legal documentation, and many find the integration process difficult. In spite of such risks, Latin American youth are increasingly seeking new opportunities and the promise of a better future beyond their own borders (Guarnizo and Díaz, 1999; Mahler, 2000; Lopes Patarra and Baeninger, 2006; International Organization for Migration, 2005).

For those migrating to other Latin American countries, Argentina, Costa Rica and Venezuela appear to be the most popular destinations. Young people comprise around 18 per cent of the population in Latin America and about 17 per cent of all intraregional migrants. (Economic Commission for Latin America and the Caribbean and Organización Iberoamericana de Juventud, 2004). Young women make up a significant proportion of intraregional migrants. In Chile, for example, young Peruvian females outnumber their male counterparts by nearly two to one (Stefoni, 2002), and a similar situation prevails in Argentina with Bolivian migrants. For many young women, intraregional migration is associated not with the chance for personal or professional development but rather with the perpetuation of their traditional roles. Young female migrants are increasingly being engaged to perform household chores and to provide care for children and senior citizens. They are locked into occupations with long workdays and low income and face the discrimination and risk of abuse that tend to go hand-in-hand with low economic status and persistent gender inequalities. The substantial participation of young women in intraregional migration in Latin America is consistent with the feminization of migration globally (United Nations Population Fund, 2006).

Massive numbers of Latin Americans have migrated to other regions; in 2001, an estimated 21 million were living in OECD countries. The United States represents the primary destination, followed by Spain, Canada, and the Netherlands (International Labour Office, 2005).

Latin American migration to the United States has increased dramatically over the past two to three decades. Between 1980 and 1990 the number of Latin American immigrants living in the country rose from about 4.4 million to 8.4 million, and by 2000 the figure had reached 14.5 million. In 2004 the United States Census Bureau placed the Latin American migrant population at about 18 million; approximately 2.9 million (16 per cent) were between the ages of 15 and 24, and the vast majority of these youth (2.5 million) were from Mexico or other countries in Central America. By 2005, the number of young Latin American migrants residing in the United States exceeded the total number of youth living in Chile and was equal to about half the youth population of Peru.

The sharp increase in Latin American migration to the United States in recent years represents a response to challenges and opportunities on a number of levels. In many Latin American countries, productive capacity has declined dramatically and opportunities for decent employment are seriously limited. More specific factors influencing youth migration include the desire to escape the stigmatization and victimization linked to gang activity and police efforts to repress it, the availability of better educational and job opportunities (not only for poor or disenfranchised youth but also for the sons and daughters of the upper-middle class), and cross-border family reunification policies. Migration to the United States is facilitated by long-standing linkages between the American Southwest and Mexico and by the extensive support networks available for newly arrived immigrants (Pizarro and Villa, 2005).

Young men are dominant in Latin American youth migration to the United States (see figure 2.3). Males constitute only a slight majority of young migrants from Caribbean and South American countries but are heavily overrepresented among Central American youth coming to the United States. One important consideration within this context is that migrants from countries closer to the United States are more likely to travel to the border and make the crossing on foot, and the extreme personal risks associated with such a journey may discourage some young women from migrating, or at least from taking this route.

Figure 2.3
Share of youth among Latin American and Caribbean migrants in the United States, by sex, 2004

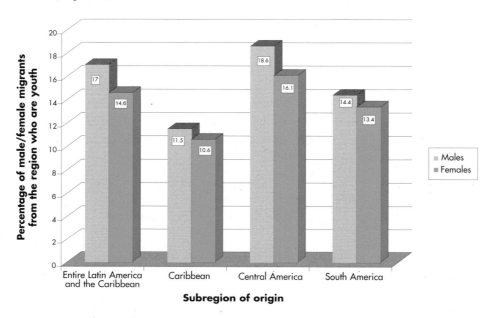

Source: United States Census Bureau, "Foreign-born population of the United States: current population survey—March 2004" (Washington, D.C.) (available from http://www.census.gov/population/www/socdemo/foreign/ppl-176/tab04-1.xls; accessed on 20 July 2006).

Migration from Latin America to Spain has gained considerable momentum in recent years. According to the national census, about 200,000 migrants from Latin America lived in Spain in 1991; various estimates place the total at between 840,000 and 1.2 million ten years later (Martínez Pizarro and Villa, 2005; Valls and Martínez, 2005). In 2001, around 15 per cent of these immigrants were between the ages of 17 and 24 (Martínez Buján, 2003). Latin American migrants living in Spain are predominantly female, with specific countries providing the bulk of this flow; there tends to be gender parity among migrants from Argentina, Chile and Ecuador, but women constitute an overwhelming majority of those coming from Bolivia, Brazil, the Dominican Republic and Peru. Latin Americans residing in Spain tend to work in low-skill occupations; some 40 per cent of the female migrants are domestic employees, and about 30 per cent of the males work in construction (Valls and Martínez, 2005).

The massive Latin American emigration to the United States and other OECD countries has raised concerns on both sides. Undocumented migrants, especially the young, are vulnerable to labour exploitation, often receive substandard health care, have fewer educational opportunities, and are reluctant to demand or assert their rights. Even legal migrants are facing increasing discrimination in an environment in which nativist sentiments are openly voiced and validated by various local and national politicians.

Human smuggling and trafficking constitute perhaps the most disturbing form of intraregional and interregional migration. The clandestine nature of such activity makes determining the precise magnitude of the problem next to impossible. However, Interpol estimates that 35,000 women are trafficked out of Colombia every year; between 50,000 and 70,000 women from the Dominican Republic are working abroad in the sex industry; about 500,000 girls are engaged in prostitution in Brazil; and some 2,000 girls, many of them migrants, work as prostitutes in Costa Rica (International Organization for Migration, 2005).

The report of the World Commission on the Social Dimension of Globalization entitled *A Fair Globalization: Creating Opportunities for All* calls for bilateral and plurilateral action at three levels to address the issues and problems associated with international migration. First, steps should be taken to build upon the foundations of existing instruments, revitalizing and extending multilateral commitments. Second, the "dialogue between countries of origin and destination on key policy issues of common interest" must be strengthened and made more productive. Finally, steps must be taken to develop a multilateral framework for governing the cross-border movement of people (International Labour Office, 2004, p. 99).

WEAK POLITICAL PARTICIPATION: APATHY OR THE ABSENCE OF AN ENABLING ENVIRONMENT?

Many young people in Latin America have limited resources and struggle simply to survive. A substantial number migrate to other countries, seeking to escape enduring socio-economic pressures at home. Forced to concentrate on basic survival and lacking the conviction that the status quo may be successfully challenged, growing numbers of Latin American youth are withdrawing from the realm of political activism.

Young people in Latin America have a rich history of political engagement, and recent events demonstrate that committed youth still constitute an effective political force. The 2006 Penguin Revolution in Chile is one example of a powerful social movement started by young people demanding educational reform. An estimated 800,000 protesters, most of them secondary and tertiary students, came together to participate in the largest social movement since the end of the military dictatorship 16 years earlier, and their actions resulted in increased educational spending and placed education at the top of the political agenda (Reel, 2006).

Recent evidence of youth engagement notwithstanding, the results of a region-wide survey conducted by the Latinobarómetro Corporation in 2004 suggest that the political fervor characterizing many Latin American societies in the past may have diminished.1 When asked whether democracy was preferable to all other forms of government, whether in some circumstances an authoritarian system was preferable to a democracy, or whether no single system was preferable to another, only about 60 per cent of the respondents favored democracy. Support for democracy averaged 56 per cent among youth in their late teens and early twenties,2 though national figures varied widely. In Uruguay, a country with strong democratic traditions, youth support for democracy exceeded 80 per cent, while in countries with weaker democratic histories, such as Ecuador, Guatemala, Honduras, Nicaragua and Paraguay, the corresponding figure was closer to 45 per cent. Only a third of the young people surveyed claimed to be "very interested" or "somewhat interested" in politics, though again, significant intercountry disparities were apparent (see figure 2.4). At least 40 per cent of the young respondents from the Dominican Republic, Mexico, Panama and Uruguay expressed an interest in politics, while the same was true for only a quarter of the youth from Brazil, Costa Rica, Ecuador, Guatemala and Nicaragua. It should be noted that all of the countries in the higher-interest group, with the exception of Mexico, were in the middle of presidential campaigns in 2004.

Figure 2.4
Level of interest in politics among Latin American youth aged 18-24 years, 2004

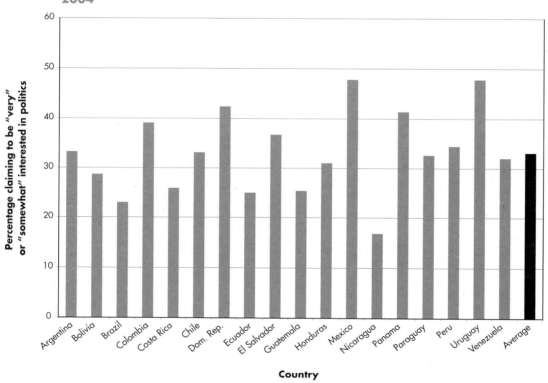

Source: Elaborated from Latinobarómetro, Banco de Datos: Latinobarómetro 2004, annual survey on politics and institutions (database available from www.latinobarometro.org).
Note: Brazil and Nicaragua: 16-24 years.

Why do young people in a region with a rich history of political activism seem to be growing increasingly apathetic? Does this trend reflect a genuine disinterest in sociopolitical participation on the part of youth or are there other factors at play? As noted previously, many young people are preoccupied with meeting their basic needs, but their political disengagement may have more to do with the changing nature of politics in their respective countries. Political structures are continuously evolving, and many of the overarching ideologies that once informed Latin American politics no longer dominate the political landscape. Elections are held more frequently, which is a positive development by any standard; however, voter fatigue may occur, and gains such as these can breed complacence. ICT developments have allowed the public to become better informed, and exposure to frequent political scandals and a growing distrust of political parties have fostered an anti-political attitude among many citizens, including youth.

It would appear that both socio-economic and political factors affect the capacity and willingness of young people to participate in the political process. In Latin America, these factors have fostered a climate in which young people are more likely to adopt non-standard approaches to participation that do not necessarily promote societal cohesion.

It is important to acknowledge the connection between young peoples' confidence in the political system and their decisions regarding political participation. Levels of satisfaction with the way democracy works largely determine the extent of support for democracy. Youth in Latin America were asked how satisfied they were with the exercise of democracy in their own countries, and less than a third indicated that they were "very satisfied" or "rather satisfied" with the efforts of the Government to apply democratic principles (see figure 2.5). Only in Chile were a (bare) majority of young respondents satisfied with the way democracy was working.

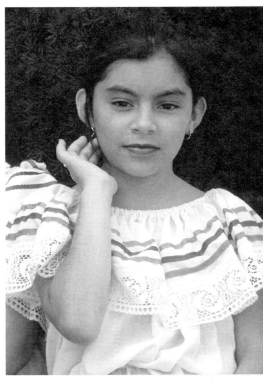

Figure 2.5
Support for and satisfaction with democracy among Latin American youth aged 18-24 years, 2004

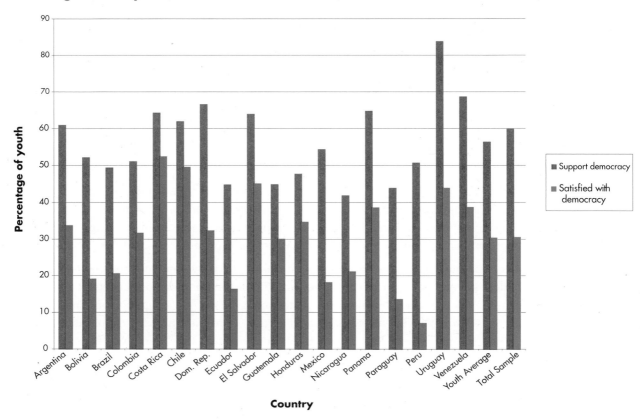

Source: Elaborated from Latinobarómetro, Banco de Datos: Latinobarómetro 2004, annual survey on politics and institutions (database available from www.latinobarometro.org).

Notes: For each country, the level of "support for democracy" reflects the percentage of respondents who chose the option "democracy is preferable to any other form of government", and the proportion of those "satisfied with democracy" derives from the combined percentages of those who said they were "very satisfied" or "rather satisfied" with how democracy was working.

Brazil and Nicaragua: 16-24 years.

In Latin America, the widespread dissatisfaction with the way democracy works coincides with very low levels of public trust in key institutions associated with democratic governance (see figure 2.6). Among those young people surveyed in 2004, only 37 per cent indicated that they had "some" or "a lot of" trust in the judicial system, and the corresponding levels of trust in the legislature and political parties were even lower, at 30 and 21 per cent respectively. The older survey respondents placed less faith in the efficacy of these institutions than did the younger group. The data in figure 2.6 suggest that political trust diminishes with age; these findings may simply reflect the expected gap between the idealism of youth and the growing realism that comes with adulthood and accumulated experience, but another possible explanation is that those youth most critical of their political institutions decided to "vote with their feet" and migrated in search of a better future.

Figure 2.6
Level of trust in key political institutions by age, 2004

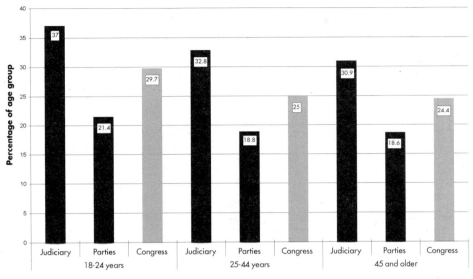

Source: Elaborated from Latinobarómetro, Banco de Datos: Latinobarómetro 2004, annual survey on politics and institutions (database available from www.latinobarometro.org).
Note: Brazil and Nicaragua: 16-24 years.

The results of the Latinobarómetro survey reveal a direct correspondence between the level of interest in politics and the level of political activism in specified areas. Figure 2.7 indicates that in all but one of the activities probed in the survey, rates of participation were lower among youth than among older respondents.3 Young people were more likely to sign petitions than to engage in any other political activity, but the only area in which their participation rates were higher than those of older groups was "illegal protests". The older respondents were far more likely to contact State officials than to participate in street demonstrations, but youth were almost equally likely to do either. The tendency to withdraw from politics is higher among Latin American youth than among their older counterparts, but when young people do participate, they are more inclined to engage in non-conventional forms of political activism. The prevalence of such behaviour may indicate the extent to which young people feel unrepresented by and unwelcome within the traditional political establishment.

Figure 2.7
Political participation in Latin America by age group, 2004

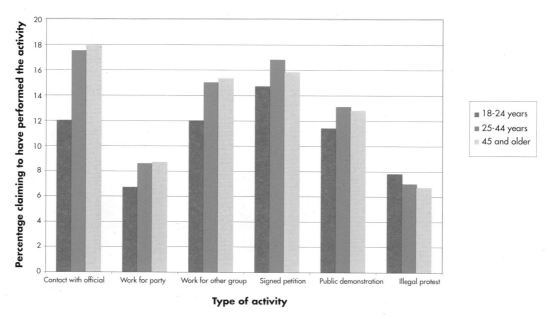

Source: Elaborated from Latinobarómetro, Banco de Datos: Latinobarómetro 2004, annual survey on politics and institutions (database available from www.latinobarometro.org).
Note: Brazil and Nicaragua: 16-24 years.

Gender disparities are evident in assessments of political participation in Latin America. Figures 2.8 through 2.13 clearly show that at all ages, men are more likely than women to be politically active. However, the gender differential is relatively small among youth, particularly the more educated segments. A number of factors discourage female political participation. Young people have more limited access to sociopolitical assets, fewer resources, and weaker ties within the social network than do older members of society, and young women are at a particular disadvantage. Females tend to have more domestic responsibilities, which limits the time they can spend on activities outside the home. Another important factor relates to gender roles and expectations; although the involvement of women in the public sphere is gaining greater acceptance in the region, traditional attitudes persist in some countries. Established customs and conventions keep women from participating in the political process, weakening the capacity of civil society to address the inequities females face in the region.

Educational gains are likely to contribute to improvements in most of the areas addressed above, with positive implications for political activism. Recent statistics indicate a positive correlation between educational attainment and political participation in Latin America (see figures 2.8-2.13). In a context of widespread political apathy, better educated youth generally have a greater awareness of their rights and are more inclined to assert them by engaging in political activism. Evidence suggests that education improves the quality of participatory democracy by encouraging greater involvement in public affairs.

Figure 2.8

Political participation in Latin America: percentage of respondents claiming to have contacted State officials, by age, sex and educational level, 2004

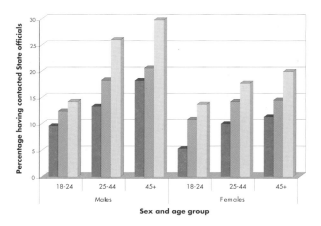

Figure 2.9

Political participation in Latin America: percentage of respondents claiming to have worked for a political party, by age, sex and educational level, 2004

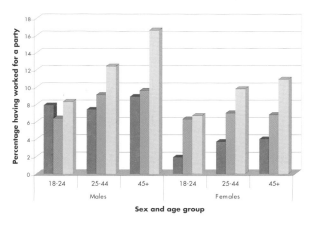

Figure 2.10

Political participation in Latin America: percentage of respondents claiming to have worked for or donated money to another group, by age, sex and educational level, 2004

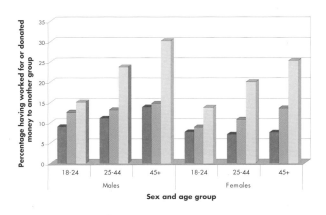

Figure 2.11

Political participation in Latin America: percentage of respondents claiming to have signed a petition, by age, sex and educational level, 2004

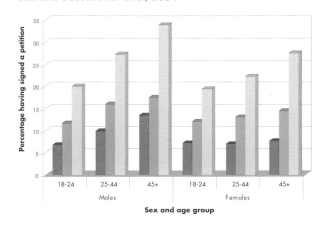

Figure 2.12

Political participation in Latin America: percentage of respondents claiming to have participated in a public demonstration, by age, sex and educational level, 2004

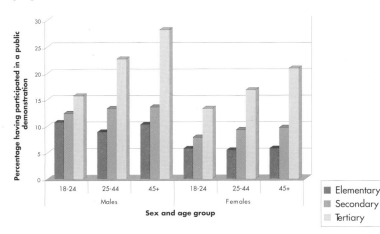

Figure 2.13

Political participation in Latin America: percentage of respondents claiming to have participated in an illegal protest, by age, sex and educational level, 2004

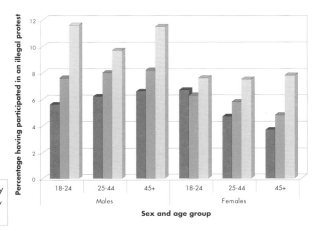

Source: Elaborated from Latinobarómetro, Banco de Datos: Latinobarómetro 2004, annual survey on politics and institutions (database available from www.latinobarometro.org).

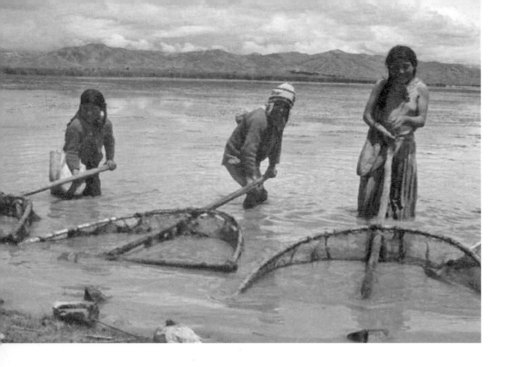

Latin Americans of all ages appear to have little trust in their political institutions, are largely unsatisfied with the way democracy works in their countries, and are not as politically active as in times past. Political frustrations and disappointments seem to be shared by most of the region's residents, regardless of age; there are few factors specific to youth that might explain the high degree of political distrust and apathy among them. Young people exhibit many of the same political attitudes and tendencies as their elders but seem to be even more reluctant to become politically involved. The growing political indifference in Latin America is largely related to frustrations over the lack of opportunities for upward social and economic mobility, the high levels of inequality, poverty and social exclusion (United Nations Development Programme, 2004a), and the lack of accountability and responsiveness among political leaders and institutions. Young people struggling to transition successfully into adulthood are particularly vulnerable to the challenges arising in connection with these issues and feel powerless to halt the seemingly inexorable decline. If they are to overcome their sense of hopelessness and political disconnectedness, young people must be given more opportunities to contribute to the decisions that affect them and society at large.

SUMMARY AND CONCLUSIONS

Various structural factors effectively prevent Latin American youth from participating fully in society. Job creation for young people remains relatively limited in spite of improved economic growth in a number of countries, and younger professionals are being absorbed more slowly into the most dynamic industries and activities. Inadequate educational preparedness and professional training are problems for many young people trying to enter the job market, and those who are able to find work must often settle for lower pay and fewer benefits (particularly in the areas of social security and health care). Increasing numbers of youth are migrating to countries perceived as having more opportunities for participation, but cross-border movement often presents new challenges that must be overcome before youth can hope to benefit from these opportunities and build a better life for themselves. While these factors are difficult to change in the short run, it is critical that Governments and civil society establish stronger foundations and effective mechanisms for the integration of youth as a long-term strategy. Within this framework, it is necessary to begin with the fundamentals; changes in education, health care, and economic policies must be based on the supposition that youth will become tomorrow's leaders and will therefore be responsible for the future development of the region.

Well-educated youth generally have better prospects for social and economic success and are more likely to become contributing members of society. Action is required on multiple levels to enhance the quality of education and increase school retention rates, especially at the secondary level. Steps should be taken to improve teacher training and learning environments and to ensure that educational content is aligned with labour force requirements. While all young people require sustained educational support, targeted policies and programmes may be needed to expand access for specific groups, including rural girls, indigenous youth, and young people living in poverty. Youth from economically disadvantaged families are more likely to drop out of school and, lacking marketable skills, are unable to secure decent, permanent employment. Effective educational retention strategies ultimately improve job prospects and therefore represent a powerful tool for poverty alleviation.

Young people are often unable to find work in their own communities. Some youth accept low-paying jobs for which they are overqualified, and rural residents may seek employment in urban centres, while other young people move elsewhere within or outside Latin America. Those who migrate face a new set of challenges relating to both social and economic integration; immigrants may experience prejudice and are particularly vulnerable to exploitation.

Young women are especially at risk. Female youth have made greater educational gains than their male counterparts, but this has not translated into greater income security in the long run. In many areas the job market is limited for women. Those who find jobs are often poorly paid and work long hours doing menial labour; young women who migrate frequently work in the domestic service or sex industries and are regularly exploited.

In order to protect the rights of workers both domestically and internationally, minimum wage requirements and laws governing working hours need to be enforced where they exist and established where they do not. Global action must be taken within a collaborative framework to deal with human trafficking and sexual exploitation. Progress in these areas will benefit all of humanity but is especially important for youth (particularly young women), who tend to be among the world's most vulnerable citizens.

To encourage Latin American youth to remain at home and make a positive contribution to their own communities, Governments and civil society institutions must work to provide social support, educational and economic opportunities, and spaces for political activism and other forms of public participation. A certain level of migration is inevitable, however, and the Governments of host countries must acknowledge that immigrants can contribute significantly to society and the economy and should provide clear rules for granting permanent residence to those who wish to establish deeper roots in their adopted countries.

Latin Americans of all ages are largely dissatisfied with the political system, public institutions, and the way democracy is (or is not) exercised in their countries. Young people in the region were once well-known for their interest and involvement in public affairs, but the youth of today seem indifferent to politics, and relatively few are engaged in conventional forms of activism. For many young people, alienation from traditional politics appears to be a consequence of their social marginalization.

Young people are unlikely to have faith in their public institutions or to support the democratic process until the Government addresses its own shortcomings and takes decisive action to satisfy the needs of citizens in general and of youth in particular. Increased transparency and accountability in public administration, a more responsive political system, and greater attention to social, economic and cultural development priorities would have a positive impact on young people's attitudes towards the political establishment and would encourage more constructive involvement among youth in public affairs.

---

[1] All the data reported in this section have been elaborated from the original 2004 Latinobarómetro dataset.

[2] The Latinobarómetro survey included interviews with Latin American citizens eligible to vote—those aged 18 and above in all but two Latin American countries. In Brazil and Nicaragua the minimum voting age is 16, so the relevant survey information for those countries relates to youth between the ages of 16 and 24.

[3] Respondents to the Latinobarómetro survey were asked whether they had ever participated in any of the political activities listed in figure 2.7. Older people had lived longer and had thus had more opportunities for participation, so it is likely that the degree of political participation among youth is underestimated when compared with that of older citizens.

References

Agüero, Felipe, and Jeffrey Stark, editors (1998). *Fault Lines of Democracy in Post-Transition Latin America*. Miami: North-South Center Press, University of Miami.

Associated Press (2007). Venezuelan youth show coordinated fight (5 June).

De Ferranti, David, and others (2004). *Inequality in Latin America and the Caribbean: Breaking with History?* World Bank Latin American and Caribbean Studies. Washington, D.C.: World Bank.

Duryea, Suzanne, Olga Jaramillo and Carmen Pagés (2003). Latin American labour markets in the 1990s: deciphering the decade. Inter-American Development Bank Working Paper No. 486. Washington, D.C.: May.

Economic Commission for Latin America and the Caribbean (1999). *Panorama Social de América Latina 1998*. United Nations publication, Sales No. S.99.II.G.4.

_____ (2002). Vulnerabilidad sociodemográfica: viejos y nuevos riesgos para comunidades, hogares y personas (síntesis y conclusiones) (LC/G.2170 [SES.29/16]).

_____ (2004a). *Boletín Demográfico: América Latina y Caribe, Estimaciones y Proyecciones de Población, 1950-2050*, vol. 37, No. 73 (January).

_____ (2004b). *Panorama Social de América Latina 2004*. United Nations publication, Sales No. S.04.II.G.148.

_____ (2005). *Panorama Social de América Latina 2005* (LC/G.2288-P/E). Santiago.

_____ (2007). *Statistical Yearbook for Latin America and the Caribbean 2006*. United Nations publication, Sales No. E/S.07.II.G.1.

_____ and Organización Iberoamericana de Juventud (2004). La juventud en Iberoamérica: tendencias y urgencias (LC/L.2180). Santiago: October.

Garretón, Manuel Antonio, and Edward Newman, editors (2001). *Democracy in Latin America: (Re)Constructing Political Society*. Tokyo: United Nations University Press.

Guarnizo, Luis, and Luz Díaz (1999). Transnational migration: a view from Colombia. *Ethnic and Racial Studies*, vol. 22, No. 2 (March), pp. 397-421.

Haggard, Stephan, and Robert R. Kaufman (1995). *The Political Economy of Democratic Transitions*. Princeton, New Jersey: Princeton University Press.

Human Rights Watch (2005). Colombia: displaced and discarded—the plight of internally displaced persons in Bogotá and Cartagena. *Human Rights Watch*, vol. 17, No. 4(B) (October).

International Labour Office (2004). *A Fair Globalization: Creating Opportunities for All*. Report of the World Commission on the Social Dimension of Globalization. Geneva.

_____ Regional Office for Latin America and the Caribbean (2005). *Panorama Laboral 2005: América Latina y el Caribe*. Lima.

International Organization for Migration (2005). *World Migration 2005: Costs and Benefits of International Migration*. Geneva.

Joint United Nations Programme on HIV/AIDS (2006a). UNAIDS fact sheet: Latin America. Geneva. Available from http://data.unaids.org/pub/GlobalReport/2006/200605-fs_latinamerica_en.pdf.

_____ (2006b). *2006 Report on the Global AIDS Epidemic*. Annex 2. Geneva.

Latin American and Caribbean Demographic Centre. Economic Commission for Latin America and the Caribbean (2007). Database on Internal Migration in Latin America and the Caribbean (available from http://www.eclac.cl).

Latinobarómetro (2004). Banco de Datos: Latinobarómetro 2004. Database available from www.latinobarometro.org.

Lopes Patarra, Neide, and Rosana Baeninger (2006). Mobilidade espacial da população no Mercosul: metrópoles e fronterias. *Revista Brasileira de Ciências Sociaís*, vol. 21, No. 60 (February), pp. 83-102.

Mahler, Sarah (2000). *Migration and Transnational Issues: Recent Trends and Prospects for 2020*. CA2020: Working Paper No. 4. Hamburg: Institut für Iberoamerika-Kunde.

Martínez Buján, Raquel (2003). *La Reciente Inmigración Latinoamericana a España*. Santiago: Economic Commission for Latin America and the Caribbean. United Nations publication, Sales No. S.03.II.G.76.

Martínez Pizarro, Jorge, and Miguel Villa (2005). International migration in Latin America and the Caribbean: a summary view of trends and patterns (UN/POP/MIG/2005/14). United Nations Expert Group Meeting on International Migration and Development, New York, 6-8 July 2005.

Merkle, Caspar (2003). Youth participation in El Alto, Bolivia. *Environment and Urbanization*, vol. 15, No. 1, pp. 205-214.

Molinas Vega, José (1999). Migración interna en Paraguay: ¿Quiénes migran? ¿Adónde? ¿Porqué? y ¿Cómo viven? Un análisis económico de la encuesta de hogares 1996. BID-BM-CEPAL, Programa MECOVI-Paraguay. April.

Moser, Caroline O.N. (2005). City violence and the poor. *In Focus* (August), pp. 10-12. United Nations Development Programme, International Poverty Centre.

Partnership for Educational Revitalization in the Americas (2007). *A Lot to Do: A Report Card on Education in Central America and the Dominican Republic*. Task Force on Education Reform in Central America.

Reel, Monte (2006). Chile's student activists: a course in democracy. *Washington Post Foreign Service* (25 November).

Rodríguez, Ernesto, and Bernardo Dabezies (1991). *Primer Informe sobre la Juventud en América Latina 1990*. Madrid: Organización Iberoamericana de Juventud.

Rodríguez Vignoli, Jorge (2004). *Migración Interna en América Latina y el Caribe: Estudio Regional del Período 1980-2000* (LC/L.2059-P). Santiago: Economic Commission for Latin America and the Caribbean. United Nations publication, Sales No. S.04.II.G.3.

Romero, Simon (2007). Chávez looks at his critics in the media and sees the enemy. *The New York Times* (1 June).

Sáinz, Pedro (2007). Equity in Latin America since the 1990s. In *Flat World, Big Gaps: Economic Liberalization, Globalization, Poverty and Inequality*, Jomo K.S. and Jacques Baudot, editors. Hyderabad, India: Orient Longman; London; New York: Zed Books; and Penang, Malaysia: Third World Network. Published in association with the United Nations.

Stefoni, Carolina (2002). Mujeres inmigrantes Peruanas en Chile. *CIEAP/UAEM Papeles de Población*, No. 33 (July-September). Toluca, Mexico: Universidad Autónoma del Estado de México.

Teichman, Judith A. (2001). *The Politics of Freeing Markets in Latin America: Chile, Argentina, and Mexico*. Chapel Hill: University of North Carolina Press.

United Nations (2007). *World Population Prospects: The 2006 Revision*. Extended Dataset. CD-ROM. New York.

United Nations Development Programme (2004a). *La Democracia en América Latina: Hacia una Democracia de Ciudadanos y Ciudadanas*. Second edition. Lima.

_____ (2004b). *Human Development Report 2004: Cultural Liberty in Today's Diverse World*. New York.

United Nations Educational, Scientific and Cultural Organization (2006). *Education for All Global Monitoring Report—Regional Overview: Latin America and the Caribbean* (ED/2007/EFA/MRT/PI/ LAC/1). Paris: UNESCO Publishing.

_____ Institute for Statistics (2007). Database. Available from www.uis.unesco.org.

United Nations Millennium Project (2005). *Investing in Development: A Practical Plan to Achieve the Millennium Development Goals.* New York.

United Nations Population Fund (2006). *State of World Population 2006—A Passage to Hope: Women and International Migration.* New York. Sales No. E.06.III.H.1.

United States Census Bureau (2004). Foreign-born population of the United States: current population survey—March 2004. Washington, D.C. Available from http://www.census.gov/population/www/socdemo/foreign/ppl-176.html (accessed on 20 July 2006).

Valls, Andreu Domingo, and Rosana Beatriz Martínez (2005). La población Latinoamericana censada en España en 2001: un retrato sociodemográfico. Paper presented at the XI Encuentro de Latinoamericanistas Españoles: La Comunidad Iberoamericana de Naciones, Tordesillas (Valladolid), 26-28 May 2005.

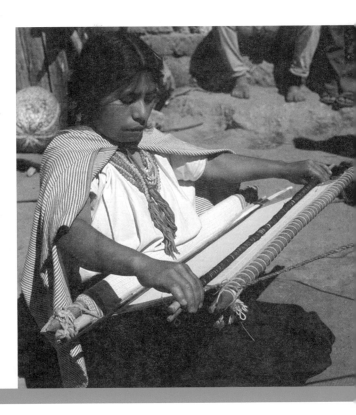

Chapter 3

Overcoming the barriers of poverty:
challenges for *YOUTH* participation
in sub-Saharan Africa

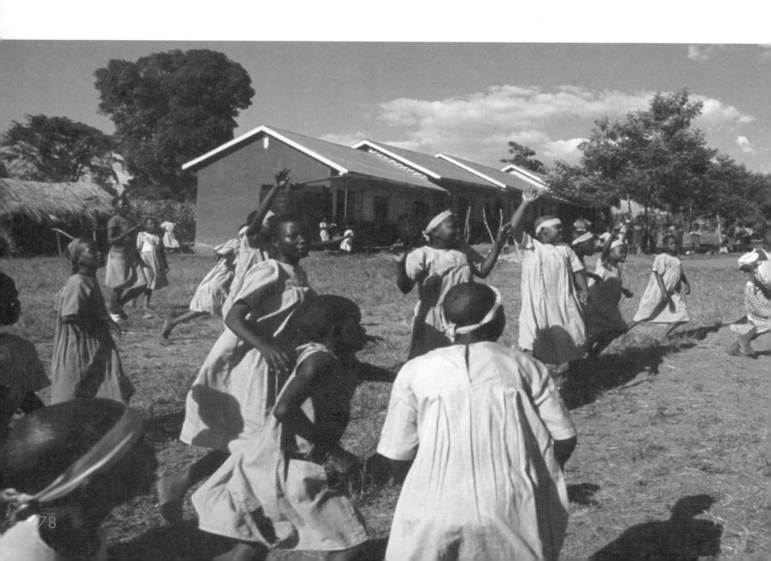

Young people in all regions of the world, experience some degree of difficulty or uncertainty as they make the transition into adulthood. However, the situation that youth in Africa face is one of the most difficult in many respects. Average life expectancy in the region is among the lowest in the world. Weak infrastructure and poor economic development have traditionally impeded youth development in the region; staying enrolled in school, finding decent and productive work, and maintaining a healthy lifestyle all present very real challenges to a large proportion of youth in the region.

The estimated 157 million young people living in sub-Saharan Africa today are by no means a homogenous group. They come from varied cultural and ethnic backgrounds, and they speak one or more of the estimated 800 languages spoken in the region. Many have qualifications that compare favourably with or exceed those of their colleagues in more developed parts of the world; however, many more fall far below global education averages. Youth in sub-Saharan Africa are adopting new techniques of learning, working and communicating with the outside world in their attempts to create meaningful lives for themselves. They are navigating the communications highway and exchanging text messages and electronic mail with colleagues, gradually overcoming social and cultural factors that previously limited their access to information. Nevertheless, poverty remains a major constraint to the achievement of the full potential of youth in the region.

The intense poverty that has long characterized the region is highly multidimensional and includes monetary and non-monetary aspects. Apart from an overall lack of material and financial resources, there are also chronic and sporadic deficiencies in the quantity and quality of basic social services, amenities and communal services. Chronic food insecurity in sub-Saharan Africa has increased substantially since 1970, with the number of malnourished people in the region soaring from 88 million to 200 million by 1999-2001; this is the only region in the world in which levels of hunger have been steadily increasing since 1990. More specifically, the number of hungry people in sub-Saharan Africa is estimated to have increased by 20 per cent between 1990 and 2005 (von Braun, 2005). Because of the extent to which poverty is entrenched in the region, the challenges of youth development cannot be adequately addressed without consideration of the poverty context and its impact on the formative years of young people. The political and social landscape of the region has also been characterized by successive changes in government and poor governance. In several countries in the region, violent conflicts have further complicated the prospects for youth development.

The chapter includes a review of these and other major constraints to national development over the past 25 years or so, as they have had an enormous impact on youth development in the region. The progress and challenges experienced by young people in sub-Saharan Africa are explored in the sections to come. The chapter begins with an overview of the demographic context, focusing on the unique status of the present youth cohort as a "bridge generation" between a past era of explosive growth in the region's youth population and a nascent era of more restrained growth. The chapter then examines the role of the macroeconomic and social milieux that have shaped youth opportunities and the capacity of young people to participate in development. The next section reviews persistent obstacles to young people's participation in economic, social and political life in the region and focuses on the constraints imposed by the HIV/AIDS epidemic, the environment of conflict in some countries, and the challenges of globalization. The final section presents an overview of areas in which the region is making progress in involving youth in development. It highlights, in particular, recent trends in youth voluntarism and regional initiatives to advance youth development.

YOUTH: A MAJOR RESOURCE IN A CHANGING DEMOGRAPHIC CONTEXT

Young people aged 15-24 years accounted for 20.4 per cent of the total population of sub-Saharan Africa in 2005 (see table 3.1). This figure reflects the United Nations definition of youth; however, when the broader definition used by the African Union (encompassing all those aged 15 to 34 years) is considered, the proportion jumps to 34.3 per cent, or 1 in 3 people. The region's population aged 15-24 years totalled almost 157 million in 2005; another 100 million would be added under the broader definition of youth (see table 3.1). By 2015, the population aged 15-24 years in sub-Saharan Africa is expected to reach some 200 million, and the population aged 15-34 years is projected to be 343 million.

Table 3.1
Size and share of the youth population in sub-Saharan Africa, 1980-2015

Year	Population by age			Youth aged 15-24 years as percentage of total population	Youth aged 15-34 years as percentage of total population
	Youth aged 15-24 years*	Youth aged 15-34 years*	Total population		
1980	73 457	124 274	388 063	18.9	32.0
1985	85 260	144 690	449 349	19.0	32.2
1990	99 418	168 292	519 391	19.1	32.4
1995	116 356	212 674	596 402	19.5	35.7
2000	136 099	228 043	679 873	20.0	33.5
2005	156 899	263 753	769 348	20.4	34.3
2010	177 255	302 591	866 948	20.4	34.9
2015	197 878	343 410	971 522	20.4	35.3

Source: United Nations, World Population Prospects (New York: 2007); data accessed online at www.unpopulation.org (11 May 2007).
Note: *The table includes figures based on the United Nations definition of youth (aged 15-24 years) and that used by the African Union (15-34 years).

Youth make up a relatively large proportion of the total population in most countries of the region. Table 3.2 shows that between 2005 and 2015, the youth share in most subregions ranged between 18 and 20 per cent. The table also indicates, however, that in most subregions the growth in the size of the youth population is not as high as it used to be. This is especially true for Southern Africa, where the HIV/AIDS epidemic is taking a heavy toll on young lives. Even with the slowdown in growth in Southern Africa, the challenge of youth development in the region is immense.

Table 3.2
Size and growth of the youth population in Africa and its subregions, 1980-2015

Region/ subregion	Year	Population aged 15-24 years (thousands)	Share of population aged 15-24 years (percentage)	Change in youth population (percentage)
Sub-Saharan Africa	1980	73 457	18.9	-
	1985	85 260	19.0	16.1
	1990	99 418	19.1	16.6
	1995	116 356	19.5	17.0
	2000	136 099	20.0	17.0
	2005	156 899	20.4	15.3
	2010	177 255	20.4	13.0
	2015	197 878	20.4	11.6
Eastern Africa	1980	27 890	19.1	-
	1985	32 579	19.2	16.8
	1990	38 172	19.4	17.2
	1995	44 299	19.8	16.1
	2000	52 159	20.3	17.7
	2005	60 586	20.7	16.2
	2010	68 597	20.7	13.2
	2015	76 815	20.5	12.0
Middle Africa	1980	10 139	18.5	-
	1985	11 833	18.7	16.7
	1990	13 897	18.9	17.4
	1995	16 729	19.3	20.4
	2000	19 373	19.8	15.8
	2005	22 499	20.0	16.1
	2010	25 848	19.9	14.9
	2015	29 361	19.8	13.6
Southern Africa	1980	6 466	19.6	-
	1985	7 402	19.8	14.5
	1990	8 487	20.3	14.7
	1995	9 698	20.5	14.3
	2000	10 633	20.5	9.6
	2005	11 185	20.4	5.2
	2010	11 528	20.4	3.1
	2015	11 743	20.3	1.9
Western Africa	1980	25 295	18.8	-
	1985	29 089	18.6	15.0
	1990	33 849	18.7	16.4
	1995	39 818	19.1	17.6
	2000	47 289	19.7	18.8
	2005	55 221	20.3	16.8
	2010	62 914	20.5	13.9
	2015	70 577	20.5	12.2

Source: United Nations, World Population Prospects (New York: 2007); data accessed online at www.unpopulation.org (11 May 2007).

Note: A hyphen (-) indicates that an item is not applicable.

Demographic realities complicate many aspects of social and economic development. For example, the provision of education for a large and growing cohort of young people has been difficult. More schools, teachers, books and other educational resources are needed every year to maintain the existing, and often inadequate, quality of instruction, and recurrent expenditures on facilities maintenance are likely to be higher because of the large sizes of youth cohorts.

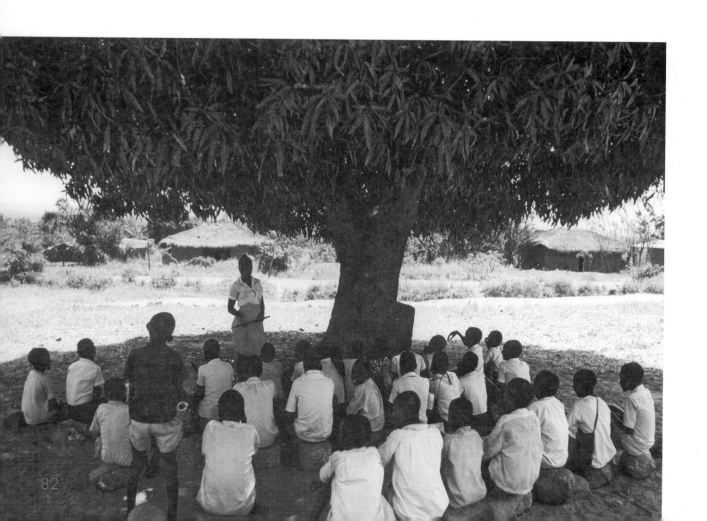

Whether the African Union definition or the United Nations definition (which is the basis for analysis in the rest of the chapter) is used, the demographic picture makes it patently evident that engaging youth fully in sub-Saharan Africa's development is not a matter of choice, but rather an imperative for national development. Young people constitute a significant share of the African population and will continue to do so for many years to come. It should be recognized that despite the challenges associated with youth development in the region and inadequate access to education, the young people of today are, on average, better educated than their parents. They are better connected to the rest of the world than any of the earlier generations of youth in the region, and they are, as a result, more determined to find options to close the gap between their limited opportunities in the region and what they perceive to be possible in the global economy. Failure to provide opportunities for African youth to build their capacity to participate in development would be a missed opportunity to harness the huge potential in human capital, and this could have enormous economic, cultural, political and social consequences.

IMPLICATIONS OF A CHALLENGING ECONOMIC ENVIRONMENT

Youth in Africa today are on the cusp of a transition to lower fertility and population growth rates in the region. They were born between the early 1980s and early 1990s, which was the beginning of a period of incipient decline in fertility rates and in annual population growth rates in the region. In many parts of sub-Saharan Africa, the first notable decline in fertility rates was registered in the early to mid-1980s, when many of today's youth were born. The young people of today have grown up in smaller families; their parents were among the first in the region to have improved access to modern methods of contraception, and the declines in fertility suggest that many used these opportunities to limit their fertility. This ostensibly opened up avenues for the children of that era, who are today's youth, to benefit from higher allocations of household resources.

However, economic difficulties arising from a combination of factors, including the global economic recession of the 1980s, domestic political and management difficulties, and prolonged droughts in many parts of the region, resulted in high levels of individual and national poverty. Therefore, between 1983 and 1992, when most of today's youth were born, the majority of sub-Saharan African countries experienced major social and economic setbacks. Investment in key areas of health and education suffered. Though fertility rates had begun to change in the 1980s, Governments still had to contend with the demands associated with the momentum and pressure created by the large birth cohorts of previous generations. These and other developments set the stage for major macroeconomic difficulties at the national level; the measures taken to promote recovery, including structural and sectoral adjustment policies that called for cost recovery in the social sectors, had equally devastating effects on young people and their families. Constraints to youth participation in African society are therefore not simply related to young people's lack of effort or disinterestedness, but to a complex interaction of household, national and global economic and social forces that impinge on their welfare.

Although the size of the youth population in sub-Saharan Africa presents major challenges to Governments in the region, the opportunity for countries to reap a dividend from the large numbers of people in the labour force cannot be overlooked. It has been emphasized in this connection that, to fully reap the demographic dividend, options must be provided for broadening opportunities to enable young people to develop skills and to use them productively; young people should be given the assistance they need to acquire the capabilities to make good decisions in pursuing those opportunities, and second chances should be offered to those who need to recover from decisions that have negatively affected their development (World Bank, 2006). There is little doubt that youth transitions in sub-Saharan Africa have been affected by the lack of capabilities and skills among young people. A majority of youth in Africa today have completed more years of schooling than their parents did but have limited opportunities in employment and other areas of development participation. Although developing capabilities and skills is undeniably important, it is also vital to address the socio-political and economic environments that have affected youth development in the region and to provide second chances to those who may have fallen through the cracks of the structural and sectoral policy shifts that defined the childhood of many of today's youth.

POVERTY: THE EFFECTS OF RECESSION, ADJUSTMENT AND LIBERALIZATION POLICIES OF THE 1980s AND 1990s

Many of today's youth in sub-Saharan Africa have suffered the consequences of severe poverty from birth. In this sense, they differ from their parents, who grew up at a time when many African countries were emerging from colonial administration, with its promise of a brighter, independent future. Unlike their parents' generation, which enjoyed many opportunities for free or State-subsidized education and health care, today's youth, from birth, have experienced the consequences of a serious global economic recession and of structural adjustment and liberalization policies that led to major retrenchment and job losses and the withdrawal of State subsidies for basic services. These changes resulted in increased poverty in the households in which young people grew up and diminished opportunities for their early development.

African countries were particularly vulnerable to the global recession of the early 1980s. This was because of a weak resource base at the time of independence, the dependence of almost all countries in the region on primary commodity production, a lack of non-aid financial capital, dependency on foreign aid and heavy indebtedness, and a lack of policy ownership resulting from many policies being imposed from outside the region by donors (Geda and Shimeles, 2007). This situation was exacerbated in a number of countries by war, civil strife and environmental disasters, as reflected in the general decline (and in some cases reversals) in major social indicators of progress. Coupled with the pressure of growing populations and worsening terms of trade for primary commodities in international markets, these factors resulted in a virtual collapse of the public sector.

Furthermore, in many countries, the cost of child-rearing rose, and the supply of many basic commodities and services was reduced. During the 1990s, malnutrition was a serious problem in Africa. Nowhere in the region was annual per capita consumption greater than US$ 500, and all countries fell far short of universal primary enrolment. The consequences of these difficulties and interventions were similar across the continent (Christiaensen, Demery and Paternostro, 2002). For most, if not all, countries, the effect on people's welfare was dramatic. In some areas, social indicators such as school enrolment ratios and trends in infant and under-five mortality, which had been improving throughout the 1960s and 1970s, reversed after 1985. Infant mortality rose during 1987 and 1991, and a higher percentage of children under the age of five were stunted or wasted in 1990 than in 1970 (McCulloch, Baulch and Cherel-Robson, 2001).

Many countries in this situation adopted structural adjustment programmes and trade liberalization policies under the leadership and guidance of the Bretton Woods institutions. Since the late 1980s, many African countries have liberalized their external regimes through a policy mix of foreign exchange allocation liberalization, realignment of exchange rates, and the removal of various tariffs. Many of these actions were associated with cutbacks in public sector investment and employment and the implementation of retrenchment and cost recovery policies, which affected the context in which the young people of today were growing up. Both the protracted and deep-rooted economic crisis that occurred before structural adjustment and the policies that were adopted to reverse those trends negatively affected the well-being of the majority of people. Real incomes and per capital social sector expenditures fell, with an adverse impact on the welfare of many (Ekouevi and Adepoju, 1995; Basu and Stewart, 1993). Structural adjustment and related retrenchments in the public sector exacerbated the situation and resulted in growing poverty and increasing inequalities in the distribution of income. Government funding for public education declined, leading to an increased focus on private education initiatives; however, these were affordable only to some, as family incomes were declining, and the share of the family budget available for education was limited (Reimers and Tiburcio, 1993). Many households experienced extreme difficulty in accessing basic goods and services, including those needed to support the education and health of their children—today's generation of youth.

Estimates of monetary poverty for sub-Saharan African youth that were presented in the World Youth Report 2003 (United Nations, 2004) have been revised for this report and are presented in the statistical annex. Table 3.3 shows an extract of those indicators for a selection of countries and provides estimates of the numbers of youth living below the minimum dietary requirements. Data are presented for a selection of countries, including some of the largest in the region.

Table 3.3
Estimates of youth living with monetary poverty and inadequate nutrition in selected countries of sub-Saharan Africa

Country	Total youth population (thousands)	Year of poverty data	Percentage of youth living on less than US$ 1 per day (PPP)	Estimate of youth living on less than US$ 1 per day (thousands)	Percentage of youth living on less than US$ 2 per day (PPP)	Estimate of youth living on less than US$ 2 per day (thousands)	Percentage of youth consuming less than dietary minimum (2003)	Number of youth consuming less than dietary minimum (thousands)
Benin	1 839	2003	30.9	568.3	73.7	1 355.3	14	257.5
Burkina Faso	2 917	2003	27.2	793.4	71.8	2 094.4	17	495.9
Cameroon	3 662	2001	17.1	626.2	50.6	1 853.0	25	915.5
Côte d'Ivoire	4 141	2002	14.8	612.9	48.8	2 020.8	14	579.7
Ethiopia	16 675	2000	23.0	3 835.3	77.8	12 973.2	46	7 670.5
Madagascar	3 856	2001	61.0	2 352.2	85.1	3 281.5	38	1 465.3
Mauritania	617	2000	25.9	159.8	63.1	389.3	10	61.7
Nigeria	28 821	2003	70.8	20 405.3	92.4	26 630.6	9	2 593.9
Rwanda	2 236	2000	51.7	1 156.0	83.7	1 871.5	36	805.0
South Africa	9 747	2000	10.7	1 042.9	34.1	3 323.7	..	..
Tanzania	8 624	2000/01	57.8	4 984.7	89.9	7 753.0	44	3 794.6
Zambia	2 701	2002/03	75.8	2 047.4	94.1	2 541.6	47	1 269.5

Sources: Population data are drawn from United Nations, *World Population Prospects: The 2006 Revision* (New York: 2007).

Percentages for those living below the poverty line are drawn from United Nations Development Programme, *Human Development Indicators 2006* (available from http://hdr.undp.org/hdr2006/statistics/indicators/ 23.html; accessed on 5 April 2007). Estimates of the numbers of youth living below the poverty line and on less than the minimum dietary requirements are calculations of the United Nations Programme on Youth.

Notes: Two dots (..) indicate that an item is not available. PPP = purchasing power parity

The estimates presented in table 3.3 suggest that the percentages of youth living in poverty are extremely high. It is estimated, for example, that over 90 per cent of the young people in Nigeria and Zambia live on less than US$ 2 per day, and the same is true for almost 40 million youth in Ethiopia and Nigeria. These high levels of poverty persist despite poverty reduction strategies and some improvement in economic growth in the region. This suggests that recent policies adopted to revitalize the economy in Africa are not having much of an impact on youth poverty. Though the estimates presented in table 3.3 are extrapolations from the proportions of the total population living in poverty in the countries shown, they are likely to be accurate estimates of youth who live in poverty, as the situation of youth in many countries is often dependent on that of adults.

The use of income poverty measures alone does not suffice in estimating poverty in a population. Human poverty is more accurately defined as unmet basic human needs; important factors within this context include nutritional adequacy, access to health care (including maternal and reproductive health care), the availability of basic facilities and infrastructure, and any other variables that may improve prospects for survival and increased longevity. Table 3.3 provides estimates relating to hunger and malnutrition. The table indicates that serious nutritional deprivation exists among youth in Ethiopia, where an estimated 7 million young people are consuming less than the dietary minimum. As with the distribution of monetary poverty across the household, it can be assumed that the availability of basic amenities is the same for all household members, including youth, who constitute about 20 per cent of the world's population.

Table 3.4 suggests that access to electricity, which is essential if youth are to benefit from modern information and communication technologies, is highly limited in the region. The data suggest that in only two countries, Gabon and Nigeria, are more than half of the households served by electricity. In almost all countries, more than 90 per cent of rural households have no electricity. In Uganda, Mozambique, Lesotho, Malawi, Rwanda and Chad, between 91 and 96 per cent of all households do not have access to electricity. Overall, access to water is much better than access to electricity. However, in this case as well, large differentials exist between urban and rural areas, and some countries are much worse off than others. If it is assumed that youth are distributed equally across households, then these data also reflect the situation of youth with respect to access to electricity and water, and they suggest a high level of deprivation.

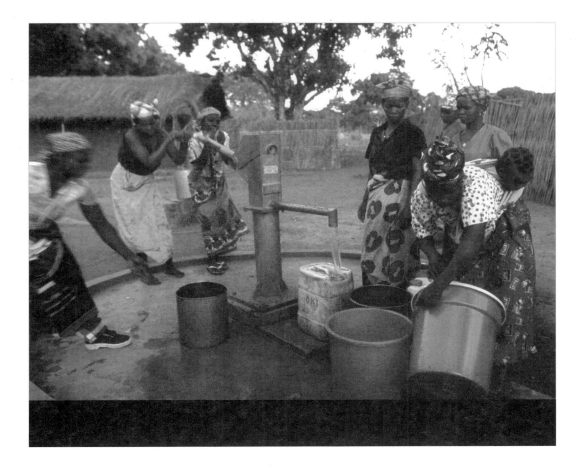

Table 3.4
Percentage of households with no electricity and with no access to water within 15 minutes of the home, ranked in ascending order based on lack of access to electricity for all households

Country	Year	Percentage of households with no electricity			Percentage of households that have no water within 15 minutes of the home		
		Total	Rural	Urban	Total	Rural	Urban
Gabon	2000	26.3	70.1	9.8	25.4	48.1	16.9
Nigeria	2003	47.7	66.0	15.0	43.7	48.6	35.1
Ghana	2003	51.6	75.8	23.1	38.2	53.5	20.2
Cameroon	2004	52.8	84.5	22.9	41.5	52.9	30.8
Senegal	2005	52.8	84.1	19.6	28.1	45.8	9.3
Namibia	2000	63.5	86.7	26.8	21.7	32.3	5.0
Congo (Brazzaville)	2005	66.2	85.1	49.2	45.3	65.6	26.9
Eritrea	2002	67.8	96.9	21.7	68.4	91.8	31.3
Mauritania	2000/01	77.4	96.9	50.1	46.2	52.9	36.8
Benin	2001	77.9	94.3	50.3	36.8	44.4	23.9
Guinea	2005	79.4	96.9	35.5	37.6	44.8	19.5
Madagascar	2003/04	79.6	89.1	47.3	33.3	35.0	27.5
Zambia	2001/02	82.6	97.0	54.9	40.3	50.1	21.6
Kenya	2003	83.9	95.2	49.8	46.8	56.9	16.2
Ethiopia	2005	85.9	98.0	14.3	66.1	73.1	24.5
Ethiopia	2000	87.3	99.6	23.8	73.7	78.8	47.3
Burkina Faso	2004	88.4	99.0	47.5	47.3	51.1	32.7
Tanzania	2004	88.4	98.2	61.0	60.2	70.4	31.9
Mali	2001	88.8	97.3	62.9	29.9	34.4	16.1
Uganda	2000/01	91.2	97.3	56.0	77.5	84.6	37.3
Mozambique	2003	91.8	98.8	74.9	64.3	75.0	38.4
Lesotho	2004	93.0	99.0	73.6	53.9	63.0	24.5
Malawi	2004	93.0	97.6	69.6	58.2	63.3	32.6
Rwanda	2000	93.7	99.0	61.1	74.6	79.9	42.3
Malawi	2000	95.0	98.8	71.2	66.6	71.7	34.6
Rwanda	2005	95.1	98.6	74.7	69.9	73.0	52.1
Chad	2004	96.2	99.5	83.3	55.4	62.7	26.1

Source: MEASURE DHS, STATcompiler (2007) (available from http://www.measuredhs.com; accessed on 15 May 2007).

The impact that lack of access to basic household facilities has on youth poverty cannot be overemphasized. Where water is unavailable in the household, young people, especially girls, may be responsible for fetching water not only for their own household, but also for others. Activities such as these detract from self-development and involve risks of exploitation. Access to electricity is essential for participation in an increasingly globalized world. Without it, there is no access to computers, which not only facilitate communication but may also offer distance-learning opportunities for young people.

EDUCATION: DESPITE PROGRESS, THERE IS MUCH YET TO BE DONE

Sub-Saharan Africa has perhaps made the greatest progress in recent years in providing access to education. Efforts towards achieving universal primary education by 2015, as called for in the Millennium Development Goals, have produced a higher number of primary education graduates in sub-Saharan Africa. Enrolment in primary education increased from 57 per cent in 1999 to 70 per cent in 2005 (United Nations, 2007). For a number of countries, household data on educational attainment also show gains over the years. Table 3.5 indicates that while many young people are not enrolled in school, the share of youth who are enrolled has generally increased over time. In Eritrea, for example, there was a 7-percentage-point increase in enrolment between 1995 and 2002. In Madagascar, the corresponding share rose from 14.6 per cent in 1992 to 21.4 per cent in 2003/04, and in Mozambique the percentage enrolled in school nearly doubled between 1997 and 2003. With regard to tertiary education, though progress has been more limited, there is also evidence of improvements in access. Successful tertiary institutions have found ways of improving their financial situation while also boosting the quality of their programmes, though often at the cost of price increases for students (Bollag, 2004).

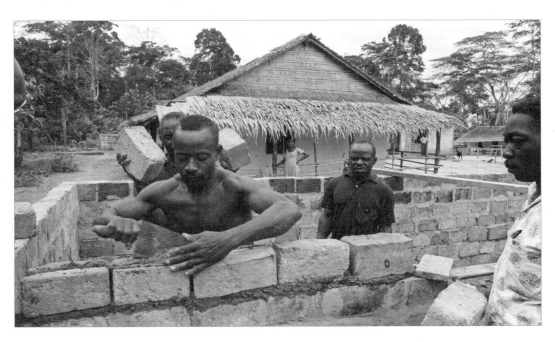

Table 3.5

Percentage of household members aged 16-20 years who are attending school, by urban/rural residence and sex, selected countries in Africa

Country	Year of survey	Both sexes			Males			Females		
		Urban	Rural	Total	Urban	Rural	Total	Urban	Rural	Total
Mauritania	2000/01	47.0	20.8	33.4	47.7	29.0	38.6	46.3	13.9	28.7
Mozambique	1997	35.3	15.2	21.1	45.0	27.3	33.4	23.3	6.0	10.3
	2003	54.9	29.3	41.2	61.2	43.5	52.2	47.6	16.0	29.9
Namibia	1992	53.2	64.2	60.9	61.8	69.0	67.1	46.5	59.2	55.1
	2000	50.7	60.4	57.3	53.0	63.1	59.9	48.4	57.6	54.6
Niger	1992	27.3	2.5	7.7	32.8	4.2	11.0	21.7	1.1	5.1
	1998	24.7	1.4	6.9	31.3	2.8	10.4	18.6	0.4	4.3
Nigeria	1990	34.9	24.3	27.2	39.4	31.8	33.9	30.4	16.8	20.5
	1999	49.7	37.2	41.0	58.3	44.7	49.1	41.1	30.9	33.9
	2003	51.3	40.6	44.2	61.7	50.9	54.8	41.1	31.9	34.9
Rwanda	1992	26.2	12.5	13.4	28.0	15.5	16.3	24.5	9.8	10.8
	2000	14.1	4.9	6.7	14.4	7.0	8.3	13.8	3.0	5.2
Senegal	1992/93	27.5	6.3	15.7	34.7	11.2	21.8	20.3	1.6	9.7
South Africa	1998	69.3	73.9	71.4	71.2	77.0	74.0	67.1	70.2	68.5
Tanzania	1992	21.4	17.0	18.1	29.3	23.7	25.1	14.6	10.5	11.6
	1996	23.7	24.3	24.1	31.1	31.1	31.1	17.6	17.8	17.8
	1999	18.7	17.2	17.6	19.8	18.9	19.1	17.8	15.8	16.4
	2004	28.7	20.8	23.0	36.2	29.0	30.9	22.2	13.2	15.8
Togo	1998	50.4	40.4	44.3	65.3	55.0	58.7	37.5	22.9	29.3
Uganda	1995	30.1	24.5	25.4	40.5	38.1	38.5	22.7	12.5	14.3
	2000/01	44.1	40.4	41.1	53.7	53.5	53.5	36.5	28.9	30.4
Zambia	1992	41.6	26.1	34.3	51.5	39.7	45.9	32.0	12.7	22.9
	1996	41.3	25.1	32.6	50.6	35.7	42.4	32.9	14.7	23.3
	2001/02	41.8	33.0	36.5	50.1	46.2	47.7	34.6	18.9	25.5
Zimbabwe	1994	31.9	37.1	35.6	40.9	45.4	44.2	25.0	27.5	26.6
	1999	35.7	39.7	38.3	42.1	47.0	45.4	30.5	31.4	31.0

Source: MEASURE DHS, STATcompiler (2007) (available from http://www.measuredhs.com; accessed on 28 January (2007).

Despite these achievements, progress in providing education to Africa's youth has been somewhat uneven, and many obstacles remain. During the latter part of the 1970s and into the 1980s, around the time the present generation of youth were set to begin their basic education, government difficulties in meeting the growing educational needs of the population became overwhelming. Although many countries in the region had policies for providing free and compulsory primary schooling, education remained expensive for the average household because of non-tuition costs such as uniforms, books and transportation. As a result, many of Africa's current youth cohorts were unable to complete a basic primary education, which is considered the minimum level required to function in society. Data published by MEASURE DHS indicate that in countries such as Burkina Faso (2003), Mali (2001) and Niger (1998), more than 50 per cent of male youth aged 15-19 years at the time of the respective surveys had not obtained a primary education. Among youth aged 20-24 years, 58 per cent of males in Burkina Faso (2003), 31 per cent in Chad (2004), 33 per cent in Ethiopia (2005), and 59 per cent in Mali (2001) had no education. The data also show that the proportions of female youth without any education are much higher than the corresponding rates for males in many countries.

Rural areas lag behind urban areas with respect to school attendance, though a surprising departure from this pattern is apparent in Kenya, where school attendance seems to be higher in rural areas than in urban areas. Youth in francophone countries are at a particular disadvantage, and gender differentials are wide, with several countries in the region registering virtually no participation of rural girls in school.

Access to post-primary education remains limited in many contexts. In comparison with other world regions, secondary school enrolment rates in sub-Saharan Africa are still very low; figure 3.1 indicates very little change between 2000 and 2004. Young people between the ages of 16 and 20 should ordinarily be enrolled in post-primary education, but table 3.5 shows that in many sub-Saharan African countries the percentage of those not attending school is quite high. This failure to progress to post-primary levels relates to poor rates of completion at lower levels of education, which may derive, in part, from the poor quality of the education system. In Burkina Faso, out of 1,000 pupils entering the sixth year of schooling, only 580 reach the ninth year, and only 373 do so without repeating a grade. In 1995/96, more than 70 per cent of the 14,784 primary school teachers in Burkina Faso were assistant teachers (with no professional qualifications), and 40.7 per cent of teachers had received only basic training (Ilboudo and others, 2001).

Figure 3.1
Secondary school enrolment by world region, 2000 and 2004

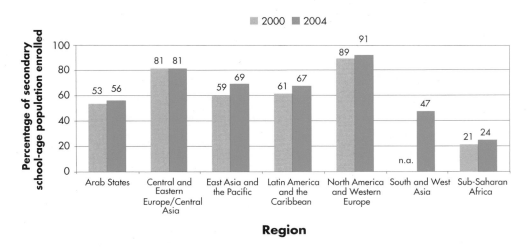

Source: United Nations Educational, Scientific and Cultural Organization, UNESCO Institute for Statistics, *Teachers and Educational Quality: Monitoring Global Needs for 2015* (Montreal: 2006) (available from http://www.uis.unesco.org/TEMPLATE/pdf/Teachers2006/TeachersReport.pdf; accessed on 5 October 2007).

In many ways, the situation with respect to tertiary access has been the most difficult for young people. Many Governments in sub-Saharan Africa were providing tertiary education at fully subsidized rates in the 1970s and 1980s, though access was frequently limited to a select group of privileged youth. By the 1990s it was becoming clear that these investments could not be sustained. As part of the adjustment programmes overseen by international lending institutions, Governments redirected funding from higher to primary education and, to make up for the shortfall, had students assume a share of the costs of their higher studies. These measures often resulted in major strikes and other forms of civil disobedience that, in turn, led to disruptions and the closure of a number of tertiary institutions across the region. In addition, lending for higher education relative to basic education dropped dramatically. In the period 1985-1989, only about 17 per cent of all education lending by the World Bank in the region was directly allocated to higher education, and this figure dropped to 7 per cent between 1995 and 1999. In contrast, for primary education, the corresponding shares for these periods were 29 and 49 per cent respectively (Bollag, 2004).

A reflection of the problems in financing quality tertiary education programmes is that tertiary graduation rates, though mixed, are relatively low throughout much of the region. Young people's prospects of entering tertiary education and remaining enrolled for a substantial period of time have not improved significantly since the early 1990s and remain remote. The lowest ratios (less than 1 per cent) are in countries such as Burundi, Chad, Madagascar, Mozambique, Niger and Tanzania, and the highest are in Mauritius, South Africa and Togo (United Nations Educational, Scientific and Cultural Organization, Institute for Statistics, 2006).

In addition to formal education, non-formal education is also important for the development of a young person's capabilities as an individual and as a responsible member of society. Non-formal education is at the heart of what many youth organizations have been doing for years. Youth organizations such as the World Scout Movement and the Young Men's Christian Association (YMCA) aim to educate young people through a non-formal system whose approach is to develop the body, mind and spirit. Many youth organizations offer volunteering programmes, peer education initiatives and community development programmes for women. These "learning by doing" approaches to education can not only help young people into work but at the same time help youth develop their leadership capacities, their life skills and draw them into civil engagement. The skills young people acquire from non-formal education can be used throughout their lives.

It is clear that to achieve the correct skill mix for poverty reduction and economic growth, all levels of education and training need to be supported so as to bring about the kinds of expected developmental outcomes associated with education (Palmer, 2006). The UNESCO Institute for Statistics (2007) notes that to ensure equity and prevent exclusion, a high share of private funding at the tertiary level can potentially be offset by government subsidies in the form of student grants or loans. Inadequate public investment in tertiary education means that spaces available for the region's large youth cohorts will remain limited, and only those who can afford to enter the fast-growing private tertiary education institutions will have access to higher education. Without renewed attention to ensuring that tertiary education receives the attention it deserves in African countries, youth will continue to seek opportunities abroad, and the promise of better salaries and work opportunities outside their countries of origin may keep many from returning to contribute to their countries' development.

Difficulties in educational access for young women

As noted above, gender inequalities in access to schooling persist in sub-Saharan Africa. Though the gender gap has been reduced at lower levels of education, it remains prevalent at the tertiary level. Those young women who are pursuing tertiary studies are less likely to graduate with degrees in science or mathematics, which are especially relevant in today's global economy. Female youth do not even prevail in those areas traditionally dominated by women in other parts of the world; in sub-Saharan Africa (and in some East and South Asian countries), men dominate in health, welfare and education studies as well as in the traditionally male-dominated fields of specialization. Few women graduate with degrees in engineering, manufacturing, construction, science or agriculture (United Nations Educational, Scientific and Cultural Organization, Institute for Statistics, 2006).

Social and cultural factors probably account for the relative absence of young women from many fields of study. Young women tend to have little say in the career they pursue and may be directed towards fields of study that are considered appropriate for females. Data from many countries in the region suggest that women have limited decision-making power over even the most routine activities (see table 3.6). In most of the countries shown in the table, young women do not make independent or joint decisions on issues relating to their health care, daily purchases, or visits to friends or family. It is possible that young women are similarly limited in their educational pursuits by societal expectations that they marry and raise a family. Whatever the cause, exclusion from the full benefits of a relevant education implies that young women in Africa are more likely than young men to face a difficult transition to the workplace and independent adulthood. This situation may further reinforce the existing tendency for young women to be excluded from decision-making.

Table 3.6
Distribution of young women with regard to their decision-making roles in households: selected countries in Africa

Country	Year of survey	Young women's participation in decision-making, by age group									
		Percentage who say they have independent or joint final say in specific decisions									
		Own health care	Making large purchases	Making daily purchases	Visits to relatives or friends	What food to cook daily	Own health care	Making large purchases	Making daily purchases	Visits to relatives or friends	What food to cook daily
		Young women aged 15-19 years					Young women aged 20-24 years				
Benin	2001	5.8	5.3	11.4	18.0	19.0	23.1	21.9	45.3	41.0	56.5
Burkina Faso	2003	7.7	7.9	11.9	16.5	24.2	16.9	18.0	29.7	28.1	56.7
Cameroon	2004	8.9	6.7	10.5	16.9	26.8	28.2	24.2	35.2	42.0	58.3
Eritrea	2002	68.3	19.6	25.4	28.8	41.6	86.9	46.5	54.6	61.2	70.7
Ghana	2003	18.1	8.8	9.4	11.5	13.1	44.7	32.8	38.4	41.4	42.3
Kenya	2003	20.8	5.5	8.5	15.7	17.3	47.2	20.1	36.1	44.3	59.3
Madagascar	2003/04	33.5	30.5	34.5	34.3	40.2	65.7	61.9	69.6	67.0	73.3
Malawi	2000	21.4	8.3	13.7	34.4	23.3	29.6	18.7	30.9	60.8	49.1
Mali	2001	9.9	9.9	12.8	19.9	26.6	12.0	13.2	19.3	26.4	47.5
Mozambique	2003	37.7	15.2	24.4	31.8	38.1	59.5	33.4	50.3	56.2	71.5
Nigeria	2003	9.7	6.3	8.3	16.1	15.5	19.7	13.3	21.0	27.1	31.2
Rwanda	2000	18.8	11.0	11.9	26.4	20.0	40.9	33.2	37.0	53.1	56.9
Tanzania	2004	32.5	10.0	14.1	21.1	23.5	52.5	27.3	37.0	42.9	62.6
Uganda	2000/01	24.9	8.4	10.7	20.3	30.4	56.6	27.5	33.9	48.2	76.8
Zambia	2001/02	26.8	11.6	..	23.2	..	41.6	28.7	..	39.8	..

Source: Demographic and Health Surveys ORC Macro, 2007.
Note: Two dots (..) indicate that data are not available or are not separately reported.

Poverty is foremost among the reasons for poor educational attainment among youth, especially young women. Table 3.7 shows that in Cameroon, Kenya, Uganda, Zambia and Zimbabwe, more than 40 per cent of today's young women did not complete primary school because they were unable to pay education costs or needed to contribute to the household income. Financial reasons also figured largely in secondary school drop-out rates. Interestingly, in many of the countries featured in table 3.7, pregnancy or marriage, though important factors, were cited less often than financial insufficiency as the primary reason for leaving school. In reality, the two reasons are probably interrelated; some of the young women who marry at an early age may see it as an opportunity to "escape" from poverty.

Table 3.7
Percentage of young women aged 15-24 years who did not complete primary or secondary school because of marriage, pregnancy or the inability to pay, selected countries in Africa

| Country | Year of survey | Level of education not completed and reason | | | |
| | | Primary | | Secondary | |
		Could not pay or needed to earn money	Married or became pregnant	Could not pay or needed to earn money	Married or became pregnant
Benin	1996	16.0	1.5	6.9	19.0
Burkina Faso	1998/99	20.0	1.7	18.0	37.0
Cameroon	1998	46.7	14.9	28.0	46.0
Central African Republic	1994/95	21.2	8.5	40.4	18.2
Chad	1996/97	13.4	23.4	71.0	10.2
Comoros	1996	12.1	9.2	31.3	7.6
Côte d'Ivoire	1998/99	26.1	0.6	14.2	30.6
Eritrea	1995	12.3	48.5	38.1	11.3
Gabon	2000	22.9	33.3	28.5	38.8
Guinea	1999	11.9	8.6	30.0	8.3
Kenya	1998	48.6	22.7	39.2	49.0
Madagascar	1997	26.2	6.7	19.0	29.0
Mali	1995/96	5.7	8.4	38.0	5.0
Mauritania	2000/01	6.1	15.1	25.3	3.5
Mozambique	1997	26.0	24.9	36.3	28.4
Niger	1998	2.2	4.2	13.7	3.3
Nigeria	1999	33.9	31.8	32.3	34.7
South Africa	1998	32.3	34.8	43.2	22.3
Tanzania	1996	15.0	19.0	16.2	14.7
Togo	1998	26.1	7.1	16.7	27.9
Uganda	1995	75.7	9.3	33.8	59.4
Zambia	1996	44.7	9.9	29.3	16.3
Zimbabwe	1994	64.0	10.6	14.5	50.6

Source: MEASURE DHS, STATcompiler (2007) (available from http://www.measuredhs.com; accessed on 28 January 2007).

Without an adequate education, youth face a difficult transition to adulthood and independence, as they are likely to experience unemployment, poverty and social exclusion. The exclusion of young people from the education system, and consequently from other opportunities later in life, is likely to persist unless policies are adopted and implemented to ameliorate the situation. The limited opportunities for youth in Africa to obtain a relevant, high-quality education leave many with no choice but to migrate. Tertiary students from sub-Saharan Africa are the most mobile in the world; the region's outbound mobility ratio of 5.9 per cent is the highest in the world and almost three times the global average. UNESCO defines the outbound mobility ratio as the share of all tertiary students in a country or region that are studying or are likely to study abroad. Statistics indicate that one in every 16 students in sub-Saharan Africa are studying abroad (United Nations Educational, Scientific and Cultural Organization, Institute for Statistics, 2006).

While the outward flow of students contributes to the shortage of well-trained and skilled labour within the region, there are positive repercussions as well. Migration trends, which often begin with student mobility, are associated with the large-scale transfer of resources through remittances. Youth who migrate in search of an education and stay to work in their host countries often become contacts or financiers for others back home who have few opportunities. Although there are no estimates of the proportion of remittances sent by youth, there are data indicating that young male migrants who are married are likely to send money regularly. Young female migrants also tend to contribute regularly to their families, particularly if their children are left behind (United Nations Population Fund, 2006).

EMPLOYMENT: POOR EDUCATION AND LIMITED JOBS UNDERLIE YOUTH UNEMPLOYMENT

Young people in Africa begin to do various forms of work and become skilled in domestic and income-generating activities at a very early age. Girls, in particular, often become adept at managing household duties and are able to assist their families with activities related to trade and various activities in the informal economy. The labour force participation rate in sub-Saharan Africa, estimated at 74 per cent in 2006, is one of the highest in the world; at the country level, the highest estimate in 2006 was 90.9 per cent for Burundi, which implies that hardly anyone of working age, male or female, was not participating in the economy (International Labour Office, 2007). It is important to note that large numbers of young people are seeking work because they are unable to continue their education for financial or other reasons. Many people in Africa, especially youth, remain unemployed or underemployed. The household and other skills acquired by young people at an early age are generally inadequate to prepare them for work in the modern economy or, more generally, for effective participation in a globalized world.

Because of limited vacancies in the job market, unemployment among youth in the region was a very high 19.5 per cent in 2005. Between 1995 and 2005, the number of unemployed youth in Africa rose by about 34 per cent. The youth to adult unemployment ratio of 3.0 in table 3.8 indicates that young people in the region are three times more likely than adults aged 25 years and above to be unemployed. Of even greater concern is that 27 per cent of youth are neither in school nor at work (International Labour Office, 2006), a situation that can lead to frustration, delinquency and social exclusion. As the fastest growing labour force in the world, sub-Saharan Africa's young labour market participants will be increasingly difficult to accommodate in the future (Economic Commission for Africa, 2005).

Table 3.8
Indicators of youth participation in the labour force: sub-Saharan Africa

Indicator	1995	2005	Percentage change
Size of the youth labour force (thousands)	74 077	96 153	29.8
Youth share of total working-age population (percentage)	35.7	36.9	3.4
Number of employed youth (thousands)	61 105	78 739	28.9
Number of unemployed youth (thousands)	12 972	17 414	34.2
Youth labour force participation rate			
Males	76.1	73.7	-3.2
Females	60.2	57.3	-4.8
Total	68.2	65.5	-4.0
Employment to population ratio	56.2	53.7	-4.4
Ratio of youth to adult unemployment	3.3	3.0	-9.1

Source: Compiled from International Labour Office, *Global Employment Trends for Youth 2006* (Geneva: International Labour Organization, August 2006).

For the region as a whole, youth unemployment is much higher in urban areas than in rural areas. In Africa, as in other regions, unemployed rural youth often assume that work opportunities are better in big cities, and many flock to urban areas where their qualifications and experience may be inadequate to meet labour market needs. Under such circumstances, youth are more likely to accept harsh or exploitative working conditions, and many remain unemployed. An important consequence of unemployment in Africa, for adults and youth alike, is that those without work often do not receive any form of formal social security allowance or insurance. This means that being unemployed often leads to absolute poverty.

There are important gender dimensions of the labour market situation for youth in Africa. Table 3.8 shows that while labour force participation rates for females were lower than those for males in both 1995 and 2005, more than one half of the young women in the region wished to work. The 2005 labour force participation rate among young women in sub-Saharan Africa, at 57 per cent, was second only to that of East Asia, where the corresponding rate was 68 per cent. These labour force statistics underestimate female participation, as large numbers of young women work in the home but are not accounted for in national accounts because they do not earn an income.

Various factors contribute to the employment difficulties of youth in Africa, including the region's sluggish economic growth and the consequent lack of progress in job creation. However, there is also an apparent preference among employers for adult workers, who have more work experience than youth. According to the International Labour Office, this preference reflects the failure to acknowledge that, "whereas young people do lack job skills and experience, they can often compensate for this with enhanced motivation and a potential for offering new ideas and insights" (2007, p. 10). Other factors that limit youth access to work include inadequate or irrelevant educational experience and limited work and career development experience during their school years. Unemployment may also be aggravated by young people's preference for certain types of jobs, especially office-based white collar work.

It has been argued that the most important reason behind the youth unemployment crisis in Africa is slow economic growth and the decline in formal sector employment. Any strategy to combat youth unemployment must include provisions for boosting labour demand on a sustainable basis through economic policies that improve the conditions for enterprises to do business and hire people. Where few decent jobs are available, young people are often compelled to accept work in which conditions are poor, hours are long, wages are low, and there are no expectations of job security, legal protection or social benefits (Kanyenze, Mhone and Sparreboom, 2000). In 2005, youth accounted for 65 per cent of the agricultural labour force. In this sector, there are few opportunities to earn a decent wage or acquire useful work experience (International Labour Office, 2007). Although agricultural workers are technically employed, many experience poverty. Sub-Saharan Africa is the only region that has registered a sharp increase in the total number of young working poor (those subsisting on less than US$ 1 per day); between 1995 and 2005, the number of such individuals rose from 36 million to 45 million (International Labour Office, 2006). The poor conditions associated with employment in agriculture have fuelled an increase in rural-urban migration.

There is a tendency at the policy level to assume that the main cause of unemployment among youth in Africa is the absence of artisanal and vocational skills. Interventions to promote youth employment in Africa must be based on a careful assessment of job opportunities and skill requirements. The continuous expansion of training and supply in such areas as carpentry, auto mechanics and bricklaying can lead to unemployment because of market saturation. These skills, especially at the rudimentary levels, are becoming increasingly irrelevant in a fast-changing, technology-driven world. It is imperative that training programmes do not produce large numbers of young people with qualifications for sectors that offer few opportunities for decent work (Kanyenze, Mhone and Sparreboom, 2000).

HEALTH: VARIOUS DISEASES, INCLUDING HIV/AIDS, CONSTRAIN YOUTH DEVELOPMENT

Young people in sub-Saharan Africa face serious health concerns relating both to infectious diseases such as HIV/AIDS, tuberculosis and malaria and to non-communicable conditions such as injuries, mental illness and environmental risks. Large numbers of the current cohort of 15- to 24-year-olds in Africa have likely experienced malnutrition and/or were exposed to diseases such as pneumonia, malaria, diarrhoea or measles as children (Keith and Shackleton, 2006). According to health surveys for the period 1988-1999, between 30 and 40 per cent of the children in sub-Saharan Africa experienced stunting due to chronic undernutrition (World Health Organization, 2006). Without proactive health care, many of the children and youth in sub-Saharan Africa today will be susceptible to reduced longevity, lower educational achievement, weakened immune systems and, ultimately, the replication of these conditions in the next generation.

Although prevalence rates appear to have levelled off in many parts of the region, the number of new cases of HIV in Africa (especially among women) and the number of people with advanced HIV infection continue to grow and are rising faster than treatment services are being scaled up (United Nations, 2007). The region has historically had the world's highest incidence and prevalence rates. The AIDS Epidemic Update published in December 2006 indicates that almost two thirds of those living with HIV in the world today reside in sub-Saharan Africa (Joint United Nations Programme on HIV/AIDS and World Health Organization, 2006). Furthermore, the region's 2.1 million AIDS-related deaths represent 72 per cent of global deaths within this context. There is evidence that the epidemic may be slowing down in some parts of the region. In most countries, the situation has stabilized, with the number of new infections roughly equivalent to the number of deaths.

Data on the prevalence of HIV among youth aged 15-24 are limited and often come from samples of young women attending antenatal clinics. Survey data from other sources, however, provide a sense of the vulnerability of young people to HIV and AIDS within the region. According to these data, HIV prevalence among young people aged 15-24 years varies widely by sex. Surveys conducted in Burkina Faso (2003), Cameroon (2004), Ghana (2003), Kenya (2003), Mali (2001), Uganda (2004/05), and Zambia (2001/02) suggest the HIV prevalence rate for young women is at least twice as that for young men.

Young sex workers, the majority of whom are female, are at high risk of HIV infection. The results of studies undertaken in major urban areas of sub-Saharan Africa indicate that rates of HIV infection among female sex workers are as high as 73 per cent in Ethiopia, 68 per cent in Zambia, 50 per cent in Ghana and South Africa, and 40 per cent in Benin (Joint United Nations Programme on HIV/AIDS and World Health Organization, 2006). Many sex workers lack information about HIV and about services that might help protect them. A study carried out along major transport routes in Africa found that the average age of sex workers was 22.8 years, and the average level of educational attainment was upper primary school. Only 33 per cent knew that they were at risk if they had unprotected sex (Joint United Nations Programme on HIV/AIDS and World Health Organization, 2006). These data underscore the need to work with specific vulnerable groups on HIV prevention using a combination of strategies (Ross, Dick and Ferguson, 2006). At present, for example, the majority of HIV interventions in this area are aimed at the sex workers themselves, with insufficient attention paid to their clients or the contexts in which they work.

HIV and AIDS have also had a major impact on other age groups, with repercussions for youth. High rates of morbidity and mortality within the workforce have seriously affected the availability of qualified teachers, particularly in those countries most affected by the epidemic. Pupil-teacher ratios are already high in many countries (see figure 3.2). The continued loss of large numbers of teachers is likely to exacerbate this situation, gradually reducing the quality of education young people receive in the region.

Figure 3.2
Pupil-teacher ratios for primary school in sub-Saharan African countries, 2005

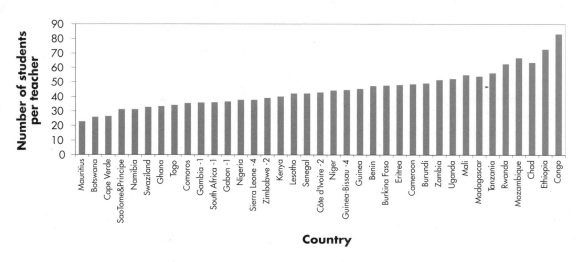

Source: United Nations Educational, Scientific and Cultrural Organization, Institute for Statistics (data accessed from www.uis.unesco.org on October 5 2007).
Notes: -1 Data refer to 2004. -2 Data refers to 2003. -4 Data refer to 2001.

The severity of HIV/AIDS in sub-Saharan Africa is apparent in the high prevalence of orphanhood (mother and/or father deceased) among children under the age of 15. Recent survey data (MEASURE DHS, 2007) reveal that at least 11 per cent of children have been orphaned in Kenya (2003), Malawi (2000), Namibia (2000), Uganda (2000/01 and 2004/05), and Zambia (2001/02). In Rwanda, 26.5 per cent of those under 15 years of age are orphaned; this figure reflects the consequences of both the HIV/AIDS epidemic and the genocide that occurred in the country in the 1990s. Virtually all of the orphaned children in sub-Saharan Africa will be poorly positioned to make the transition to youth and later to adulthood.

The prospects for alleviating the epidemic's burden on youth are uncertain. Research undertaken during the period 2000-2005 indicated positive trends in young people's sexual behaviour (increased use of condoms, delayed first sexual experience, and fewer sexual partners) in 8 of 11 high-prevalence countries, including Botswana, Burundi, Côte d'Ivoire, Kenya, Malawi, Rwanda, Tanzania and Zimbabwe. However, for responses to keep pace with the epidemic, life-saving prevention efforts and HIV treatment programmes need to be intensified. In the 2006 five-year assessment of progress towards achieving the goals of the Declaration of Commitment on HIV/AIDS, not even one country was able to report that it had reached the target of ensuring that 90 per cent of youth aged 15-24 years were able to correctly identify ways of preventing HIV transmission and rejected major misconceptions about HIV transmission (Joint United Nations Programme on HIV/AIDS and World Health Organization, 2006).

Other causes of illness, disability and death

While HIV/AIDS has been devastating to Africa's youth, there are other causes for concern as well. Some of the leading causes of death for those aged 15-29 years in the region are tuberculosis, violence, lower respiratory infections, road traffic accidents, war, unsafe abortion and malaria (World Health Organization, 2006). There are an estimated 2.4 million new tuberculosis cases in Africa every year, and the incidence of this disease has increased in tandem with the HIV/AIDS epidemic. The World Health Organization notes that tuberculosis is increasingly occurring in younger, economically productive members of society, especially girls and women, closely resembling the trend in HIV prevalence. Africa also accounts for over 90 per cent of an estimated 300 million to 500 million clinical cases of malaria that occur in the world every year (World Health Organization, 2006).

Injury, especially that resulting from motor vehicle accidents, is a leading cause of death and disability in sub-Saharan Africa for those under 29 years of age. Road traffic deaths are 40 per cent higher in the countries of this region than in all other low- and middle-income countries. A study in Kenya showed that more than 75 per cent of road traffic casualties were economically active young adults, and that those most at risk of death were pedestrians and users of motorized two-wheelers. Alcohol is an important factor in causing crashes. A study in South Africa found that around 29 per cent of non-fatally injured drivers and over 47 per cent of fatally injured drivers had been drinking (World Health Organization, 2006). As the numbers of vehicles on the roads increase, more and more young people in Africa will be at greater risk of road traffic injury and death.

A growing threat to youth transitions in sub-Saharan Africa is the increase in the drug trade. In the *World Drug Report 2007*, published by the United Nations Office on Drugs and Crime, it was found that drug traffickers were increasingly exploiting Africa as a transit point for drugs trafficked into Europe. Trafficking has greatly increased the availability of illegal drugs, and there are troubling signs pointing to the emergence of new markets for narcotics in a number of countries throughout Africa. Significant increases were reported in the use of cannabis, cocaine, heroin and various amphetamine-type stimulants. Among the youth population, cannabis was reported as the most widely used illicit drug, followed by amphetamine-type stimulants such as Ecstasy. Widespread unemployment and underemployment in the region make youth a prime target for traffickers. Apart from the threats to health posed by the use of these substances, the increased abuse of these drugs by youth, particularly in rapidly expanding urban areas, has raised concern over the links between drug abuse and criminal behaviour (United Nations, 2000). To prevent youth from turning to drugs, economic and healthy leisure opportunities must be provided.

ARMED CONFLICT: LINGERING EFFECTS ON YOUTH POVERTY AND WELFARE

Sub-Saharan Africa has been the site of numerous armed conflicts in which young people have been both victims and perpetrators of violence. It has been noted that the period 1990-2000 alone saw 19 major armed conflicts in Africa, ranging from civil wars to the 1998-2000 war between Eritrea and Ethiopia. Angola, Guinea-Bissau, and Mozambique all experienced chaotic transitions from colonial rule (Addison, 2003).

Box 3.1
WHY DO THEY CHOOSE TO FIGHT?

While there is widespread condemnation of children fighting in conflict zones, a recent study by the International Labour Organization (ILO) found that two thirds of child soldiers served under their own initiative in armed forces. One reason for this is because older youths are more reactive to political ideologies, and are more likely to join armed groups. One former young combatant and current Ugandan activist, Okwir Rabwni, said "I joined as a volunteer. I had been exposed to politics and I was ready to join the struggle when I was 15. This is common in Africa. … Young people are politically idealistic and ambitious, and attracted to quick solutions to their problems." Unrest in the Horn of Africa and State of Somalia has seen youths fighting on both sides of the conflict: the Ethiopian-backed Transitional Federal Government (TFG) and the Union of Islamic Courts (UIC). Libya, Eritrea and Egypt have been used as training grounds for these young soldiers, who have been implicated in a number of assassinations and attacks against foreigners in Somalia, according to the International Crisis Group. The breakdown of normal social structures prevents young people from making the natural transition to adulthood with its accompanying identities. In times of conflict and poverty, young people are attracted to the military as it offers them an identity they are otherwise deprived of. Caught between childhood and adulthood, youths can be drawn into armed groups as it gives them a fast-track to adulthood. Adolescence and youth are a critical stage in a person's development. It is a time of rapid transformation which can see young people taking risks as they try on their new roles and responsibilities. This period is intensified during times of conflict when the social norms and means of support are removed, stopping young people from making a normal evolution to becoming an adult.

Source: Excerpt from Integrated Regional Information Networks, *IRIN In-Depth—Youth in Crisis: Coming of Age in the 21st Century* (special series, February 2007) (available from http://newsite.irinnews.org/pdf/in-depth/Youth-in-crisis-IRIN-In-Depth.pdf; accessed on 13 May 2007).

Children and youth are increasingly participating in armed conflicts as active soldiers. Various reasons account for their involvement (see box 3.1). Some are being forcibly recruited, coerced and induced to become combatants and are often manipulated by adults (United Nations, 1996). Many young people who engage in armed conflict do so because of poverty. In one study, crippling poverty and hopelessness were unanimously identified as key motivators for the 60 combatants interviewed (Human Rights Watch, 2005). Research has indicated that drug use is associated with crime and violence, and it has been alleged that cannabis is being produced to finance armed rebellions in West Africa. Many young people in urban areas are being recruited to sell these drugs in the cities (Wannenburg, 2005). Factors such as these make youth living in poverty especially vulnerable to the combined effects of illicit drug use and armed conflict.

It is becoming increasingly recognized that non-economic aspects of poverty, such as the absence or inadequacy of essential services, the lack of livelihood and educational opportunities, and the non-participation of youth in decision- and policy-making, are conditions that promote the involvement of young people in conflict. Quite often, these conditions are worse during and after conflicts, as there is a further breakdown in family, community and State mechanisms that would ordinarily be in place to protect and support young people (McIntyre, 2003). Conflict prevents children from obtaining a decent education and learning useful skills; lacking any real social capital, many feel excluded from mainstream society and seek to become part of an armed militia, where they feel accepted (Integrated Regional Information Networks, 2007).

There are direct and indirect health consequences associated with conflict, including the displacement of populations, the breakdown of health and social services, and the heightened risk of disease transmission. Young people are often among the victims of the violence and brutality that occurs in periods of conflict (see box 3.1). Even in countries that have not experienced armed conflict, there is a heavy toll from firearms injuries and other types of interpersonal violence that can lead to physical disability (World Health Organization, 2006).

Whatever the cause, conflict causes heavy losses in resources, deepening poverty. It is estimated that in Rwanda, owing to the genocide of 1994, the proportion of households below the poverty line rose from 53 per cent in 1993 to 70 per cent in 1997 (International Monetary Fund and World Bank, 1999). Combined with poverty, conflict deepens the alienation of young people from society and hampers their ability to participate fully in development even after the conflict is over. In a culture where youth often have no voice, and no opportunities to develop themselves, recruitment of young people into militias has been easy, especially when it comes with the promise or prospects of some meagre remuneration or power.

OVERCOMING THE CHALLENGES: YOUTH, GOVERNMENTS AND OTHER STAKEHOLDERS RESPOND WITH NEW DETERMINATION

After decades of major youth development challenges in sub-Saharan Africa, the tide has begun to turn. Governments are increasingly recognizing the importance of building youth capacities so that young people can contribute meaningfully to national development. More and more, young people are being viewed as having a major role to play, and Governments, in conjunction with youth-led organizations and other civil society institutions, are beginning to devise and implement new sets of youth development policies and strategies that, unlike those of the mid-twentieth century, reflect the perspectives and collaboration of adults and young people. Regional development and cooperation initiatives also include emphasis on youth development goals. Young people in sub-Saharan Africa are becoming increasingly involved in voluntary activities that promote the development of their own potential and that of their communities. Opportunities such as these give youth the chance to gain labour market skills while also contributing to national and community development.

At the regional level, the New Partnership for Africa's Development (NEPAD), with its vision of eradicating poverty and promoting sustainable growth and development on the continent, recognizes the key role that young people should play in socio-economic development and the promotion of peace and security (New Partnership for Africa's Development, 2004). Adopted as the economic programme of the African Union, NEPAD has become a tool for achieving good governance and a criterion for assessing the performance of African Governments within this context. NEPAD provides an advisor and a "youth desk" that offer direct entry points for young Africans wishing to participate in the new development framework for Africa. Young people are contributing to the peer review mechanism process designed to strengthen the implementation of NEPAD; the African Youth Parliament is working to ensure that youth are meaningfully involved in this process.

The African Union recognizes that "Africa's future cannot be mapped out, and the African Union's mission fulfilled, without effectively addressing youth development, empowerment and the preparation of young people for leadership and the fulfilment of their potential" (African Union, 2006). In July 2006, the Heads of Member States of the African Union adopted the African Youth Charter as a framework for Governments to create supportive policies and programmes for youth (see box 3.2).

Box 3.2

THE AFRICAN YOUTH CHARTER: A REGIONAL COMMITMENT TO YOUTH PARTICIPATION IN DECISION-MAKING

Adopted in July 2006, the African Youth Charter provides a platform for youth to assert their rights and execute their responsibility to contribute to the development of the continent (African Union, 2006).

The Charter notes that "every young person shall have the right to participate in all spheres of society" and proposes the following measures to promote active youth participation in society:

a. Guarantee the participation of youth in parliament and other decision- making bodies in accordance with the prescribed laws;

b. Facilitate the creation or strengthening of platforms for youth participation in decision-making at local, national, regional, and continental levels of governance;

c. Ensure equal access to young men and young women to participate in decision-making and in fulfilling civic duties;

d. Give priority to policies and programmes including youth advocacy and peer-to-peer programmes for marginalised youth, such as out-of-school and out-of-work youth, to offer them the opportunity and motivation to re-integrate into mainstream society;

e. Provide access to information such that young people become aware of their rights and of opportunities to participate in decision-making and civic life;

f. Institute measures to professionalize youth work and introduce relevant training programmes in higher education and other such training institutions;

g. Provide technical and financial support to build the institutional capacity of youth organisations;

h. Institute policy and programmes of youth voluntarism at local, national, regional and international levels as an important form of youth participation and as a means of peer-to-peer training;

i. Provide access to information and services that will empower youth to become aware of their rights and responsibilities;

j. Include youth representatives as part of delegations to ordinary sessions and other relevant meetings to broaden channels of communication and enhance the discussion of youth-related issues.

The creation of the West African Youth Network (WAYN), a subregional youth network established in 2001 with membership in 12 West African countries, was an initiative developed in direct response to the rise in violent conflicts in West Africa. The network aims to serve as an umbrella group for youth organizations in West Africa to ensure participation of young people in local and regional decision-making bodies. The Network also provides technical support to youth organizations to empower them to address regional issues and become involved in efforts geared towards peace-building, the recognition and assertion of human rights, conflict resolution, promoting good governance, and HIV/AIDS prevention. The Network has proved effective in implementing several regional projects for young people, including the Mano River Union Youth Peace Initiative (West African Youth Network, 2005).

The Southern African Development Community (SADC) Youth Movement, an extensive network for youth development encompassing the 14 SADC member countries, has been particularly effective in developing strategic partnerships with institutions and organizations working on similar objectives in the region. Both the WAYN and the SADC Youth Movement are working to create effective, youth-driven platforms from which greater participation in subregional and regional processes can take shape. In particular, these two regional youth networks and many other youth organizations are emphasizing the fact that democracy, human rights and good governance should be cornerstones of African strategies and programmes such as NEPAD.

Various activities are also taking place at the country level in recognition of the importance of youth contributions to development. National youth organizations are active across the continent, and young people are pushing the boundaries to be included in national and global decision-making. The National Association of Youth Organizations in Uganda (NAYOU) was established in 1999 and consists of 43 member organizations and a network connecting approximately 11,300 youth throughout the country. The main focus of NAYOU is to develop a strong and democratic youth institution that will link youth organizations throughout the country to leverage the sharing of information and skills. It also seeks to promote democracy and human rights and to contribute to poverty eradication.

Among the most significant developments in the region is the emergence of volunteerism as a way to overcome the barriers imposed by shrinking options in the labour market, but also as an option for youth who seek to help develop their communities. Youth volunteering for development is a strategy for engaging young men and women in a range of activities that can improve their participation and positively direct their energy, vigour and innovation towards the realization of national and global development goals. In this connection, the 2006 African Youth Charter makes a regional commitment to the development of policies and programmes for youth volunteerism at the local, national, regional and international levels through its provisions for developing an Africa Youth Corps as a component of the African Union Volunteers (AUV) programme established by the AU Executive Council Decision on Post-Conflict Reconstruction and Development.

The Economic Community of West African States (ECOWAS) Youth Ambassadors for Peace, a subregional volunteer programme started in Guinea Bissau, Togo, Sierra Leone, Liberia and Côte d'Ivoire, is responding to some of these needs. The programme is part of the larger Peace and Development Programme (PADEP) of ECOWAS, which seeks to develop and consolidate peace-building in West Africa. The United Nations Volunteers (UNV) programme is supporting the development of ECOWAS capacity to manage and sustain the Youth Ambassadors programme, which is aimed at strengthening the capacity of non-governmental organizations working in conflict prevention and peace-building in participating countries, as well as providing valuable professional experience for youth in the region.

The nurturing climate provided by the African Union and ECOWAS for volunteerism is also evident in a number of country-level initiatives. Increasingly, Governments in Africa are promoting youth participation in development by creating an enabling environment for youth volunteering and by establishing structured volunteer programmes. Examples of these initiatives include the Scout Volunteers against HIV/AIDS programme in Benin (see box 3.3); the Volunteers for Development programme in Burkina Faso (see box 3.4); Férias Desenvolvendo o Distrito, a volunteer-based initiative set up in Mozambique to attract youth into districts (see box 3.5); the Youth Engagement and Job Creation through Agriculture programme in Sierra Leone (see box 3.6); and the Partnership for Community-based Volunteering programme in Tanzania (see box 3.7).

Box 3.3
BENIN: SCOUT VOLUNTEERS AGAINST HIV/AIDS

The Ministry of Youth, Sports and Leisure of Benin has come up with an original and effective idea to help address the HIV/AIDS pandemic. It is tapping into an available pool of human resources through the Scout movement, an organization with the spirit of volunteering at its core.

The programme focuses on building the skills of Scout leaders and young Scouts in planning and organizing education and sensitization sessions on HIV/AIDS, using radio programmes, workshops, meetings, and consultations for advocacy on HIV/AIDS. Trained Scout leaders now constitute a permanent pool of resource people in communication and training for youth against HIV/AIDS and can begin to spread the word to their Scouts, who in turn can sensitize other youth.

The programme aims at:

- Sensitizing thousands of young people to the danger of HIV/AIDS and how to prevent it;

- Making local Scout structures a potential reference point in the HIV/AIDS eradication process;

- Making every Scout an HIV/AIDS fighter.

The programme is implemented by the Ministry of Youth, Sports and Leisure in partnership with the Ministry of Health, through the National Programme Against AIDS, and is supported by UNDP and UNV. The programme is making inroads into mobilizing youth volunteering through scouting and contributing to reducing stigmatization among HIV/AIDS victims.

Box 3.4

BURKINA FASO: VOLUNTEERS FOR DEVELOPMENT

How does a country get its youth to take voluntary action for development when the tradition of volunteering itself needs to be revitalized? This is a challenge that the Government of Burkina Faso is addressing in its efforts to eradicate poverty and improve governance.

In 2006, a programme was launched aimed at enabling young Burkinabe to become Volunteers for Development. During the first year, the following steps were taken to establish a legal and operational volunteer infrastructure:

- Legislation on national volunteering was drafted and is now being considered by Parliament;

- An independent committee (*Groupement d'Intérêt Public*) was set up to facilitate an innovative partnership between counterpart ministries, civil society organizations, the private sector and other stakeholders, for which proposed by-laws and a list of members were prepared;

- A country-level coordination mechanism was established for the National Volunteer Programme, which is to be integrated in the Ministry of Youth and Employment;

- A regional volunteer centre was set up in each of six pilot regions selected through a call for proposals from civil society organizations. They will promote volunteering and will support the "Volunteers for Development" who join the programme;

- The operational procedures and management tools were defined for the National Volunteer Programme.

The first wave of National Volunteer Corps activity will begin in 2008 with the assignment of 100 Volunteers for Development to institutions working in priority sectors such as health, education, environment, economic development, and local community capacity-building. Each volunteer will enter into a tripartite contract signed by the volunteer, the host institution and the National Volunteer Programme and will serve for a period of 12 to 24 months. The contract is intended to ensure adequate training, integration and monitoring of the volunteers.

The lessons learned from the first wave will shape the further development of the programme. The spirit of volunteerism is already being widely promoted through campaigns. An annual National Volunteer Day has been designated, volunteers are being given media exposure, and a logo and a website about volunteering have been created. This initiative will provide young people in Burkina Faso one channel among others through which they can contribute to the achievement of national development goals.

Box 3.5
MOZAMBIQUE: ATTRACTING YOUTH INTO DISTRICTS

One of the key development issues for Mozambique is the need for skilled people to live and work in rural areas. Like young people in many countries, the skilled youth in Mozambique are attracted to the towns and cities, where they hope to find interesting jobs and a comfortable lifestyle.

Through an initiative called *Férias Desenvolvendo o Distrito* (meaning "youth developing districts"), the National Youth Council and the University Students' Association have devised a means of addressing this issue. Supported by the Ministry of Youth and Sports and various United Nations agencies, they are using volunteering as a means of building up the skills of graduates while opening up possible alternative employment paths for them. Graduate students have the opportunity to volunteer at district offices (where working conditions are normally deemed not to be good) through volunteer vacation programmes. The initiative helps the Government of Mozambique fill posts that have been vacant and works to improve the level of service provision for development at the district level.

The programme began in 2006 with the placement of 200 undergraduate and postgraduate students from all public universities in Maputo in 18 district offices that deal with issues such as agriculture, education, health, social action, fishing, public administration, decentralized planning, environment and justice. Before their placement, the volunteers were trained in community-based participation and public administration. The programme was repeated in 2007 and included participants from all over the country.

This programme has been successful in at least three ways: it has ensured that skills are brought to offices that are otherwise under-resourced; it has taken some steps towards addressing the major problem of youth unemployment in Mozambique by giving young people skills and practical experience and opening up opportunities they may not have previously considered; and it has helped change young people's perceptions of working in district offices. Surveys indicate a significant decrease in the percentage of students expressing discontent with working and living conditions at the district level.

Box 3.6
SIERRA LEONE: YOUTH ENGAGEMENT AND JOB CREATION THROUGH AGRICULTURE PROGRAMME

Food insecurity, skill deficiencies, and problems associated with population growth and increasing urbanization are all challenges faced by large numbers of youth in Sierra Leone. One volunteer programme addresses all of these issues in one go.

Through a programme called Youth Engagement and Job Creation through Agriculture, some 15,000 young men and women between the ages of 15 and 35 are involved in a major effort to improve food security. At the same time, they are improving their own skills and gaining access to resources, which in turn ensures sustainable livelihoods. The Ministry of Youth and Sports, with assistance from UNDP and UNV, is meeting three goals simultaneously:

- *Youth empowerment and employment.* Many subsistence farmers are young people; training and resources that have been passed on to the youth provide them with the means to sustain their businesses and livelihoods, which in turn contributes to their sense of empowerment;

- *Food security.* The programme has proved that young people can manage crops and animals effectively;

- *Rural-urban migration.* The programme demonstrates that there are viable livelihood alternatives outside the cities.

By supporting young people in farming activities, the community-based programme also empowers youth to organize themselves for microenterprise development; facilitates the process of youth empowerment by organizing and supporting various voluntary group projects; establishes networks between engaged youth groups for voluntary experience and best-practice sharing; and provides for self-employment for mixed groups of youth farmers in vegetable gardening, food-processing, other agricultural activities, and marketing, which will promote recognition of their volunteer actions in the districts.

The programme has been successful in proving that young people can be positively engaged in their own development as well as in the development of the nation.

Box 3.7
TANZANIA: PARTNERSHIP FOR COMMUNITY-BASED VOLUNTEERING

The Ministry of Labour, Employment and Youth Development of Tanzania has set up youth camps as a mechanism for mobilizing youth and engaging them in community activities. The camps are encouraging young people to get involved in volunteering within their community and are supporting the delivery of social services.

The programme began in June 2006 with 30 male and female volunteers in the Moshi district. The original plan, which provided for four camps, has been expanded to allow the establishment of ten camps in various districts by December 2007. The volunteers assist with "cleaning up" and preserving the environment, construction activities (schools, dispensaries, and road rehabilitation), and tree planting. The camps also provide spaces where community youth can meet the volunteers to discuss issues and to learn through seminars. Seminar topics include:

- The concept of development and volunteerism;
- The National Strategy for Growth and Reduction of Poverty (MKUKUTA);
- HIV/AIDS education;
- The formation and registration of community-based and non-governmental organizations;
- The formation of Savings and Credit Cooperative Societies (SACCOS);
- The National Youth Policy;
- Environment conservation.

A key lesson from this Tanzanian initiative is that a range of partners can contribute to the success of a youth volunteer programme. This programme draws strength through its partnership with the local government structure. This helps to ensure that community members are aware of the camps and are willing to participate in them. In addition, the youth department liaises with district youth offices to ensure that the programme is well supported through access to infrastructure and equipment. The programme has also aligned itself with the National Strategy for Growth and Reduction of Poverty (MKUKUTA) and receives international support from UNDP and UNV.

The youth camps in Tanzania have shown that if young people are given opportunities and adequate facilitation, they are often willing to participate actively in structured community activities that support local social services. The involvement of local citizens with youth in community activities has helped to revitalize the spirit of volunteering and self-help, breaking down the notion that development is to be delivered only by the Government.

These initiatives, along with others in the region, help to develop the capacities of Africa's youth and equip them with skills they will use throughout their lives. They also enable youth to see themselves as active agents of development within their communities. In the process, youth are perceived not only as assets to their communities, but also as individuals who have acquired practical experience. Through their involvement in such programmes, young people are helping to broaden public awareness of volunteering, and helping to shape the direction of civic engagement policies and interventions. According to a consensus statement of the Economic Commission for Africa and the African Union, "since the heroic contributions of youth to the independence movements in Africa, young people's enthusiasm has underpinned the most energetic and effective social movements. The idealism and commitment of youth have the potential to enact far-reaching social change and to build up effective institutions for humanitarian action, social development and political change. It is essential, therefore, that African Governments, working with their development partners, foster the spirit of volunteerism among young people" (Economic Commission for Africa and African Union, 2006).

SUMMARY AND CONCLUSIONS

In spite of the many positive developments, the challenges to the development of the youth population in sub-Saharan Africa and to their participation in national development remain monumental. Young people in Africa today are at a crossroads. On the one hand, they have endured major health, economic, and social crises, which have left them in a weaker position in terms of participating fully in development. On the other hand, because they have survived these difficulties, they are perhaps more determined than any previous generation to overcome the challenges of youth and to make up for opportunities they lacked in their childhood in order to enjoy a poverty-free life.

Sub-Saharan youth do not lack determination; however, because they are starting out in a weaker position than most of their contemporaries around the world, they will need major institutional and social support to achieve their full potential in society. They will need Governments that are committed to overall development but that also recognize the unsustainability of development efforts that exclude a critical one fifth of their populations. For the current generation of young people, there is a pressing need to provide the second chances that are called for by the World Bank (2006), especially through efforts to overcome deficiencies in literacy, education, health, and preparedness for a competitive labour market. Governments must adopt policies and programmes specifically designed to meet the needs of today's youth and to remove obstacles that stand in the way of their full development and participation. In an increasingly competitive world, youth need to obtain much more than a basic education to secure decent work. Both young men and young women require access to the full spectrum of health services, as health challenges are growing and becoming more complex with globalization.

Although relevant age-disaggregated data are scarce, there is no doubt that many young people in sub-Saharan Africa are poor. Poverty among youth can lead to exclusion not only from opportunities in the global economy but also from community relationships. Young people who feel excluded are often drawn to membership in armed militias and other antisocial groups that give them greater visibility and power. Traditional African societies are known for their elaborate extended family systems and for the tendency to include even the poorer members of the family in decision-making. However, most residents of the region are plainly aware of the exclusionary power of poverty, as evidenced by the popular African adage "poor-no-friend". If poverty is associated with exclusion from one's peer group or "circle of friends", by implication it also strips individuals of the right to be listened to, to be heard, and to be seen. Young people, whose age alone often denies them many rights in African society, are much more likely to be completely alienated by poverty in all its aspects.

There are no quick-fix solutions to the youth development challenges in the region. Efforts to address the problem of poverty among youth in Africa will be most effective if carried out through partnerships with all stakeholders—especially young people themselves. Youth in general are dynamic and therefore need support policies and programmes that can harness their energy and innovative spirit. Their sheer numbers, as well as their ability to learn quickly and to adapt to new situations and developments, gives young African men and women the right to a place at the table and the right to contribute to their own development and that of their communities.

It should be emphasized that many of the region's development problems are systemic; they affect entire national populations and determine the welfare of the household in which youth spend their formative years. As the issues are deeply rooted in a combination of factors, including poor economic performance, low levels of education and skills mismatch, the inadequacy of health care for the large numbers of young people living with HIV/AIDS, and gender discrimination, a multi-pronged approach that mainstreams youth development policies in broader national growth strategies is required. In the absence of a comprehensive approach, youth will continue to be left behind, unable to build the capacities that will allow them to contribute meaningfully to national development. ████████

References

Addison, Tony (2003). *Africa's Recovery from Conflict: Making Peace Work for the Poor.* Helsinki: United Nations University, World Institute for Development Economics Research (UNU/WIDER). Available from http://www.wider.unu.edu/publications/pb6.pdf (accessed on 23 September 2007).

African Union (2006). African Youth Charter (AU/YF/YOUTH/2). Adopted at the Conference of African Ministers in Charge of Youth, Addis Ababa, 26-28 May 2006.

Basu, Anuradha, and Frances Stewart (1993). Structural adjustment policies and the poor in Africa: an analysis of the 1980s. Discussion Paper in Development Economics, Series No. 10. University of Reading, Department of Economics.

Bollag, Burton (2004). Improving tertiary education in sub-Saharan Africa: things that work! Report of a regional training conference held in Accra, Ghana, on 22-25 September 2003. Washington, D.C.: World Bank. Available from www.worldbank.org/afr/teia.

von Braun, Joachim (2005). The world food situation. Paper prepared for the CGIAR Annual General Meeting, Marrakech, Morocco, 6 December 2005. Available from http://www.ifpri.org/pubs/agm05/jvbagm2005.asp (accessed on 29 September 2007).

Christiaensen, Luc, Lionel Demery and Stefano Paternostro (2002). *Growth, Distribution and Poverty in Africa: Messages from the 1990s.* World Bank Policy Research Working Paper Series, No. 2810. Available from http://ssrn.com/abstract=636093 (accessed on 7 May 2007).

Economic Commission for Africa (2005). *Economic Report on Africa 2005: Meeting the Challenges of Unemployment and Poverty in Africa.* Addis Ababa. Sales No. E.05.II.K.9.

_____ and African Union (2006). Consensus statement. Fifth African Development Forum (ADF V): Youth and Leadership in the 21st Century, Addis Ababa, 16-18 November 2006.

Ekouevi, Koffi, and Aderanti Adepoju (1995). Adjustment, social sectors, and demographic change in sub-Saharan Africa. *Journal of International Development,* vol. 7, No. 1 (January-February), pp. 47-59.

Geda, Alemayehu, and Abebe Shimeles (2007). Openness, trade liberalization, inequality and poverty in Africa. In *Flat World, Big Gaps: Economic Liberalization, Globalization, Poverty and Inequality*, Jomo K.S. and Jacques Baudot, editors. Hyderabad, India: Orient Longman; London; New York: Zed Books; and Penang, Malaysia: Third World Network.

Government of Rwanda, International Monetary Fund and World Bank (1999). Rwanda: Enhanced Structural Adjustment Facility Policy Framework Paper for 1998/2000 – 2001/02. Available from http://www.internationalmonetaryfund.com/external/np/pfp/1999/rwanda/index.htm#VIA (accessed on 13 May 2007).

Human Rights Watch (2005).Youth, poverty and blood: the lethal legacy of West Africa's regional warriors. *Human Rights Watch*, vol. 17, No. 5 (A) (March).

Ilboudo, E.K., and others (2001). *Review of Education Sector Analysis in Burkina Faso, 1994-1998*. ADEA Working Group on Education Sector Analysis. Available from http://www.adeanet.org/wgesa/en/doc/bfeng/chapter3.htm (accessed on 7 May 2007).

Integrated Regional Information Networks (2007). *IRIN In-Depth—Youth in Crisis: Coming of Age in the 21st Century*. Special series. February. Available from http://newsite.irinnews.org/pdf/in-depth/Youth-in-crisis-IRIN-In-Depth.pdf (accessed on 13 May 2007).

International Labour Office (2006). *Global Employment Trends for Youth 2006*. Geneva: International Labour Organization, August.

_____ (2007). *African Employment Trends, April 2007*. Available from http://www.ilo.org/public/english/employment/strat/download/getaf07.pdf (accessed on 14 July 2007).

Joint United Nations Programme on HIV/AIDS and World Health Organization (2006). *AIDS Epidemic Update: December 2006* (UNAIDS/06.29E). Geneva.

Kanyenze, Godfrey, Guy C.Z. Mhone and Theo Sparreboom (2000). *Strategies to Combat Youth Unemployment and Marginalisation in Anglophone Africa*. Harare: International Labour Organization, Southern Africa Multidisciplinary Advisory Team (ILO/SAMAT).

Keith, Regina, and Peter Shackleton (2006). *Paying with Their Lives: The Cost of Illness for Children in Africa*. London: Save the Children.

McCulloch, Neil A., Bob Baulch and Milasoa Cherel-Robson (2001). Poverty, inequality and growth in Zambia during the 1990s. Discussion Paper No. 2001/13. Helsinki: United Nations University, World Institute for Development Economics Research (UNU/WIDER).

McIntyre, Angela (2003). Rights, root causes and recruitment: the youth factor in Africa's armed conflicts. *African Security Review*, vol. 12, No. 2, pp. 91-99.

MEASURE DHS (2007). STATcompiler. Available from http://www.measuredhs.com (accessed on 15 May 2007).

New Partnership for Africa's Development (2004). The African Peer Review Mechanism (APRM) Support Mission to Kenya, 26th to 27th July 2004. Communiqué.

Palmer, R. (2006). Beyond the basics: balancing education and training systems in developing countries. *Journal of Education for International Development*, vol. 2, No. 1 (March). Available from http://www.equip123.net/JEID/articles/2/BeyondBasics.pdf (accessed on 18 September 2007).

Reimers, Fernando, and Luis Tiburcio (1993). *Education, Adjustment and Reconstruction: Options for Change*. UNESCO Policy Discussion Paper. Paris.

Ross, David A., Bruce Dick and Jane Ferguson, editors (2006). Preventing HIV/AIDS in Young People: A Systematic Review of the Evidence from Developing Countries—UNAIDS Inter-agency Task Team on Young People. WHO Technical Report Series, No. 938. Geneva: World Health Organization.

United Nations (1996). Promotion and protection of the rights of children: impact of armed conflict on children. Note by the Secretary-General (A/51/306). Report of Graça Machel, Expert of the Secretary-General of the United Nations. Available from http://www.unicef.org/graca/ (accessed on 30 May 2007).

_____ (2000). World situation with regard to drug abuse, with particular reference to children and youth. Note by the Secretariat (E/CN.7/2001/4).

_____ (2004). *World Youth Report 2003: The Global Situation of Young People.* Sales No. E.03.IV.7.

_____ (2007). Africa and the Millennium Development Goals: 2007 update (DPI/2458). June. Available from http://www.un.org/millenniumgoals/docs/MDGafrica07.pdf (accessed on 7 May 2007).

United Nations Educational, Scientific and Cultural Organization. Institute for Statistics(2006). *Global Education Digest 2006: Comparing Education Statistics Across the World* (UIS/SD/06-01). Montreal. Available from http://www.uis.unesco.org/TEMPLATE/pdf/ged/2006/GED2006.pdf (accessed on 7 October 2007).

_____ (2007). *Global Education Digest 2007: Comparing Education Statistics Across the World* (UIS/SD/07-01). Montreal. Available from http://www.uis.unesco.org/template/pdf/ged/2007/EN_web2.pdf (accessed on 3 November 2007).

United Nations Office on Drugs and Crime (2007). *World Drug Report 2007.* Vienna. Sales No. E.07.XI.5.

United Nations Population Fund (2006). Sending money home. *Moving Young—State of World Population 2006: Youth Supplement.* Sales No. E.06.III.H.2. Available from http://www.unfpa.org/swp/2006/moving_young_eng/stories/stories_Rajini.html.

Wannenburg, Gail (2005). Organised crime in West Africa. *African Security Review*, vol. 14, No. 4.

West African Youth Network (2005). Annual report 2004. Freetown, Sierra Leone. Available from www.waynyouth.org (accessed on 20 October 2006).

World Bank (2006). *World Development Report 2007: Development and the Next Generation.* Washington, D.C.

World Health Organization (2006). *The Health of the People: The African Regional Health Report.* Brazzaville: WHO Regional Office for Africa.

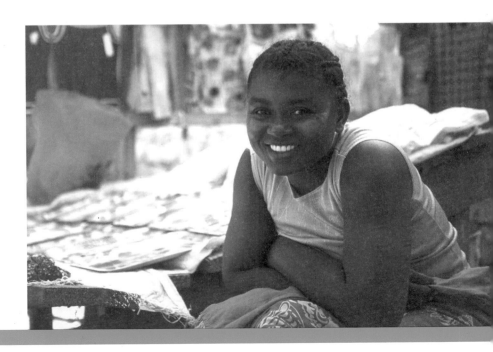

Chapter 4

Labour market participation among

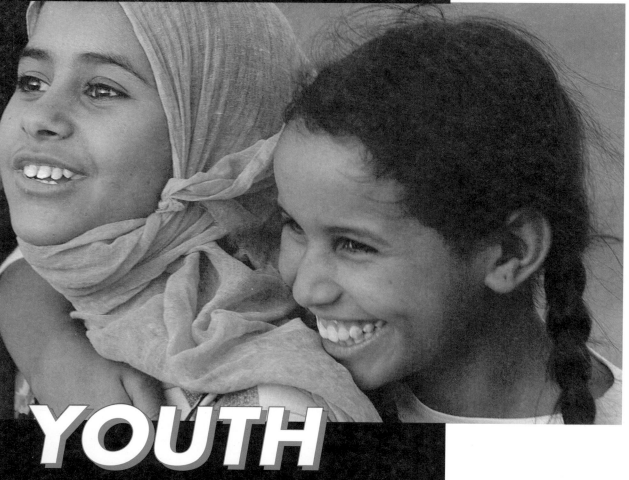

YOUTH

in the
Middle East and **North Africa**
and
the special challenges faced
by young women

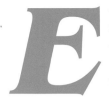conomic participation represents one of the most fundamental and rewarding ways in which young people can become involved in their communities and make a positive contribution to development. Earning an income through paid employment fosters independence and is an essential part of the transition to responsible adulthood. In the Middle East and North Africa, the shift from school to work is fraught with difficulties that at times seem insurmountable; youth face a relatively high degree of socio-economic exclusion and often find it hard to secure decent employment with competitive wages and adequate benefits, largely because they lack the appropriate skills and experience.

Young women in the region are doubly disadvantaged, as both age and gender considerations tend to limit their employment opportunities. Some women are able to find jobs, often after overcoming serious obstacles, but a relatively large number choose not to participate in the labour market at all. Female labour force participation has increased in many parts of the world over the past two generations, but in the Middle East and North Africa the gender gap in employment has remained wide; in 2005, the labour force participation rate of 25.1 per cent for young women was one of the lowest in the world and well below the rate of 54.3 per cent for young men in the region (International Labour Office, 2006b). These percentages represent the proportions of young people actively seeking employment. Only a quarter of the region's female youth are looking for work, and a significant share will not be able to find jobs; unemployment rates for this group in 2004 stood at 26.4 per cent in the Middle East and at 46.8 per cent in North Africa (International Labour Office, 2005).

An effort is made in this chapter to identify some of the key labour market constraints faced by young people in the Middle East and North Africa and to examine their causes and consequences, especially as they relate to the participation of young people in society and the process of development. The second part of the chapter focuses on the special challenges faced by young female labour force participants in the region. Interventions and policies aimed at strengthening youth participation in the labour market are explored. The situation in the Middle East and North Africa (a region defined in the present chapter based on World Bank criteria) varies considerably. For analytical purposes, the countries under review are generally grouped together on the basis of geographic and/or economic considerations, as shown in table 4.1. It should be noted, however, that the analyses presented in this chapter relate mostly to the Arab States and may be less applicable to other countries such as Israel and Malta.

Table 4.1
Middle East and North Africa: subregional configurations used in this chapter

North Africa	Gulf Cooperation Council (GCC) States	South-West Asia (Non-GCC States)
Algeria	Bahrain	Islamic Republic of Iran
Djibouti	Kuwait	Iraq
Egypt	Oman	Israel
Libyan Arab Jamahiriya	Qatar	Jordan
Malta	Saudi Arabia	Lebanon
Morocco	United Arab Emirates	Syrian Arab Republic
Tunisia		Occupied Palestinian Territory
Yemen		

THE UNEMPLOYMENT GAP
BETWEEN YOUTH AND ADULTS

Youth unemployment rates are high throughout much of the Middle East and North Africa, both in absolute terms and relative to the corresponding rates for adults (see figure 4.1). Statistics suggest that unemployment among young people is lowest in the Gulf Cooperation Council (GCC) States, but the gap between this subregion and others virtually disappears when expatriate workers—who typically have work visas and are seldom unemployed—are excluded from the analysis; in Bahrain, Qatar and Saudi Arabia, unemployment rates are higher for "nationals only" than for the population as a whole. In all countries, youth unemployment rates far exceed those for adults, which are typically below 10 per cent.

Figure 4.1
Unemployment rates for youth aged 15-24 years and adults aged 25-64 years in selected countries of the Middle East and North Africa

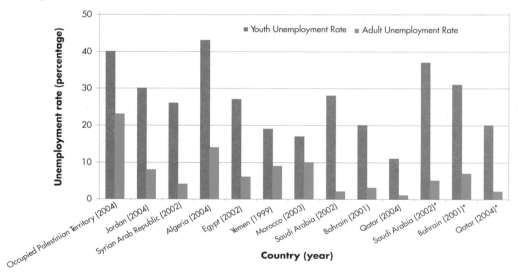

Sources: International Labour Office, LABORSTA database (2006); Bahrain Central Informatics Organization (2002); Planning Council of Qatar (2005); and Saudi Arabia Central Department of Statistics (2003).
Note: Statistics are based on the most recent available data.
* Nationals only.

Young people constitute one third of the working-age population in the Middle East and North Africa but account for almost half (49.7 per cent) of the unemployed, which suggests that joblessness is in many respects a youth issue rather than a generalized population issue (International Labour Office, 2006b). Since opportunities for labour force participation appear to increase after the age of 25, there may be structural factors that militate against the employment of youth. Alternatively, the process of acquiring marketable job skills may not be complete for many until they reach adulthood.

FACTORS LIMITING OPPORTUNITIES FOR ECONOMIC PARTICIPATION AMONG YOUTH

The labour market situation in the Middle East and North Africa has evolved over many decades and is the product of demographic, economic, social, political and cultural factors. This section focuses on three critical areas, examining how demographic changes, the complex dynamic between education and employment, and macroeconomic developments have affected opportunities and prospects for youth employment in the region.

Demographic factors

In the Middle East and North Africa, as in other regions of the world, high fertility and low infant mortality during the 1960s and 1970s were responsible for major demographic shifts, the impact of which is apparent today. The average fertility rate in the Middle East and North Africa was 7.2 births per woman in 1960, compared with 4.6 worldwide; this regional figure held relatively steady for more than two decades but declined sharply thereafter, falling to 3.3 births per woman by 2000. During the same period, infant mortality rates dropped by an average of 2.3 per cent annually, compared with an average decrease of 1.6 per cent at the global level (World Bank, 2005b). The population of the Middle East and North Africa more than tripled between 1960 and 2005 (see table 4.2) and is now estimated at nearly 350 million. Although the population has grown rapidly in all of the subregions under review, the rate of expansion has been most dramatic in the GCC States, where the number of residents has increased nearly seven-fold since 1960 (United Nations, 2007). The exceptionally high and volatile population growth in this subregion is partially attributable to the unique migration patterns prevailing in the area. These overlapping trends have translated into extremely high labour force growth rates over the past several decades (Kabbani and Kothari, 2005); as part of this dynamic, the youth labour force grew by 30 per cent between 1995 and 2005 (see table 4.3).

Table 4.2
Population statistics for the Middle East and North Africa, 1960-2005

Region/Country	1960	1980	2000	2005	Percentage change 1960-1980	Percentage change 1980-2000	Percentage change 1960-2005
National population (thousands)							
North Africa	61 455	100 618	160 073	174 525	63.7	59.1	184.0
Algeria	10 800	18 811	30 506	32 854	74.2	62.2	204.2
Djibouti	85	340	730	804	300.0	114.7	845.9
Egypt	27 840	43 674	66 529	72 850	56.9	52.3	161.7
Libyan Arab Jamahiriya	1 349	3 063	5 346	5 918	127.1	74.5	338.7
Malta	312	324	389	403	3.8	20.1	29.2
Morocco	11 626	19 567	28 827	30 495	68.3	47.3	162.3
Tunisia	4 221	6 458	9 564	10 105	53.0	48.1	139.4
Yemen	5 222	8 381	18 182	21 096	60.5	116.9	304.0
GCC States	5 209	13 757	29 951	34 444	164.1	117.7	561.2
Bahrain	156	347	650	725	122.4	87.3	364.7
Kuwait	278	1 375	2 228	2 700	394.6	62.0	871.2
Oman	565	1 187	2 402	2 507	110.1	102.4	343.7
Qatar	45	229	617	796	408.9	169.4	1 668.9
Saudi Arabia	4 075	9 604	20 807	23 612	135.7	116.6	479.4
United Arab Emirates	90	1 015	3 247	4 104	1 027.8	219.9	4460.0
Western Asia	38 555	71 168	122 343	132 558	84.6	71.9	243.8
Islamic Republic of Iran	21 704	39 330	66 125	69 421	81.2	68.1	219.9
Iraq	7 332	14 093	25 052	27 996	92.2	77.8	281.8
Israel	2 114	3 764	6 084	6 692	78.1	61.6	216.6
Jordan	896	2 225	4 799	5 544	148.3	115.7	518.8
Lebanon	1 888	2 785	3 772	4 011	47.5	35.4	112.4
Syrian Arab Republic	4 621	8 971	16 511	18 894	94.1	84.0	308.9
Occupied Palestinian Territory	1 101	1 476	3 149	3 762	34.1	113.3	241.7
Regional total	105 219	185 543	312 367	341 527	75.7	68.2	223.1

Source: United Nations, *World Population Prospects: The 2006 Revision* (New York: 2007).

As not enough jobs have been created in either the public or the private sector to accommodate the growing cohorts of young job-seekers, unemployment rates have soared, and many young people have dropped out of the labour force entirely. Consequently, the region now holds the distinction of having both the highest rate of youth unemployment in the world and the lowest rate of labour force participation among young people (see table 4.3). As noted previously, the vast majority of young women in the Middle East and North Africa are neither working nor seeking employment. The labour force participation rate for female youth has risen a couple of percentage points over the past decade but remains far below that for young men. Largely due to the low participation rates of young women, the youth employment to population ratio of 29.7 per cent is the lowest in the world. This means that only every third youth in the region has a job. This figure may not seem encouraging, but it does represent an increase over the 1995 ratio of 28.5 per cent; the Middle East and North Africa represents the only region in the world in which the share of employed youth in the total working-age population has increased over the past decade (International Labour Office, 2006b).

Table 4.3
Indicators of youth participation in the labour force: Middle East and North Africa

Indicator	1995	2005	Percentage change
Youth labour force (thousands)	25 086	33 174	32.2
Youth as a proportion of the total working-age population (percentage)	33.5	32.6	-2.7
Number of employed youth (thousands)	17 876	24 649	37.9
Number of unemployed youth (thousands)	7 209	8 525	18.3
Youth labour force participation rates			
Males	56.2	54.3	-3.4
Females	23.2	25.1	8.2
Total	40	40	—
Youth employment to population ratio	28.5	29.7	4.2
Ratio of youth to adult unemployment	3.0	3.1	3.3

Source: Compiled from International Labour Office, *Global Employment Trends for Youth 2006* (Geneva: International Labour Organization, 2006).
Note: A dash (—) indicates that the amount is nil or negligible

As mentioned previously, population growth was exceptionally high in the 1960s and 1970s but slowed down considerably in subsequent decades with the sharp decline in fertility from 1980 onward. At the subregional level, differences in the timing of the demographic transition are apparent (see figure 4.2). In North Africa and Southwest Asia the proportion of youth in the total population peaked around 2004, while in the GCC States the already lower youth share dipped briefly between 1985 and 1995 but began to decline steadily around 2000. Figure 4.2 projects a degree of subregional convergence in the youth share by 2020.

Figure 4.2
Youth aged 15-24 years as a share of the total population in subregions of the Middle East and North Africa

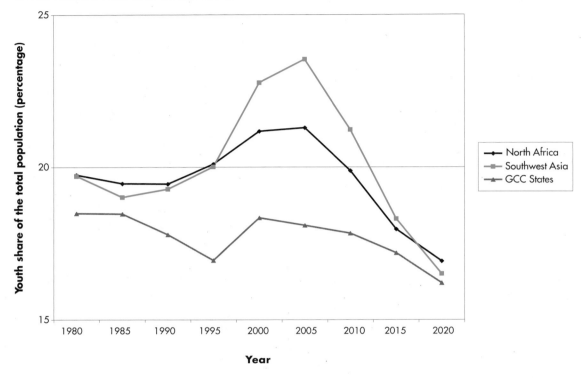

Source: United Nations (2007), *World Population Prospects: The 2006 Revision* (New York).

Youth employment prospects are likely to improve somewhat with the gradual easing of demographic pressures, but the potential gains may be offset by other factors that continue to impede labour force participation among young people in the Middle East and North Africa.

The failure to translate educational gains into gainful employment

Since the 1970s, the share of GDP spent on education has been higher in the Middle East and North Africa than in any other developing region. Educational expenditures have averaged around 5 per cent of GDP annually since 1975, compared with 2-3 per cent in other developing regions and 4 per cent worldwide. This investment has paid off in terms of educational attainment, particularly among girls. It is apparent from figure 4.3 that the average years of schooling have increased significantly across the region and that disparities among countries have narrowed over the past several decades; the regional average rose from just over one year of schooling in 1960 (the lowest in the world) to 5.4 years in 2000 (well above the corresponding figures for South Asia and sub-Saharan Africa). Progress has also been achieved in narrowing the gender gap in education; by 2000, the average years of schooling for females was 80 per cent of that for males (Barro and Lee, 2000).

Figure 4.3
Average years of schooling for those aged 15 years and above in selected countries of the Middle East and North Africa

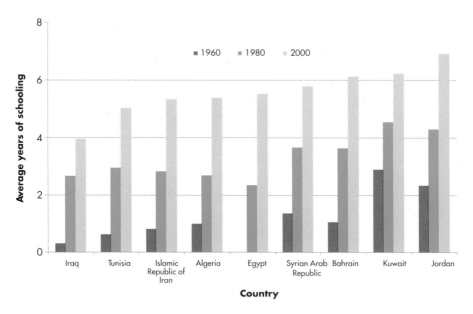

Source: Robert J. Barro and Jong-Wha Lee, "International data on educational attainment: updates and implications", Center for International Development at Harvard University (CID) Working Paper No. 42 (Cambridge: Harvard University, April 2000).

With increased school enrolment, illiteracy rates for youth declined to less than half of those for adults (UNESCO Institute for Statistics, 2007). In North Africa, gender disparities persist, with illiteracy rates for young females twice as high as those for young males. The gender gap in literacy is almost the same for youth as for adults in the subregion, which suggests that illiteracy patterns may extend across generations.

It is unclear whether educational attainment is directly correlated with employment in the Middle East and North Africa, as the relationship between the two factors is complex (see figure 4.4). In most of the countries in the region, unemployment is lowest among those who have not completed primary schooling; individuals from low-income households cannot afford to remain jobless for long. Unemployment rates are also relatively low among university graduates in the GCC States, where the public sector is a major employer, and in the Islamic Republic of Iran. In Jordan, Morocco and Tunisia, unemployment among university graduates is quite high. In 2006 around 27 per cent of Moroccan degree-holders were without work, compared with a national average of 12 per cent. In 1991, the Government offered tax breaks to private sector enterprises hiring university graduates, but this initiative yielded limited returns. High unemployment among youth has contributed to increased poverty—and to a sense of desperation exemplified by a protest incident in 2005 in which six unemployed graduates attempted to burn themselves alive (World Education Services, 2006).

Figure 4.4
Unemployment rates by level of education completed for selected countries in the Middle East and North Africa

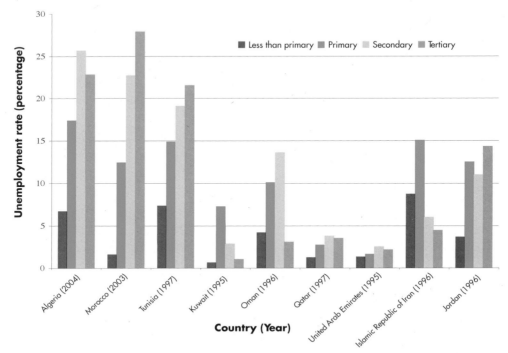

Source: International Labour Office, *Global Employment Trends*, estimation model (Geneva: 2005); and International Labour Office, LABORSTA database (Geneva: 2006).
Note: Statistics are based on the most recent available data

One reason employment prospects are poor for graduates might be that the significant increases in educational attainment do not appear to have had much of an impact on worker productivity (Pritchett, 1999). Such poor returns suggest low educational quality, a lack of correspondence between student training and the needs of the labour market, or a lack of awareness among graduates of how to apply their skills in the workplace. It has been observed that in several countries in the region, educational curricula do not incorporate those technical and occupational components that are currently in high demand in the job market (Alissa, 2007).

Though school enrolment rates have risen or remained steady in the Middle East and North Africa, chronic underinvestment in higher education and in science and technology development has made it virtually impossible for most countries to build a robust and internationally competitive private sector and achieve broader economic diversification (United Nations Millennium Project, 2005). A number of countries have identified areas in which traditional education is incompatible with the demands of the global marketplace; many have introduced courses or curricula designed to expose students to modern business practices and have begun setting up work experience and mentorship programmes and developing entrepreneurial skills through competitions. These initiatives are often jointly run by Governments, non-governmental organizations, and local business communities and centre around private sector participation. A Junior Achievement programme known as

INJAZ is currently being implemented in several countries in the region; secondary school students, guided by teachers and volunteers from the business community, create and run genuine small businesses and participate in local and national competitions at the end of the school year (Junior Achievement, 2006). In Algeria, the National Agency for the Support of Youth Employment (ANSEJ) provides assistance to young entrepreneurs (see box 4.1). The increased investment in enterprise development targeting youth represents a step in the right direction, but efforts such as these have not been enough to provide young people with the knowledge and skills they need to participate fully in their communities.

Box 4.1
PROMOTING YOUTH ENTREPRENEURSHIP IN ALGERIA

Structural adjustment and public sector downsizing have made it difficult for young people to find jobs in Algeria. In 1996, the Government created the National Agency for the Support of Youth Employment (ANSEJ). The Agency provides counselling and other forms of support for young entrepreneurs and assists them in project implementation. The programme mainly targets unemployed individuals between the ages of 19 and 35 who possess the necessary professional qualifications and/or practical experience in their respective fields and can contribute 5 to 10 per cent of the investment amount. ANSEJ helps young entrepreneurs financially by providing zero-interest lines of credit and interest subsidies on bank loans.

The Agency's decentralized network extends across the country. In 2007, around 750 agents arranged for young entrepreneurs to receive funding totalling 4.5 billion Algerian dinars (US$ 64 million). The network has been electronically linked since 2002, and a database has been set up with information on young entrepreneurs and their businesses. ANSEJ published directories on microenterprises in 2002 and 2004 and organized three national exhibitions (in 1998, 2000 and 2003) as well as several regional salons. These events are intended to promote the products and services of microenterprises, to facilitate the establishment of direct links (and the creation of business networks) between them, and to encourage the development of a culture of entrepreneurship among unemployed youth by showing them what other young people have been able to achieve. In 2000, the Agency launched a website that provides extensive information on microenterprise creation and expansion.

By the middle of 2005 over 300,000 files had been submitted to the Agency and more than 65,000 microenterprises had been created, and by 2007 the investment total had reached around 114 billion dinars (US$ 6 billion); these small businesses are believed to have generated more than 186,000 direct employment opportunities.

Source: Jean-Paul Barbier, *L'Intermédiation sur le Marché du Travail dans les Pays du Maghreb: Etude Comparative entre l'Algérie, le Maroc et la Tunisie* (Geneva: International Labour Office, 2006).

Macroeconomic, policy and other constraints

Apart from the labour market pressures caused by demographic trends and the mismatch between education and work skills, slow growth in many of the economies in the region has constrained opportunities for job creation. Weak labour demand, low wages in the private sector (especially the informal economy), lack of knowledge about how to find work, as well as lack of access to capital for entrepreneurial projects have all contributed to the poor labour market participation of youth in the Middle East and North Africa.

Faster GDP growth is seen as essential for job creation to accommodate the more than 1 million young people entering the region's labour markets annually (World Bank, 2000). Strengthening the economy requires a sustained commitment to private sector development, but many countries in the region have been somewhat reluctant to abandon what is generally perceived to be a reasonably supportive public sector system. The development model adopted by many countries of the region during the 1960s and 1970s reflected a strong public sector orientation, and new job opportunities were created with the expansion of the civil service, but a parallel trend towards over-regulation of the private sector limited enterprise growth and economic development (World Bank, 2004b). Since the 1960s, the Government has been one of the major employers in the Middle East and North Africa, especially for the highly educated. In the 1990s, public sector employment accounted for 17.5 per cent of total employment in the region—the highest proportion in the developing world. In this region, unlike other regions, wages were 30 per cent higher in the public sector than in the private sector (Schiavo-Campo, de Tommaso and Mukherjee, 1997a; 1997b). With non-wage benefits and job security factored in, it is not surprising that the region's youth have gravitated towards public employment (World Bank, 2004b). This is especially true for young females, who benefit from generous maternity leave policies, less discrimination, and more flexible work hours in the public sector.

The dynamics of the job market are changing. In recent years, many Governments in the region have implemented rationalization and retrenchment programmes and have privatized State enterprises, and young people are being encouraged to seek jobs in the private sector. However, because there are still bureaucratic obstacles to the development of private enterprise (only in sub-Saharan Africa is the cost of doing business higher), private sector expansion has been too sluggish to offset reductions in the public sector and accommodate the steady influx of new entrants to the labour market (World Bank, 2005a). As long as wages and benefits are better in the public sector than in the private sector, many youth, especially females, will elect to wait (often unemployed) for a civil service position. Many of those who cannot afford to be unemployed are compelled to work in the informal economy, where working conditions are poor, wages are low, and benefits are virtually nonexistent (Schneider, 2006). At present, the informal economy is something of a refuge for youth. In order to develop and take full advantage of the economic potential of young people in the region, greater effort must be invested in strengthening the formal economy and creating higher-quality job opportunities. Many youth consider their work in the informal economy temporary, biding their time until more attractive opportunities materialize. While this may be an effective strategy at the individual level, it ultimately represents an enormous loss in productivity for Governments that are unable to harness the full potential of youth in the labour force.

Because job opportunities are limited, young people in the Middle East and North Africa have increasingly resorted to internal and international migration in search of work. Urbanization trends are apparent throughout the region and are expected to continue (see figure 4.5). Urban residents already constitute the majority in every country except Egypt and Yemen, and throughout most of the region the rural population is either declining or growing more slowly than the urban population (United Nations, 2004; 2005b). Moving to the city carries no guarantee of finding a job. More than a third of the young people looking for work in the urban centres of Morocco remained unemployed in 2002; the same year, youth unemployment in rural areas was only 6.2 per cent, though this figure fails to reflect the (probably high) prevalence of underemployment and working poverty (El Aoufi and Bensaïd, 2005). Amid these uncertainties, many young Moroccans will choose to migrate to urban areas as long as wages and living standards are perceived to be higher.

Figure 4.5
Current and projected share of urban residents in the total population: Middle East and North Africa (percentage)

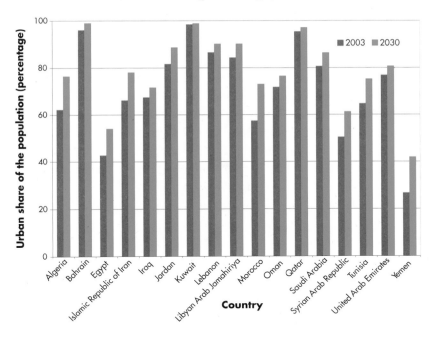

Source: United Nations, *World Population Prospects: The 2006 Revision* (New York: 2007).

With the limited employment opportunities available, it is not surprising that the region registered an annual net migration rate of -0.8 per thousand between 2000 and 2005 (United Nations, 2005b). A reverse trend prevailed only in the GCC States, where annual net migration was 8 per thousand over the same period; recent policy changes designed to encourage the hiring of young nationals in the subregion could change these dynamics, however. Although migration can expand opportunities for youth, the resulting brain drain takes a heavy toll on labour-sending countries, which are unable to benefit from the returns on their human capital investment. By 2000, 39 per cent of Lebanon's highly educated were living in OECD countries (Docquier and Marfouk, 2005).

THE SITUATION OF DISADVANTAGED YOUTH

In the Middle East and North Africa, as in other regions, access to adequate health services and opportunities to obtain a quality education, participate in the job market, and earn a decent income are linked to socio-economic status. Certain groups are particularly vulnerable to exclusion and are unable to enjoy the full benefits of development; in the region under review, those facing the greatest challenges include youth in conflict situations, youth with disabilities, and young women. Cultural and religious traditions have had an enormous impact on the status of female youth and their prospects for personal and professional growth; in many parts of the region they constitute the largest disadvantaged group. The special situation of young women is explored in the second part of this chapter.

Youth in conflict situations

The countries of the Middle East and North Africa have experienced considerable conflict over the years. The region hosts the largest refugee population in the world and has also accommodated a substantial number of internally displaced persons (Roudi, 2001). Palestinians constitute the largest refugee group and are concentrated mainly in South-West Asia, though there is also a sizeable number of Afghans in the Islamic Republic of Iran, and the Iraqi refugee population is growing. Refugees often work in their host countries, increasing labour pressures. In many cases, however, they are prohibited from working, which places them in a precarious socio-economic position. Countries that have experienced conflict have sizeable internally displaced populations; recent statistics indicate that in Iraq alone some 1.2 million residents have been displaced (United Nations High Commissioner for Refugees, 2006a). Large-scale displacement creates imbalances in the population distribution and labour market structure, typically leading to higher unemployment. Internally displaced youth and young refugees are especially vulnerable in the labour market, as they may be forced to work under difficult or dangerous conditions.

In some areas, entire generations of youth have lived through conflict, suffering psychosocial trauma and enduring sustained economic insecurity; many have been internally displaced or forced to live as refugees. Violence against females has escalated in some countries experiencing social or political instability. Youth living in such volatile conditions are often extremely vulnerable and are unable to access important opportunities at a critical time in their lives.

Many factors that increase the risk of prolonged conflict are present in the Middle East and North Africa, including a relatively large youth population, a wealth of natural resources, a history of armed conflict, large numbers of displaced persons and refugees, negligible participation in public affairs, political exclusion, poor social protection, and a large informal economy. There is evidence to suggest that large youth cohorts with poor labour market prospects are more likely to participate in activities that undermine social peace and stability. With the region's youth bulge and the expansion of higher education, growing numbers of qualified young people are unable to find gainful employment. Under such circumstances there may be an increased risk of political violence (Urdal, 2005). Excluding education and employment variables, research on civil war suggests that simply doubling the proportion of males aged 15-29 in the population can increase the risk of conflict from 4.7 to 32 per cent (Collier, Hoeffler and Rohner, 2006).

Added challenges for youth with disabilities

An unfortunate corollary of conflict in the region is physical and psychological injury, including post-traumatic stress disorder. During periods of hostility within or between countries, young people may experience trauma resulting in temporary or lifelong disability (Caffo and Belaise, 2003). The stresses of war can trigger anxiety, sleep, conduct, learning and attention problems. A study on the war experiences of children and adolescents in Lebanon found that many had experienced repeated trauma, defined as specific incidents or activities related to conflict such as the development of a physical handicap, exposure to shelling and bomb explosions, torture, the destruction of one's home, and death in the family (Macksoud and Aber, 1996).

Disabilities—whether present at birth or occurring afterward—greatly increase the already substantial challenges young people face as they struggle to become active participants in society. Their difficulties may begin within the family, but pressures can intensify when it comes to schooling and employment. Illiteracy rates tend to be much higher among young people with disabilities; in Lebanon, for example, the rate is 23 per cent, compared with 3.7 per cent for all youth (Thomas and Lakkis, 2003). Because of physical or psychological challenges or because few opportunities have been available to develop marketable skills, young people with disabilities are often inadequately prepared for the workplace and are more likely than other youth to end up in low-paying jobs, to experience long periods of unemployment, to be laid off, and to face social prejudice; for young women with disabilities, these problems are magnified (Roggero and others, 2005). Many youth with disabilities will never be able to find employment and will therefore remain dependent on others, which is likely to affect their ability to function as equal participants in society.

A number of steps have been taken by Governments in the Middle East and North Africa to improve the situation of persons with disabilities, including the adoption of anti-discrimination legislation and the establishment of hiring quotas. Egypt instituted an employment quota of 1 per cent for persons with disabilities in 1975 and raised it to 5 per cent in 1982. In 2002, Tunisia introduced legislation to ensure that all students with special needs are provided with equal educational opportunities by 2015. In some countries, promising "social business" models based on public-private partnership have been introduced to assist disadvantaged youth. These efforts represent a step in the right direction, but much remains to be done to integrate persons with disabilities in the development process. While a number of countries have adopted appropriate legislation and policies, enforcement and implementation are often weak (World Bank, Human Development Department/Middle East and North Africa Region, 2005).

For all youth, but especially for those with disabilities, vocational education and training programmes are required to provide a structured link between school and the labour market. Fewer than 10 per cent of secondary school students in the region receive vocational or technical training, and the corresponding figure for youth with disabilities is even lower.

YOUNG WOMEN AND THE LABOUR MARKET: PROGRESS AND REMAINING CHALLENGES

Young women in the Middle East and North Africa are engaged in diverse types of work. Because of the structure of the family and its place within the community, rates of labour force participation among the women of the region have long been the lowest in the world. Female labour force participation rates changed little between 1960 and the late 1980s; since the early 1990s, however, they have increased by an average of 1.5 per cent annually (World Bank, 2005b). This shift is linked to a number of factors, including reduced fertility rates, higher levels of educational attainment among both sexes, and the general trend towards increased recognition of women's rights. While the aggregate labour supply pressures exerted by rising female participation rates are weaker than those deriving from demographic trends, they do affect female-dominated occupations and may have contributed to the gender disparities in unemployment.

Young women in the region have traditionally been expected to withdraw from the labour force upon marriage, when childbearing begins, or to engage in unremunerated work in family-run businesses or agricultural activities (Cairoli, 1999). This trend continues, though growing numbers of women are pursuing professional and technical careers alongside the more conventional cadre of women holding administrative, clerical and service-oriented jobs. According to the United Nations Economic and Social Commission for Western Asia, women are most strongly represented in the service sector (18.1 per cent) and agriculture sector (13.2 per cent), but account for only 6.8 per cent of those employed in industry (United Nations Economic and Social Commission for Western Asia, 2004). In rural areas, substantial numbers of women are involved in family poultry enterprises, subsistence field work, and milk and cheese processing—informal economic activities that contribute significantly to the household income on family farms (El-Fattal, 1996). There are clear indications of increased female labour force participation, but change takes time in paternalistic societies with well-defined intergenerational hierarchies, and at this point the nature and extent of young women's participation still tends to be defined and constrained by their family roles and responsibilities. The economic empowerment of young women requires action on several fronts; for a start, steps should be taken to address such issues as job segregation, income inequality, and the relative lack of opportunities for advancement.

The role of the family

The centrality of the family in the Middle East and North Africa cannot be underestimated. Families, rather than individuals, are considered the building blocks of society and are largely responsible for shaping the norms that define the roles of young women at home and in the workplace. Family pressures and expectations intensify as a girl approaches puberty; she is brought up to assume a nurturing role and is often expected to marry and have children at a relatively young age. Issues of concern to the young women of today—including the focus and duration of their education, the transition from school to work, and the appropriateness and availability of different employment options—are regarded as variables influencing family honour and social status.

Gender roles and power imbalances both in the household and in the public sphere work together to perpetuate the dependency of women and to limit their options and opportunities for participation in society. Although the boundaries between the public and private spheres may be porous and flexible, the hierarchies of gender and age that permeate the family, social, political and economic structures are constant, and they define the nature and breadth of female citizenship and participation. Women's economic citizenship is determined by the State but is mediated by the family (or more specifically, by one or more of its male members); the legal definition of citizenship may differ from the practice of citizenship (Joseph, 2002; Kawar, 2000). The preservation of female modesty and the family honour is considered part of the male domain, so many of the choices and life decisions faced by young women are controlled by male relatives and reinforced by older females in the family. The dynamics of these relationships determine the extent of young women's participation in society; more practically, they serve to limit economic, political and other opportunities.

Marriage, childbearing and early workforce departure

Household survey data on the age distribution of female workers reveal that in most regions of the world, married women are far more likely than unmarried women to participate in the labour force, but in the Middle East and North Africa the opposite is true; the data indicate that female labour force activity in the region peaks in the mid-twenties, around the average age for marriage, while in much of the rest of the world this peak occurs during the late thirties or forties (Mensch, Singh and Casterline, 2005; Rashad, Osman and Roudi-Fahimi, 2005). In the Middle East and North Africa, single women are better represented in the labour force than any other category of women (World Bank, 2004b).

Youth-oriented sexual and reproductive health services are not widely available in most countries of the region (DeJong and Shepard, 2006). Nevertheless, fertility rates have generally declined since the 1990s, coinciding with the increased participation of young women in the labour force. Some women join the workforce in pursuit of a long-term career, but many others view their employment as temporary and as part of a long-term investment in marriage. Research indicates that in Egypt, for example, female wage-earners work partly to prepare financially for marriage, amassing funds that will fortify their families' contributions to their future households (Amin and Al-Bassusi, 2003). As noted previously, many women drop out of the labour force once they get married or start having children, their targeted employment objectives apparently having been met.

The age at marriage has major implications for a person's work situation—especially for young women, whose educational and employment opportunities have traditionally been limited by early marriage and childbearing. In the Middle East and North Africa, the age at marriage is rising for both sexes, though the male average is about four years higher than the female average (United Nations, 2000). Economic setbacks and stagnation are partly responsible for the decline in early marriage, as it often takes families some time to accumulate savings for a dowry, trousseau, and other costs associated with a wedding and setting up a household. Advances in education are also important, as higher educational attainment is positively correlated with a higher age at marriage (Mensch, Singh and

Casterline, 2005). Most families place a high value on education, as it represents a source of security for sons and, increasingly, for daughters; in many parts of the region it is becoming increasingly common for marriage to be delayed until after a young woman has completed her tertiary studies. Women's advocacy groups have been successful in getting the legal age of marriage for females changed to 18 years (equal to the minimum age for males) in Jordan and Morocco, and this has had an impact on the discourse surrounding early marriage (DeJong and Shepard, 2006).

The increase in the average age at marriage, in and of itself, is not likely to have much of an impact on young women's opportunities for participation. Persistent gender-based inequalities effectively limit economic prospects even for educated young women. Whether women marry early or relatively late, their mobility, autonomy, and decision-making authority within both the household and the workplace will be restricted as long as the present family system and social structure remain in place (Mensch, Singh and Casterline, 2005).

Progress in women's education is unmatched by opportunities

In parts of the Middle East and North Africa, the gender gap in education among youth has almost disappeared. In Egypt, for example, the differential in average years of schooling for men and women between the ages of 20 and 24 is 0.2 years (MEASURE DHS, 2006). In Jordan, the overall level of educational attainment is higher among young women than among young men; daughters are often the best educated members of their households (Rashad, Osman and Roudi-Fahimi, 2005; Kawar, 2000). It is generally acknowledged that those who are highly educated bring specialized skills to the market and can enhance overall productivity and the quality of goods and services in a country; throughout much of the Middle East and North Africa, however, educational gains have not necessarily translated into more or better jobs for young women. Although female education is increasingly being regarded in a positive light, employment opportunities for young women remain limited (Kawar, 2000; United Nations Millennium Project, 2005). Nonetheless, long-term prospects appear promising. Education exposes young men and women to new ideas, gives them greater access to certain kinds of opportunities, increases social mobility, and facilitates the political and economic integration of youth within the community. As growing numbers of girls and young women are given the chance to expand their knowledge and broaden their horizons as part of their educational experience, their confidence and sense of empowerment are likely to increase, leading to higher aspirations and greater autonomy. The Ishraq programme in Egypt exemplifies what can be achieved within this context (see box 4.2).

Box 4.2
THE EMPOWERMENT OF DISADVANTAGED GIRLS IN RURAL EGYPT

Ishraq is a multifaceted programme designed to strengthen functional literacy, life skills, health knowledge and civic participation among girls, and to challenge prevailing gender norms and community perceptions about the roles of females in society. Ishraq was implemented in four rural villages in Upper Egypt, targeting out-of-school teenage girls. The programme was launched in 2001 by four non-governmental organizations (Caritas, the Center for Development and Population Activities, the Population Council and Save the Children) in partnership with the Egyptian Ministry of Youth and the National Council for Childhood and Motherhood.

Ishraq provided development and support services for 277 girls aged 13-15 years, 84 per cent of whom had never attended school. In addition to literacy classes, the programme offered participants life-skills training, community engagement opportunities, and sports activities. Young female secondary school graduates from the community were recruited and trained as pro-gramme leaders. Each group of around 25 girls met four times a week for three-hour sessions. The meetings were set up to accommodate the girls' schedules, as they often had domestic duties and other work obligations. An important feature of the programme was the involvement of boys, parents, and community leaders, whose perceptions of gender roles became more progressive over time.

Ishraq benefited from rigorous evaluation; a pre-test/post-test design was used for partici-pant assessments, and control groups were set up in two other villages. Two thirds of the girls who participated in Ishraq from beginning to end had entered middle school by the time the 30-month programme drew to a close, while none of the girls in the control villages had done so. Among the participants who took the government literacy exam, 92 per cent succeeded in pass-ing it. The programme strengthened the girls' self-confidence, autonomy and negotiation skills and encouraged their involvement in public life. By the end of their Ishraq experience, the girls indicated an increased preference for delaying marriage and reduced support for female geni-tal mutilation. Cooperation with local authorities helped ensure that girls would be able to obtain identification cards, an important step towards limiting under-age marriage and promoting active citizenship.

The Ishraq experience offers a number of important insights for enhancing the prospects of disadvantaged young women around the world. A second phase is under way, and programme leaders who were trained in the first phase will be involved in the second. Consideration is also being given to the establishment of a fund to provide Ishraq graduates with additional schooling and training opportunities. Collaboration with local non-governmental organizations will allow the replication of the programme in other localities.

Mobility restrictions affect employment prospects for women in the Middle East and North Africa. Although many young women hold the necessary academic qualifications, their job choices may be limited because they are unable to commute long distances or migrate for work. It is not unusual for males to leave their villages or countries in pursuit of employment, but female mobility often occurs only in conjunction with marriage. In Morocco, for example, work is the single most important reason men move from rural to urban areas (44 per cent), while a relatively small proportion (27 per cent) migrate inter-nally for family reasons; in contrast, only 2 per cent of women move from rural to urban areas for employment, compared with 89 per cent for family reasons (Kabbani and Kothari, 2005). Social norms, including perceptions regarding the vulnerability of women and the need to protect them from danger, are largely responsible for limiting the international mobility of women from the region. Sex-specific customs and regulations are built into the structure of the family and public institutions and can make women less flexible as workers (World Bank, 2004a). For example, women may be required to find work that is close to home or may not be allowed to drive. In Egypt, commuting times for male workers have increased in recent years, but female workers have been unable to participate in this trend, which places them at a disadvantage in terms of looking for employment (Assaad and Arntz, 2005).

Although women in the Middle East and North Africa are increasingly well-educated and highly qualified for various types of employment, their work is typically assigned less value than that of males; women who have the same qualifications, experience or job responsibilities as men are often paid substantially less (World Bank, 2004b). This is partly because men are still viewed as the breadwinners of the family. The gender pay gap is negatively correlated with the participation of women in the workplace. Though women's involvement in the labour force has increased in every country in the region since 1990, the educational choices of girls and young women often limit their access to certain types of employment, further entrenching wage differentials. Gender inequalities in education, training and recruitment are a major cause of persistent gender wage gaps, but qualifications are not always a factor.

For sociocultural reasons, the model of the sole male breadwinner informs the welfare and social security regimes of most States in the Middle East and North Africa, so the social safety net for the vast majority of women is either non-existent or dependent on the employment of others (United Nations Development Fund for Women, 2004). In more than half of the countries in the region, men and women are not equally entitled to non-wage benefits (World Bank, 2004a). Discrimination comes in a variety of forms, including differentials in allowances for housing, children and dependant spouses (offered only to a man for a wife) and the unequal treatment of unmarried female versus unmarried male employees (Akeel, 2005). The unfair distribution of entitlements affects the well-being of women in the workplace, and broader social policies favouring males reinforce the vulnerability of widows and non-working or unmarried women, who must rely mainly on the family for their social and economic security.

Females perform most of the agricultural work on family-owned land and/or in subsistence farming situations in the Middle East and North Africa; some are old and widowed, but most are poor, young and unmarried. Women's work in family-based agriculture represents 22.8 per cent of all agricultural labour in Jordan, and in the Syrian Arab Republic and Tunisia the corresponding proportions are 20.5 and 22.4 per cent respectively (El-Fattal, 1996). These figures are indicative of the significant, though largely undocumented, role that young women play in the economy. This situation is particularly compelling, and somewhat ironic, as women residing and working in rural agricultural areas perform a crucial function within the family and the national economy but generally have less control over decision-making, household revenue and family property than do women in urban areas.

The primacy of the family must be factored into any reform efforts aimed at improving the situation of youth in the Middle East and North Africa. Policy interventions designed to enhance the participation of young people in development must be undertaken concurrently with changes in the home. One of the most effective ways to facilitate the integration of youth in society is to provide them with opportunities for active participation in the labour market. The enforcement of policies that address gender inequalities and the situation of disadvantaged groups will contribute to the achievement of this goal and the broader objective of achieving "a society for all".

Young people in the Middle East and North Africa find it difficult to secure decent employment and are therefore unable to participate fully in society. Proactive policy interventions are essential for helping youth gain entry to the labour market. Early intervention is needed to discourage the practice of tracking girls into traditionally female specializations and occupations and to help open up new areas of study and employment for young women, fuelling their confidence and ambitions. Teachers, along with well-trained guidance and vocational counsellors, may be helpful in reducing gender stereotyping, allowing young women to pursue lifelong learning and career development. For those who stop working when they marry or have children, there should be more opportunities to re-enter the workforce at a later stage. Vocational education in fields not traditionally pursued by women should also be expanded. These and other changes should help to address the discrimination in compensation caused by horizontal labour force segregation and discourage the undervaluation of women's work.

Investment in education is important to ensure that young people acquire the skills they need to navigate the changing global economy. In the context of political and social conflict in the region, educational institutions must be provided with adequate support and protection to enable them to continue to meet the growing demand for schooling so critical to enhancing the participation of young people in development. It is also necessary to include young people, especially women, in the review and revision of curricula and training programmes to ensure that their increasingly diverse educational needs are met. Similarly, they should be included in efforts to develop and implement measures aimed at reconciling family and work responsibilities, focusing particularly on child-care arrangements, safe transportation, and increased flexibility in work hours. For these efforts to be successful at both the interpersonal and policy levels, the exclusion of young women from political and other decision-making processes must be addressed. Young people must be given the opportunity to voice their concerns and to become more involved in the development of economic, social and labour market policies.

At a much broader level, economic and structural reforms are needed to create a more favourable environment for poverty eradication and job creation in the region. Steps must be taken to further stimulate labour demand, especially in the private sector, so that the economy can better absorb new entrants to the labour market. Even though demographic pressures on the labour market are gradually easing, stagnant labour demand may keep youth unemployment rates high. Governments should continue working to improve the business climate in their countries, removing barriers to private sector development and encouraging entrepreneurial activity. It is also necessary to have effective social protection systems in place to meet the needs of those who for various reasons are unable to find decent employment.

Action must be taken to ensure that young labour market entrants possess the skills necessary to secure employment and function optimally in the workplace. Aligning labour force capabilities with market demands is especially important. Interventions in the form of vocational education, apprenticeships, and career guidance services can begin before youth leave school. Programmes should also target youth who have completed school but are struggling with the transition to work; for this group, interventions may include job-search assistance and occupational counselling.

With appropriate guidance and support, young people are more likely to secure employment in which they can make best use of their skills. Ideally, occupational counselling should begin when young people are still in school. Guidance counsellors and community mentors can help students better understand the realities of work, the opportunities available in the marketplace, and the benefits of continuing their education. After students leave school, occupational counselling can be provided concurrently with job-search or job-placement assistance. In some parts of the region, public employment offices help match unemployed workers with registered job vacancies. Occupational counselling and job-search assistance generally produce positive results and can be delivered at low cost, especially when compared with formal training (Van Reenen, 2003).

Public works programmes can create short-term jobs during periods of high unemployment, especially cyclical downturns, and can thus act as a safety net. Such programmes have been used extensively throughout the region as a means of combating unemployment. In Egypt, for example, a public infrastructure project provides work for out-of-school youth in poor rural areas; between 1991 and 1997, the project created over 42,000 jobs, 90 per cent of which were temporary.

It is important that Governments in the Middle East and North Africa do not lose sight of the special needs of society's more vulnerable members, many of whom are young. Programmes targeting internally displaced persons are necessary to improve livelihoods and social stability, which can be very important in areas experiencing ongoing conflict. Continued educational gains are likely to open up opportunities for women to participate more fully in development at both the household and community levels. Only with increased participation in decision-making and full access to financial services and other forms of support can youth accumulate the social capital necessary to navigate the political, institutional and social networks currently closed to them. All young people in the region will benefit from policies that promote and facilitate their social, political and economic inclusion. Because young people hold the future in their hands, the region will benefit as well. ▬▬▬▬▬▬▬▬▬▬▬▬

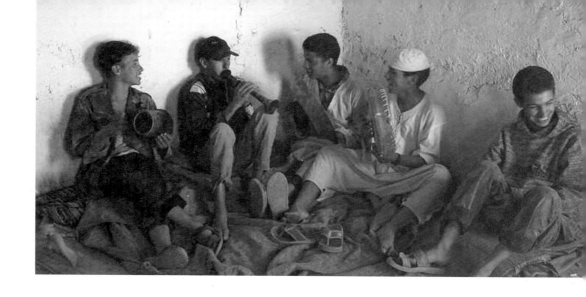

References

Akeel, Randa (2005). Gender and development in the Maghreb. Background paper for the Maghreb Roundtable, 24-25 May 2005.

Alissa, Sufyan (2007). Strengthening the private sector is a prerequisite for dealing with unemployment in the Arab world. *Dar Al-Hayat* (7 March 2007). Washington, D.C.: Carnegie Endowment for International Peace.

Amin, Sajeda, and Nagah H. Al-Bassusi (2003). Wage work and marriage: perspectives of Egyptian working women. Paper prepared for the Annual Meeting of the Population Association of America, Atlanta, Georgia, 9-11 May 2002. Cairo: Population Council/Policy Research Division, Paper No. 171.

El Aoufi, Noureddine, and Mohammad Bensaïd (2005). Chômage et employabilité des jeunes au Maroc. Employment Strategy Paper No. 2005/6. Geneva: International Labour Office.

Assaad, Ragui, and Melanie Arntz (2005). Constrained geographical mobility and gendered labor market outcomes under structural adjustment: evidence from Egypt. *World Development*, vol. 33, No. 3, pp. 431-454.

Barbier, Jean-Paul (2006). *L'Intermédiation sur le Marché du Travail dans les Pays du Maghreb: Etude Comparative entre l'Algérie, le Maroc et la Tunisie*. Geneva: International Labour Office.

Barro, Robert J., and Jong-Wha Lee (2000). International data on educational attainment: updates and implications. Center for International Development at Harvard University (CID) Working Paper No. 42. Cambridge: Harvard University, April.

Bennell, Paul (1999). Learning to change: skills development among the economically vulnerable and socially excluded in developing countries. Employment and Training Papers, No. 43. Geneva: International Labour Office.

Brady, Martha, and others (2007). *Providing New Opportunities to Adolescent Girls in Socially Conservative Settings: The Ishraq Program in Rural Upper Egypt*. New York: Population Council.

Brewer, Laura (2004). *Youth at Risk: The Role of Skills Development in Facilitating the Transition to Work*. Skills Working Paper No. 19. Geneva: International Labour Office.

Caffo, E., and C. Belaise (2003). Psychological aspects of traumatic injury in children and adolescents. *Child and Adolescent Psychiatric Clinics of North America*, vol. 12, No. 3, pp. 493-535.

Cairoli, M. Laetitia (1999). Garment factory workers in the city of Fez. *The Middle East Journal* (winter), pp. 28-43.

Carrero-Perez, Elena, and Guillermo Hakim (2006). *Reforming Technical and Vocational Education and Training in the Middle East and North Africa: Experiences and Challenges*. European Training Foundation/World Bank. Brussels: European Communities.

Collier, Paul, Anke Hoeffler, and Dominic Rohner (2006). Beyond greed and grievance: feasibility and civil war (CSAE WPS/2006-10).

DeJong, J., and B. Shepard (2006). Youth gender and family in the Arab world. *Arab Youth Strategizing for the Millennium Development Goals*. New York: United Nations Development Programme, Regional Bureau for Arab States.

Docquier, Frédéric, and Abdeslam Marfouk (2005). International migration by educational attainment (1990-2000). Policy Research Working Paper Series, No. 3381, Washington, D.C.: World Bank.

Evans, Leslie (2004). UCLA World Internet project finds gaps between rich and poor, young and old, men and women. Article published on 9 February 2004. UCLA International Institute. Available from http://www.international.ucla.edu/article.asp?parentid=7488.

El-Fattal, Lamia (1996). Women in agriculture in West Asia and North Africa: a review of literature. CGIAR Gender Program, Working Paper No. 10. Washington, D.C.: World Bank, April.

Hugo, Graeme (2006). Globalisation and Asian youth: a demographic perspective. Paper presented at the United Nations Regional Expert Group Meeting on Development for Young People in Asia, Bangkok, 28-30 March 2006.

International Foundation for Election Systems (2002). *Arab Election Law Compendium*. Available from www.arabelectionlaw.net/ (accessed on 20 October 2006).

International Labour Office (2005). *Global Employment Trends*, estimation model. Geneva.

_____ (2006a). Economically active population estimates and projections: 1980-2020. LABORSTA dataset. Geneva.

_____ (2006b). *Global Employment Trends for Youth 2006*. Geneva: International Labour Organization.

_____ (2006c). LABORSTA database. Geneva.

International Labour Office. Youth Employment Programme (2006). *Regional Labour Market Trends for Youth: Africa*. Geneva: September.

International Labour Organization (2006). Facts on youth employment. Fourteenth Asian Regional Meeting. Bangkok: August.

International Organization for Migration (2006). *2005: Turkey, Trafficking and Trends*. Ankara.

International Telecommunication Union (2004). Data obtained from http://www.itu.int/ITU-D/ict/statistics/at_glance/Internet04.pdf.

Joint United Nations Programme on HIV/AIDS (2006). *2006 Report on the Global AIDS Epidemic*. Geneva.

Joseph, Suad (2002). Gender and citizenship in the Arab world. Concept paper presented at the Mediterranean Development Forum, Amman, 8 April 2002.

Junior Achievement (2006). Information obtained from www.ja.org (accessed on 1 October 2006).

Kabbani, Nader, and Ekta Kothari (2005). Youth employment in the MENA region: a situational assessment. Social Protection Discussion Paper No. 0534. Washington, D.C.: World Bank, September.

Kawar, Mary (2000). Gender and household labour supply in Jordan. West Asia and North Africa Regional Paper No. 43. Cairo: Population Council.

Khoury, Rami (2006). Arab youth, globalization, and the media. In *Arab Youth Strategising for the Millennium Development Goals*. New York: United Nations Development Programme, Regional Bureau for Arab States.

Lloyd, Cynthia B., editor (2006). *Growing Up Global: The Changing Transitions to Adulthood in Developing Countries*. National Research Council and Institute of Medicine of the National Academies. Washington, D.C.: National Academies Press.

_____ and Barbara Mensch (1999). Implications of formal schooling for girls' transitions to adulthood in developing countries. In *Critical Perspectives on Schooling and Fertility in the Developing World*, C. Bledsoe and others, editors. Washington, D.C.: National Academy Press.

Macksoud, M.S., and J.L. Aber (1996). The war experiences and psychosocial development of children in Lebanon. *Child Development*, vol. 67, No. 1, pp. 70-88.

Mazurana, Dyan, and Kristopher Carlson (2006). The girl child and armed conflict: recognizing and addressing grave violations of girls' human rights (EGM/DVGC/2006/EP.12). Paper presented at the Expert Group Meeting on the Elimination of All Forms of Discrimination and Violence against the Girl Child, Florence, Italy, 25-28 September 2006.

MEASURE DHS (2006). STATcompiler. Available from http://www.measuredhs.com (accessed on 2 June 2006). Information for Sudan is from 1990, that for Egypt from 2000, and that for Yemen from 1997.

Mensch, Barabara S., and others (2003). Gender-role attitudes among Egyptian adolescents. *Studies in Family Planning*, vol. 34, No. 1 (March).

Mensch, Barbara S., Susheela Singh and John B. Casterline (2005). Trends in the timing of first marriage among men and women in the developing world. Paper No. 202. New York: Population Council.

Pritchett, Lant (1999). Has education had a growth payoff in the MENA region? MENA Working Paper Series, No. 18. Washington, D.C.: World Bank.

Radwan, Samir, Nivin Al-Arabi and Ghada Nadi (2006). Youth unemployment problems in the ESCWA region (E/ESCWA/24/4(Part II)/Rev.1). Paper presented at the twenty-fourth session of the Economic and Social Commission for Western Asia, Beirut, 8-11 May 2006.

Rashad, Hoda, Magued Osman and Farzaneh Roudi-Fahimi (2005). *Marriage in the Arab World*. Policy brief. Washington, D.C.: Population Reference Bureau, September.

Roggero, P., and others (2005). Employment and youth with disabilities: sharing knowledge and practices. Report of the E-discussion on Youth and Disabilities. Washington, D.C.: World Bank, October.

Roudi, Farzaneh (Nazy) (2001). *Population Trends and Challenges in the Middle East and North Africa*. Policy brief. Washington, D.C.: December.

Schiavo-Campo, Salvatore, Giulio de Tommaso and Amitabha Mukherjee (1997a). Government employment and pay in global perspective: a selective synthesis of international facts, policies and experience. Based on the same authors' Policy Research Working Paper No. 1771. Washington, D.C.: World Bank.

_____ (1997b). An international statistical survey of government employment and wages. Policy Research Working Paper No. 1806. Washington, D.C.: World Bank, August.

Schneider, Friedrich (2006). Shadow economies of 145 countries all over the world: What do we really know? Discussion paper. Linz-Auhof, Austria: University of Linz, May.

Shumer, Robert (2005). School disaffection in countries of conflict. In *International Journal on School Disaffection*, Reva Klein, editor. Staffordshire, United Kingdom: Trentham Books Ltd. Available from http://www.dropoutprevention.org/resource/journal_dis/archive/03_01Shumer.pdf (accessed on 20 April 2007).

Thomas, Eddie, and Sylavana Lakkis (2003). Disability and livelihoods in Lebanon. Paper presented at the international conference Staying Poor: Chronic Poverty and Development Policy, University of Manchester, 7-9 April 2003.

United Nations (2000). *World Marriage Patterns 2000*. Wall chart. Population Studies Series, No. 188. Sales No. 00.XIII.7.

_____ (2004). World Urbanization Prospects: The 2003 Revision. Sales No. E/04/XIII.6.

_____ (2005a). Report of the Commissioner-General of the United Nations Relief and Works Agency for Palestine Refugees in the Near East: 1 July 2004 - 30 June 2005 (A/60/13). *Official Records of the General Assembly, Sixtieth Session, Supplement No. 13*.

_____ (2005b). World Population Prospects: The 2004 Revision. New York.

_____ (2006a). *The Millennium Development Goals Report 2006*. Sales No. E.06.I.18.

_____ (2006b). Trends in total migrant stock: the 2005 revision (POP/DB/MIG/Rev.2005/Doc). New York: February.

_____ (2007). *World Population Prospects: The 2006 Revision*. New York.

_____ Statistics Division (2005). Progress towards the Millennium Development Goals, 1990-2005.

United Nations Children's Fund (2006). Nutrition, survival and development. *Progress for Children: A Report Card on Nutrition*, No. 4 (May). Available from http://www.unicef.org/progresforchildren/2006n4/index_survivalanddevelopment.html.

United Nations Development Fund for Women. Arab States Regional Office (2004). *Progress of Arab Women 2004*. Amman.

United Nations Economic and Social Commission for Western Asia (2004). Arab women: trends and statistics, 1990-2003. Executive summary.

_____ (2005). Women in decision-making in the Arab region (EGM/EPWD/2005/OP.1). Paper prepared for the Expert Group Meeting on Equal Participation of Women and Men in Decision-Making Processes, with Particular Emphasis on Political Participation and Leadership, Addis Ababa, 24-27 October 2005.

United Nations Educational, Scientific and Cultural Organization. Institute for Statistics (2007). Data available from uis.unesco.org. Paris.

United Nations High Commissioner for Refugees (2006a). *Global Refugee Trends 2005*. Geneva: 9 June.

_____ (2006b). *Refugees by Numbers*, 2006 edition (UNHCR/MRPI/B.1/ENG 1). Geneva.

United Nations Millennium Project (2005). *Investing in Development: A Practical Plan to Achieve the Millennium Development Goals*. New York.

United Nations Office on Drugs and Crime (2006). Trafficking in persons: global patterns. April. Available from http://www.crin.org/docs/unodc_trafficking_persons_report_2006.pdf.

Urdal, Henrik (2005). A clash of generations? Youth bulges and political violence. Paper presented at the Workshop on Conflict Research, Hurdal, Norway, 5-7 January 2005.

Van Reenen, John (2003). Active labour market policies and the British New Deal for the young unemployed in context. NBER Working Paper No. 9576. Cambridge, Massachusetts: National Bureau of Economic Research, March.

Wheeler, Deborah L. (2003). The Internet and youth subculture in Kuwait. *Journal of Computer Mediated Communication*, vol. 8, No. 92 (January), pp. 148-163.

World Bank (2000). Middle East and North Africa. *The World Bank Annual Report 2000*. Available from http://www.worldbank.org/html/extpb/annrep2000/pdf/regions/wb_mna.pdf.

_____ (2004a). *Gender and Development in the Middle East and North Africa: Women in the Public Sphere*. MENA Development Report. Washington, D.C.

_____ (2004b). *Unlocking the Employment Potential in the Middle East and North Africa: Toward a New Social Contract*. MENA Development Report. Washington, D.C.

_____ (2005a). Doing Business database. Washington, D.C. Available from http://www.doingbusiness.org/.

_____ (2005b). *05 World Development Indicators*. Washington, D.C. Available from http://devdata.worldbank.org/wdi2005/Cover.htm.

_____ (2006). *06 World Development Indicators*, table 2.16. Washington, D.C. Available from http://devdata.worldbank.org/wdi2006/contents/Section2.htm.

_____ Human Development Department/Middle East and North Africa Region (2005). A note on disability issues in the Middle East and North Africa. Washington, D.C.: June.

World Education Services (2006). Regional news: Middle East and North Africa. World Education News and Reviews, vol. 19, No. 5 (October). Available from http://www.wes.org/ewenr/06oct/middleeast.htm (accessed on 15 March 2007).

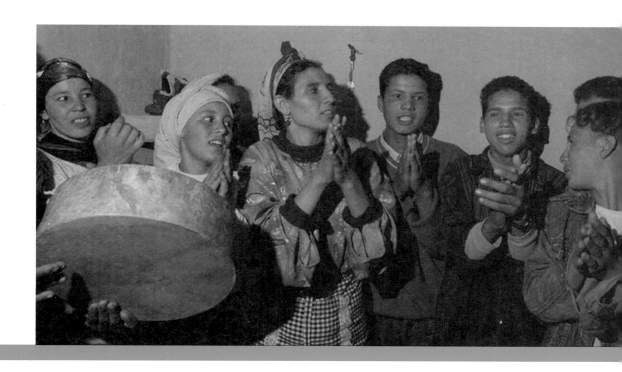

Chapter 5

Tackling the poverty of opportunity
in small island developing States

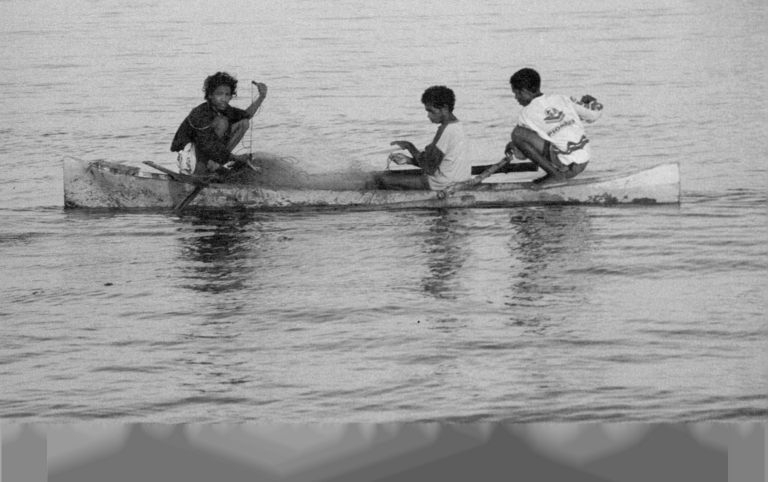

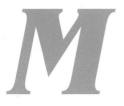Most small island developing states are known to the world as idyllic holiday destinations. However, these States face a number of challenges that constrain economic and social development, with serious implications for their national youth populations. Although many of these States have an abundance of natural beauty, most have small formal labour markets and few resources suitable for industrial development. Business development is constrained by the small size of markets resulting from small population sizes, and from the fact that small island developing States are separated from one another and the rest of the world by vast distances. The Federated States of Micronesia, for example, consist of over 600 islands scattered over nearly 3 million square kilometres of ocean (Pacific Islands Trade and Investment Commission and Asian Development Bank, 2001). Cellular phone use, Internet access, and personal computer use are limited compared with developed countries, and science and technology transfer has occurred at a slow pace. Small island developing States are susceptible to natural disasters such as hurricanes and floods and are further threatened by the uncertainties of climate change and environmental degradation. These factors, combined with high population growth rates, have constrained economic and social development in many of the States.

Most small island developing States have traditionally relied on agricultural and mineral exports and tourism. The small size and openness of the States have made their economies vulnerable to fluctuations and developments within the global economy. In the Caribbean States, export crops such as sugar and bananas have declined as a result of the global trend towards trade liberalization. Similar problems are seen in other sectors, with the exception of tourism, which has thrived despite the vulnerability of the industry. The geographical characteristics of small island developing States, combined with the effects of globalization and a shift from a traditional to a modern lifestyle, have greatly affected the vulnerability of youth in these countries.

The present chapter analyses the challenges faced by young people living in small island developing States. It begins by reviewing population statistics and notes that youth make up a considerable share of the population living in these States. Young people therefore constitute an important force for development. However, their potential is seriously undermined by "poverty of opportunity" in the form of socio-economic obstacles, which are examined in the chapter. The educational and employment situation of youth in these States is reviewed, as is the incidence of poverty. The chapter examines internal and international migration as a coping mechanism. The disillusionment of youth in the light of changing societal values is also considered. Health issues and risky behaviour resulting from this situation are highlighted as well.

YOUTH: A CONSIDERABLE FORCE IN SMALL ISLAND DEVELOPING STATES

Youth make up a significant share of the population in all small island developing States. The proportion of youth aged 15-24 years in the total population ranges from about one eighth in the Netherlands Antilles to almost one fourth in the Maldives (see table 5.1). Some countries, notably those in the Caribbean, use an expanded definition of youth that includes individuals up to the age of 30; within this framework, the proportions regarded by Governments as "youth" are even greater than those reported in table 5.1. Population growth has been high in many of these States, and youth populations are expected to increase significantly between 1995 and 2015, particularly in the African, Asian and Pacific island States (see table 5.1).

Table 5.1
Youth as a percentage of the total population in selected small island developing States

Major area, region, country or area*	Youth as percentage of total population	Projected percentage change, 1995-2015
Africa	20.4	37.7
Cape Verde	22.5	37.5
Comoros[a]	20.3	37.9
Guinea-Bissau	18.8	46.2
Mauritius[b]	15.5	-0.5
Sao Tome and Principe	21.8	30.1
Asia	18.1	12.1
Bahrain	16.0	30.6
Maldives	24.5	32.3
Timor-Leste	19.8	46.3
Latin America and the Caribbean	18.1	11.6
Caribbean[c]	17.3	9.3
Aruba	12.7	23.0
Bahamas	17.2	12.6
Barbados	14.2	-24.9
Cuba	13.8	-23.9
Dominican Republic	18.1	17.7
Grenada	21.5	18.5
Haiti	21.5	32.0
Jamaica	18.8	10.5
Netherlands Antilles	12.1	-35.7
Puerto Rico	14.8	-6.1
Saint Lucia	19.7	2.9
Saint Vincent and the Grenadines	20.7	-17.5
Trinidad and Tobago	20.3	-21.0
United States Virgin Islands	16.3	10.1
Central America	18.4	11.5
Belize	20.2	33.5
South America[d]	18.0	11.9
Guyana	15.9	-22.2
Suriname	18.7	2.0

(continued on following page)

Major area, region, country or area*	Youth as percentage of total population	Projected percentage change, 1995-2015
Oceania	15.0	17.5
Melanesia	19.5	34.6
Fiji	19.3	11.0
New Calédonia	16.9	19.8
Papua New Guinea	19.5	37.3
Solomon Islands	20.2	35.1
Vanuatu	20.7	42.6
Micronesia[e]	18.7	26.0
Guam	16.0	26.5
Micronesia, Federated States	22.8	15.3
Polynesia[f]	19.3	19.2
French Polynesia	19.2	17.4
Samoa	18.7	18.4
Tonga	21.6	15.9

Source: United Nations, World Population Prospects: The 2006 Revision (New York: 2007). CD-ROM edition: extended dataset.

Notes: *Countries or areas listed individually are only those with 100,000 inhabitants or more in 2005; the remainder are included in the regional groups but are not listed separately.

[a] Including the island of Mayotte.

[b] Including Agalega, Rodrigues, and Saint Brandon.

[c] Including Anguilla, Antigua and Barbuda, British Virgin Islands, Cayman Islands, Dominica, Montserrat, Saint Kitts and Nevis, and Turks and Caicos Islands.

[d] Including the Falkland Islands (Malvinas).

[e] Including Kiribati, the Marshall Islands, Nauru, Northern Mariana Islands, and Palau.

[f] Including American Samoa, Cook Islands, Niue, Pitcairn, Tokelau, Tuvalu, Wallis and the Futuna Islands.

These large current and future youth generations can be a crucial force for development in small island developing States. Providing young people with access to a quality education and opportunities to obtain decent work will bring these countries closer to achieving the Millennium Development Goals. Youth who are highly qualified and productive can contribute meaningfully to national development. At present, however, young people are confronted by major obstacles that hinder their effective participation in education, the economy, and society. In many cases, past and current population growth has outstripped the capabilities of these States to provide employment and education to young people, and poverty is widespread. Youth without opportunities can become disillusioned and resort to risky or antisocial behaviour as a coping mechanism. In the final analysis, large numbers of unemployed youth represent a tragic loss of opportunity for small island developing States. It is essential that Governments take urgent action to address this crisis.

EDUCATION: HIGH ENROLMENT RATES BUT PERSISTENT PROBLEMS WITH QUALITY AND RETENTION

Small island developing States as a whole have a youth literacy rate of 85.3 per cent, and gender parity has been achieved in this area. Subregional disparities exist, however; in the Pacific Islands, 92 per cent of youth are literate, while in the Caribbean the corresponding rate is only 76 per cent. Almost one in four youth living in the Caribbean cannot read and write; statistics show that literacy rates for girls in this group of island States are slightly higher than those for boys (UNESCO Institute for Statistics, 2006b).

Most small island developing States are close to achieving universal primary education and have net primary enrolment rates of 92 per cent or higher. Sao Tome and Principe and Saint Lucia have the highest net enrolment rates (98 per cent). In some countries, however, more progress is needed if future generations of youth are to have the same opportunities as their peers in other countries. The Dominican Republic has a net primary enrolment rate of 86 per cent, and it is estimated that in the Solomon Islands only 63 per cent of children of primary age are attending school (UNESCO Institute for Statistics, 2007a).

High enrolment rates are important, but mere enrolment in school is not enough. Data on primary school completion rates in small island developing States are scarce, but available statistics suggest wide variation. In Comoros, only 55.9 per cent of children complete the primary cycle. In Sao Tome and Principe the rate is also quite low, at 60.3 per cent, but girls are more likely than boys to finish primary school (63.0 versus 57.7 per cent, respectively). At the other end of the spectrum is Barbados, where 99.5 per cent of girls and 95.7 per cent of boys complete primary school (UNESCO Institute for Statistics, 2007a). Many small island developing States have remote, isolated rural communities and outer-island populations and find it difficult to ensure universal access to primary education for children outside urban areas. Few rural children attend secondary school. Nevertheless, gross secondary enrolment has generally increased since the late 1990s, with wide variation in individual country rates (see figure 5.1). With the exception of Comoros and Vanuatu, all of the small island developing States for which data are available have achieved gender parity in secondary education or have even more girls than boys enrolled in secondary education (UNESCO Institute for Statistics, 2007a). Where differentials exist, the challenge is to rectify the disparity without undermining the gains of females.

Figure 5.1

Gross secondary enrolment rates in selected small island developing States, 2004

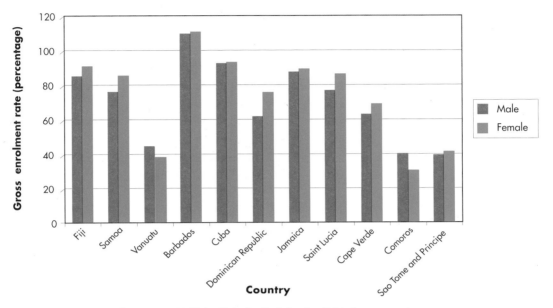

Source: Data obtained from the UNESCO Institute for Statistics (available from www.uis.unesco.org; accessed on 2 April 2007).

Many young people completing their secondary education would like to pursue higher studies. However, they are frequently obliged to travel abroad to obtain a tertiary education, as many small island developing States, with their small populations and lack of suitably trained teaching staff, are unable to establish national universities. To respond to this challenge, some small island developing States have set up joint universities through subregional partnerships. For example, the University of the South Pacific is located in Fiji but is based on a partnership between the Cook Islands, Fiji, Kiribati, the Marshall Islands, Tokelau, Tonga, Tuvalu and Vanuatu. The University of the West Indies is an autonomous regional institution supported by and serving 15 island States (UNESCO Institute for Statistics, 2006a).

Poverty keeps many young people from taking advantage of educational opportunities. In Jamaica, for example, the rate of enrolment in formal education is 85 per cent for all 15- to 16-year-olds, but enrolment among poor youth of the same age group is 68 per cent. The probability of obtaining a post-secondary education is even more dependent on economic status. At age 18, the wealthiest Jamaicans are three times more likely than the poorest residents to be enrolled in school, and the differential increases to eight times for those in the age group 19-24. Lack of money is given as the main reason for absences, with lack of interest in school and pregnancy listed as other major reasons (Government of Jamaica and United Nations Children's Fund, 2004).

Equipping those students who are able to attend school with skills that will enable them to participate meaningfully in a volatile labour market is a major challenge for the education sector in most small island developing States. The relatively poor quality of education in the Pacific States is negatively influencing employment prospects and has forced these countries to rely on expatriates to fill high-skill positions. Some countries in the region are finding it difficult to keep pace with the rapid changes and technological developments resulting from globalization, and have stressed the need for curriculum reform (CARICOM Secretariat, 2004). In the Caribbean, some of the major concerns in the education sector include the poor performance of students, low levels of attendance (owing to child labour obligations and truancy during school hours), and unsatisfactory levels of achievement among certain vulnerable groups (including children of single parents and child guardians as well as rural students). High non-completion and repetition rates, poor examination performance, gender disparities in school performance (girls outperforming boys), unequal access to educational opportunities, insufficient access to early childhood education and secondary education, and issues related to special education also pose problems. Adequate regulatory frameworks are needed to address these concerns (CARICOM Secretariat, 2004).

Improving the quality and reach of education is critical to improving the socio-economic prospects of future generations of youth. Schooling has an important impact on the behaviour of youth. Feeling connected to school (through a teacher or by working hard) reduces the likelihood of risky behaviour, including using drugs and alcohol and engaging in violent activities or early sexual activity. Research indicates that among school-going adolescents, the probability of sexual activity is 30 per cent lower for boys and 60 per cent lower for girls who are connected to school. This is likely associated with positive home and community support as well (Cunningham and Correia, 2003). Conversely, the school system can have a devastating effect on young people with low academic achievement, making them feel out of place in an academic environment and, as a corollary, socially excluded and "worthless" (Cunningham and Correia, 2003).

UNEMPLOYMENT
Quantifying youth unemployment

In small island developing States, as in other regions, the probability of unemployment is higher among youth than among adults. Youth-to-adult unemployment ratios in the Caribbean range from 2.0 to 3.6. Higher ratios are found in the Asian and African island States. In some countries, youth-to-adult unemployment ratios are exceedingly high. In the Maldives, for example, the ratio is 4, and in Mauritius, youth are almost five times more likely than adults to be unemployed; both figures are considerably higher than the global youth-to-adult unemployment ratio of 3 (International Labour Office, 2004).

In the Caribbean, youth unemployment declined from 23.8 per cent in 1995 to 20.7 per cent in 2004 (International Labour Office, 2006). Nevertheless, joblessness among young people continues to be a significant problem in the subregion (see figure 5.2).

Figure 5.2
Youth unemployment rates in selected Caribbean small island developing States, 2004 or most recent year

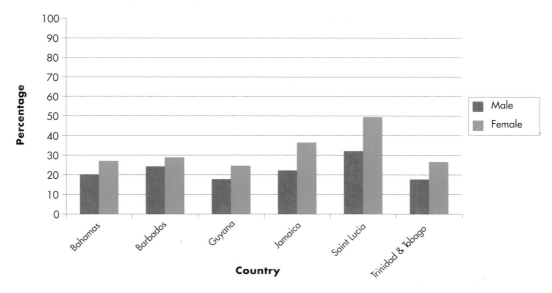

Source: International Labour Office, *Key Indicators of the Labour Market*, third edition (Geneva: 2004).

The figure clearly illustrates that unemployment is far more prevalent among young women than among young men in Caribbean countries. At the time the surveys were undertaken, 36.3 per cent of young women in Jamaica were unemployed, compared with 22 per cent of young men, and in Saint Lucia, the figures were 49.2 and 31.8 per cent respectively. The higher educational attainments of young women (relative to those of young men) do not appear to translate into improved employment prospects.

Deriving precise estimates of the extent of youth unemployment in Pacific small island developing States is difficult, as the quality of data tends to be poor, and definitions of economic activity vary from one country to another (McMurray, 2001). Table 5.2 presents youth unemployment rates for selected States within this subregion. "Unemployment" is not consistently defined in the Pacific States; it usually refers to the number of those in the labour force who do not have jobs in the formal sector, but in some countries it also includes the number of people without subsistence or informal work. The countries showing low youth unemployment rates in table 5.2 define employment as "formal, informal and subsistence work". The unemployment rate of almost 63 per cent for the Marshall Islands is extremely high by any standards. A serious shortage of employment opportunities for those of working age is evident in most Pacific countries, though unemployment rates are highest for 15- to 24-year-olds. Statistics indicate that in the year 2000, there were five people of working age available for every formal sector job in Fiji. In Solomon Islands, the corresponding ratio was 7.9, with 9.2 projected for 2010. It is estimated that in Samoa, around 4,500 students graduate from secondary school each year, but only about 1,000 of them find wage work in the formal sector or continue on to higher education (McMurray, 2001). In Papua New Guinea, it is projected that there will be almost 4 million available workers by 2015, but only 6 per cent will be able to find jobs in the formal sector (Gregory, 2006).

Table 5.2
Youth unemployment in selected Pacific small island developing States

Country	Unemployment among youth aged 15-24 years (percentage)
Fiji Islands	14.1[a]
Kiribati	2.2
Marshall Islands	62.6
Micronesia, Federated States	35.3
Papua New Guinea	3.7
Samoa	12.3
Solomon Islands	11.1[b]
Timor-Leste	5.3[b]
Tonga	13.0
Tuvalu	25.0
Vanuatu	36.0

Source: David Abbot and Steve Pollard, "Hardship and poverty in the Pacific: a summary" (Manila: Asian Development Bank, 2004).
Note: a Adult unemployment rate (for those aged 15 years and above) as per the 2002 urban household income and expenditure survey (HIES).
b Adult unemployment rate as per the national census.

Causes of youth unemployment

The high rates of youth unemployment in the small island developing States represent a significant waste of productive resources and are at the root of an array of socio-economic problems in these countries. Devising remedial solutions requires, first and foremost, that the sources of youth unemployment be identified. In the small island developing States, there are both structural and youth-specific problems that must be addressed within this context.

Small island developing States face a variety of structural problems that limit employment opportunities for all age groups. Most of these States have scarce resources and limited capital. Relatively high wage rates combine with low productivity to undermine the competitiveness of labour-intensive manufacturing. The small size and remoteness of the Pacific States has made it difficult for them to compete with world prices in any major industry, including tourism in some cases. Those small island developing States with natural resources mainly concentrate on the export of raw materials rather than on local manufacturing and services. Extraction is frequently undertaken by foreign firms, which repatriate profits and rarely invest in any local firms (McMurray, 2001).

The business sector is also relatively undeveloped, particularly in the small island developing States of the Pacific. Pacific islanders have generally been reluctant to engage in entrepreneurial activities, perhaps because there are inadequate systems to protect their earnings from family demands (McMurray, 2001). The lack of qualified employees is also an important constraint.

There are a number of other factors, including sustained population growth, that affect employment prospects for youth in particular. In many Pacific island countries, the annual increase in the labour force greatly exceeds the rate of job creation in the formal sector. Population growth and improved secondary enrolment, combined with limited job creation, have led to a situation in which large numbers of graduates are competing for a relatively small number of jobs in the formal sector. Adding to this are the high rates of urbanization in many of the small island developing States.

It has become increasingly apparent that education systems in many small island developing States are not adequately preparing youth for the existing job market. The quality of education is often poor, and young people who have completed secondary school frequently lack marketable skills. Despite the large number of graduates, expatriates dominate high-skill occupations.

Young people who are not able to obtain employment in the formal sector often experience a sense of failure. Any income-generating activities they might undertake in the informal or traditional sectors will always be seen as a second-best option (McMurray, 2001). This perception contributes to the high rates of international migration found in many small island developing States.

The limited opportunities available for youth to obtain work experience also help to explain the high unemployment rates among young people in small island developing States. In most countries, youth tend to gather experience by undertaking simple jobs that require a relatively low level of skill. Because of the general lack of employment opportunities in small island developing States, however, youth are competing with older, more experienced workers for the same kinds of jobs (McMurray, 2001). In addition, many formal sector jobs in these States are provided by the public sector, which values seniority. Entry level positions for youth are therefore limited (World Bank, 2006a). The last resort of self-employment is often not an option for youth in these countries owing to constraints such as financing limitations.

Vocational education offers small island developing States a chance to address some of the employment difficulties they are facing. However, facilities for vocational training are frequently insufficient. For example, vocational schools in Solomon Islands have only 1,200 places available for a youth population of over 90,000 (Chevalier, 2001). In addition, there is a need for more realistic career education that portrays different work options more equally (McMurray, 2001). In the absence of formal employment opportunities, participation in multiple small-scale activities in the informal sector can help youth to generate income, develop skills, and find an alternative to the disenchantment that frequently arises from idleness. It is critically important, however, for solutions to be found to increase formal employment options while keeping cultural specificities in mind.

POVERTY

Globally comparative country-level data on the prevalence of poverty, specifically among youth in small island developing States, are scant, but it is clear that poverty constitutes a major challenge across the region. In all of the Caribbean States, poverty is considered a critical social issue and a root cause of a wide spectrum of other socio-economic problems (CARICOM Secretariat, 2004). In Trinidad and Tobago, 39 per cent of the people live on less than US$ 2 per day. In Haiti, the situation is particularly worrisome; almost 54 per cent struggle to survive on less than US$ 1 a day, and as many as 78 per cent live on less than US$ 2 a day (United Nations Development Programme, 2006).

The poverty landscape is also stark in the Pacific. One fifth of the people living in the Marshall Islands and Timor-Leste survive on less than US$ 1 per day, and the corresponding proportions are even higher in Kiribati (38 per cent) and Papua New Guinea (39.6 per cent) (Asian Development Bank, 2006). According to economic studies of the Pacific Islands, many people in these countries have difficulty sustaining a reasonable standard of living (Asian Development Bank, 2003). Table 5.3 provides estimates of the proportions of those living below the basic-needs poverty line in various Pacific small island developing States, based on national household income and expenditure surveys undertaken since 2001. The table indicates that in several of these States, large numbers of residents are unable to meet their basic needs.

Table 5.3
Poverty in selected Pacific small island developing States, in ascending order

Country	Percentage of population below the basic-needs poverty line		
	National	Urban	Rural
Cook Islands	12.0	..	..
Marshall Islands	20.0	..	..
Samoa	20.3	23.3	17.9
Tonga	22.3	23.6	22.8
Fiji	25.5	27.6	22.4
Micronesia, Federated States	27.9	29.5	32.9
Tuvalu	29.3	23.7	23.4
Papua New Guinea	37.5	..	..
Timor-Leste	39.7	25.0	44.0
Vanuatu	40.0	..	..
Kiribati	50.0	51.0	50.0

Source: David Abbot and Steve Pollard, "Hardship and poverty in the Pacific: a summary" (Manila: Asian Development Bank, 2004).
Note: Two dots (..) indicate that data are not available or are not separately reported.

The insularity and structural vulnerability of small island developing States affect their productivity and exacerbate their susceptibility to poverty in a variety of ways. It has been noted, for example, that frequent extreme weather events and the long-term rise in sea levels seriously affect agriculture, food security, and overall poverty reduction in these States. The working poor and the rural poor make up much of the population living in poverty, and poverty can quickly intensify in times of natural disaster.

Research carried out in the Caribbean found that young people in disadvantaged situations often have few options. Poor parents—particularly those who are single parents—are more likely to be absent from the household, leaving children and youth unattended and unsupervised. Young girls in some countries, sometimes at the encouragement of their parents, sell sex to relieve poverty and to contribute to the household income. In countries such as Jamaica, childbearing is still used as a strategy to gain economic support (Cunningham and Correia, 2003).

The high unemployment rates in many small island developing States are certainly a factor contributing to widespread poverty. However, since many of the poor cannot afford to be unemployed, the phenomenon of the working poor is an even larger challenge in many countries. In St. Kitts and Nevis, the lack of decent work that pays a living wage is particularly evident. The country has an unemployment rate of only 5.3 per cent, suggesting that unemployment is not the main cause of poverty. The working poor appear to join the labour force at an earlier age than the non-poor, in part because those who are poor tend to spend fewer years in formal education than those who are not (Federation of St. Kitts and Nevis, 2004).

The data presented above are not youth-specific; however, it is clear that the high incidence of poverty crucially affects youth engagement in society. With job opportunities frequently available only in sectors that do not meet young people's expectations, the lack of income and scarcity of positive leisure activities drive some disillusioned and idle youth to migrate elsewhere or to engage in crime. The income inequality made obvious by the presence of foreign tourists and the media encourages youth to engage in "easy money" activities such as drug sales and prostitution (Cunningham and Correia, 2003).

MIGRATION

Internal migration

Many rural youth seek job opportunities and a more exciting life in urban areas. Urbanization is rising in all of the Pacific island States, with annual rates of growth ranging from 0.4 per cent in the Federated States of Micronesia to 6.2 per cent in Solomon Islands. Between 13 per cent (Solomon Islands) and 100 per cent (Nauru) of the total population of the Pacific Islands are now living in urban areas (Ware, 2004).

This movement of people is a response to real and perceived inequalities in socio-economic opportunities between rural and urban areas and increasing rural impoverishment in many countries (Connell, 2003; Monsell-Davis, 2000). Employment opportunities and services (especially education) are concentrated in the urban centres in most small island developing States. Along with improved prospects for work and schooling, cities offer better access to entertainment activities and consumer goods (Ware, 2004). In countries where people are forced to travel substantial distances (at great expense) for medical assistance and education, ready access to these services is also an important reason for moving.

The exodus of large numbers of people, especially youth, from rural to urban areas destabilizes village economies. It causes schools and other services to shut down, which affects the lives of other young people who may need these services. It also undermines the traditional social order in which the chiefs, the church, and families maintain law and order. Informal urban settlements, which do not have a stable social order, can be dangerous, and within these settlements, young people, particularly males, are at high risk of becoming involved with gangs, crime, alcohol and drugs. In poor urban areas, young women are often at high risk of being sexually assaulted and exploited in the sex industry (HELP Resources and United Nations Children's Fund, 2005).

Young people who move to urban areas tend to reside with relatives, where accommodation is free, and relatives are traditionally obliged to look after them. In turn, however, youth are expected to abide by traditional family rules and practices, and there is great potential for family conflict when traditional and modern views clash. Such conflict often escalates into violence. Moving in with relatives in urban areas is not always safe for young females, as it exposes them to a high risk of (sexual) abuse by family members (United Nations Children's Fund, 2004a-c; 2005a-b; Government of the Republic of the Marshall Islands and United Nations Children's Fund, 2003; Government of the Cook Islands and United Nations Children's Fund, 2004). In Fiji, a survey of female youth who were living with their extended families while attending secondary school revealed that, among the girls who dropped out of school, 26 per cent reported having been sexually abused by male relatives while living away from home (Save the Children, 2004). Sexual abuse can also lead female youth into prostitution, as those who have been abused often flee the home and, with no alternative means of support, survive by selling sex. There are even reports of girls who have remained at home being prostituted by a family member (HELP Resources and United Nations Children's Fund, 2005).

International migration

Migration rates for youth in small island developing States are among the highest in the world (World Bank, 2006a). Tourism and the expansion of modern information and communication technologies (ICT) have brought about a heightened awareness among youth from these States of better opportunities beyond their shores, and such exposure has increased their expectations for their own lives. The mismatch between their expectations and immediate situation may strengthen the desire in young people to pursue a new life abroad. For many youth from small island developing States, the possibility of a better social life is an important reason to migrate (World Bank, 2006a). At a more fundamental level, migration is inextricably tied to unemployment and the search for improved job prospects. The demand for skilled workers among the top labour-receiving countries in North America and Europe, combined with the economic vulnerabilities of most small island developing States, may trigger movement to countries or regions with more opportunities (United Nations, 2006). Inter-State agreements, such as the Compact of Free Association allowing Micronesians increased access to residency in the United States, have also encouraged youth to seek permanent residence abroad (United Nations Economic and Social Commission for Asia and the Pacific, 2003).

Youth from small island developing States and other small countries are particularly likely to pursue a tertiary education abroad. Of the eight countries in the world that have more students studying abroad than at home, five (Belize, Cape Verde, , Guinea-Bissau and Tonga) are small island developing States. More than 33 per cent of the students from Mauritius are studying in other countries, and around 14 per cent of the tertiary-age population from Bermuda, British Virgin Islands, Cayman Islands, Dominica and Montserrat are attending university abroad. Figure 5.3 clearly illustrates the strong tendency among young people from small island developing States to migrate for educational purposes. The high outbound mobility ratios shown in the figure reflect a strong interest in international studies and/or deficiencies in educational provision at home. Though youth are likely to value the experience of studying and living abroad, the main reason for migration among youth from small island developing States is the lack of opportunity to obtain a quality tertiary education at home. As noted previously, with the small size of the population in most of these countries, the costs of establishing national universities often cannot be justified, and there is a general lack of suitably trained nationals capable of teaching a full range of tertiary courses (UNESCO Institute for Statistics, 2006a).

Figure 5.3
The likelihood of studying abroad:
Which countries have the most or least students studying abroad?

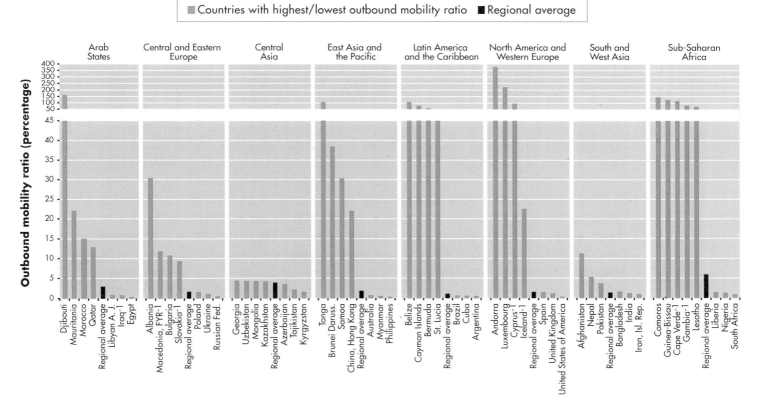

Source: UNESCO Institute for Statistics database, statistical table 10 (Montreal: 2007) (available from www.uis.unesco.org; accessed on 2 April 2007).

Notes: The outbound mobility ratio is defined as mobile students coming from a country as a percentage of all tertiary students in that country. Data on mobile students from a given country are compiled using data from multiple host countries. Therefore, data from different reference periods may be combined.

1 Data refer mainly to 2003.

Coverage: Countries reporting mobile students represent 77 per cent of global tertiary enrolment in 2004. The countries with high enrolment that are not covered are China (15 per cent of world tertiary enrolment), Egypt (1.7 per cent), Nigeria (1.0 per cent), Colombia (0.9 per cent) and Peru (0.7 per cent).

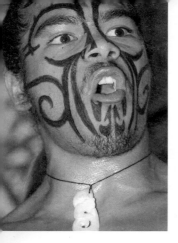

Among the Pacific small island developing States, rates of migration vary. The residents of Polynesia have been particularly mobile, with between 30 and 50 per cent of the population migrating internationally. New Zealand has been the major destination for Polynesians, but many have also migrated to the United States (Appleyard and Stahl, 1995). Between the 1950s and the 1970s, New Zealand sought migrants from its former territories and associated States in the Pacific to work in its expanding industry and service sectors. Until the 1990s, significant numbers of Polynesians migrated to New Zealand and now account for more than 5 per cent of the country's population (Statistics New Zealand, 2002). Over the past two decades, however, New Zealand has gradually imposed greater restrictions on immigration and has instituted quotas. Along with other popular destination countries such as Australia and the United States, New Zealand favours highly skilled, experienced workers. Many Pacific Islanders, especially young people, still hope to migrate to New Zealand or elsewhere, but it is becoming increasingly difficult. While not as migration-prone as Polynesia, Micronesia has also experienced significant migration, particularly in recent years. For the Federated States of Micronesia, Guam, the Marshall Islands, the Northern Marianas and Palau, migration has been mainly to the United States as a result of historical ties. Migration from Fiji has increased markedly in recent years owing to a downturn in the textile and sugar industries and the upheaval brought about by military coups in 1987 and 2000; these developments have particularly affected the migration patterns of Fijians of Indian descent.

As table 5.4 illustrates, small island developing States in other parts of the world are also experiencing significant migration. In the African island States, between 3.2 and 18.7 per cent of the population migrate, and the same is true for between 17.5 and 38.5 per cent of Caribbean nationals.

Table 5.4
Total population of selected small island developing States and the share living abroad

Region/Country	Population (thousands)	Migrants living abroad (percentage)	Main destination
Africa			
Cape Verde	470	18.7	Portugal
Comoros	600	3.2	France
Mauritius	1 222	6.9	France
Sao Tome & Principe	157	8.5	Portugal
Seychelles	84	8.7	United Kingdom
Caribbean			
Antigua & Barbuda	79	28.9	United States of America
Dominica	71	32.0	United States of America
Grenada	195	23.8	United States of America
St. Kitts & Nevis	47	38.5	United States of America
St. Lucia	161	17.5	United States of America
St. Vincent & Grenadines	109	31.1	United States of America
Trinidad and Tobago	1 313	18.8	United States of America
Pacific			
Fiji	835	13.5	Australia
Kiribati	96	2.4	United States of America
Marshall Islands	53	13.0	United States of America
Micronesia, Federated States	125	12.2	United States of America
Palau	20	20.2	United States of America
Samoa	178	35.1	New Zealand
Solomon Islands	457	0.5	Australia
Tonga	102	31.1	New Zealand
Vanuatu	210	1.0	Australia
South Asia			
Maldives	293	0.8	India

Source: David J. McKenzie, "Remittances in the Pacific", a paper presented at the Werner Sichel Lecture-Seminar Series 2005-2006: Immigrants and Their International Money Flows, held at Western Michigan University, Kalamazoo, on 15 February 2006.

In many countries, remittances from international migrants have become an important supplement not only to household income, but also to GDP. Of the 20 countries with the highest remittances as a percentage of GDP, seven are small island developing States. In Tonga, remittances account for 31 per cent of GDP—the highest proportion in the world. In Haiti, remittances represent almost one fourth of GDP, and in Jamaica the share is 15 per cent (United Nations, 2006a). While poverty remains a major challenge in the region, many small island developing States are receiving a sizeable income supplement that benefits individuals, households and communities. Reliance on remittances is deepening in the Pacific States; it is not uncommon for families to groom their youth for employment overseas. Many do not return. More than 60 per cent of the highly educated population from Haiti, Fiji, Jamaica, and Trinidad and Tobago live in OECD countries; in Guyana, the corresponding figure is 83 per cent (United Nations, 2006). This loss of skilled individuals comes at a considerable cost to their countries of origin, and remittances do not counterbalance the negative consequences of the massive brain drain (United Nations Economic Commission for Latin America and the Caribbean, 2006). A particularly serious concern is that some small island developing States are relying excessively on remittances rather than developing their own manufacturing and service industries (McMurray, 2001).

A recent report by the World Bank (2006b) argues that destination countries, rather than trying to attract the best and brightest Pacific islanders, should develop programmes that bring in unskilled workers from the Pacific Islands to work on temporary contracts. This approach would purportedly provide an outlet for the excess supply of unskilled labour in the Pacific and address labour shortages in the agriculture and service sectors of destination countries such as Australia and New Zealand. Temporary worker programmes could benefit young people in a number of ways; unskilled youth would have the opportunity to earn higher incomes than would be possible for similar work at home, and they would be able to meet family expectations by sending a share of their income home while also satisfying their desire to live a more Western lifestyle.

THE IMPACT OF SOCIAL CHANGE

Traditionally, males and females were assigned discrete social roles in the small island developing States, particularly in the Pacific. Youth were guided by these roles and led step-by-step into adulthood. In Melanesia, for example, boys were taken into men's houses or men's groups at around the age of 10 or 12, where they were initiated and socialized by the older men of the community to take on male roles and skills. Girls remained with their mothers, grandmothers and sisters, where they learned female roles and skills. Modern education systems, widely introduced in the 1950s, supplanted traditional modes of educating youth and created new aspirations.

In many small island developing States, young people experience the tensions between modern ideas and traditional norms on multiple levels. Traditional male roles, such as that of "warrior", and activities such as canoe-building, sailing and fishing have largely become obsolete, but for those without access to secondary studies or employment, such roles and activities often have not been replaced by viable alternatives. There are also limited options and opportunities for constructive activities such as sports (Asian Development Bank, 2005). In many settings, young women continue to fulfil their traditional roles, becoming wives, mothers and caregivers. Modernity has thus created far greater discontinuity between youth and adulthood for young men than for young women in the Pacific small island developing States. The elusiveness of a positive role for these disaffected young men has led to the development of a negative subculture in both urban and rural areas. This subculture defines masculinity in terms of idleness, aggression, alcohol intoxication, and the use of drugs such as marijuana and kava (a mildly narcotic traditional drink) and, increasingly, pseudoephedrine and methamphetamines (Booker, 2006).

HEALTH AND RELATED CHALLENGES

Teenage pregnancy, HIV/AIDS, and drug abuse are some of the major health issues affecting young people in the small island developing States. The causes of youth morbidity and mortality in the region are largely preventable; the majority of deaths among young people occur as a result of road accidents, suicide, HIV/AIDS and, in some island countries, homicide and violence. For girls between the ages of 15 and 19, pregnancy-related illnesses are a common cause of death, with complications from unsafe abortions being a contributing factor. These and other issues, including drug use and sexual trends, are linked to a number of considerations, including the economic situation of young people, disillusionment brought on by the lack of opportunities, and the inadequacy of health services and information.

Sexuality and teenage pregnancy: a problem of alarming dimensions

Teenage pregnancy is a major health problem in many small island developing States and is likely related to poverty and the lack of opportunities for youth. Of all the regions for which data are available, the Caribbean has been identified as the area in which residents have sex at the earliest age. Research in nine Caribbean Community (CARICOM) countries revealed that one third of school-age youth were sexually active. Of these, a quarter of the girls and half of the boys interviewed said that their first experience of intercourse had occurred at age 10 or younger. In Saint Lucia, nearly 45 per cent of sexually active adolescents had had sexual intercourse before the age of 10. The results of the reproductive health survey undertaken in Jamaica in 1997 indicated that, by the age of 11 or 12, almost 20 per cent of girls and boys in the general population had had sexual intercourse. In many cases, this early sexual activity is due to forced intercourse. In a study of nine Caribbean countries, 48 per cent of adolescent girls and 32 per cent of boys who had had intercourse reported that their first sexual intercourse had been forced. Although sexual abuse among girls is also a problem in other countries, the high incidence among boys is unusual (Cunningham and Correia, 2003).

Despite high levels of sexual activity, rates of contraceptive use are low in many of the small island developing States (Cunningham and Correia, 2003). Data on contraceptive use are generally scant, but those available suggest that male youth, when compared with female youth, more commonly report the use of a condom the last time they had sex with a non-regular partner. In Barbados, 78 per cent of males reported using a condom, compared with only 33 per cent of females. In the Dominican Republic, 48 per cent of young males and only 12 per cent of young females reported condom use (Joint United Nations Programme on HIV/AIDS, 2006). In the countries of the Caribbean Community, only a quarter of school-going sexually active teenagers used some form of birth control, with only

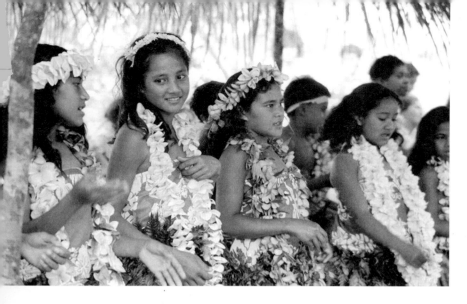

slightly more showing concern about getting pregnant or getting someone pregnant. In Jamaica, more than 40 per cent of sexually active adolescent girls said they had not used a contraceptive at last intercourse, and 87 per cent of teenage pregnancies had not been planned (Cunningham and Correia, 2003). Family planning services are generally available in many communities, but research has shown that these services are not fully utilized by the poor.

The fact that male youth are more likely to use condoms than female youth suggests a need to explore techniques such as empowerment training that may lead to a higher incidence of condom usage among young females, especially in light of the fact that, globally, young women living with HIV outnumber young men living with HIV by 1.6 to 1 (United Nations Population Fund, 2005). There is also a need for aggressive education campaigns that offer young people access to information services and dialogue in an environment free of the stigma associated with being sexually active. Accurate information delivered at the right age within an appropriate context tends to encourage responsible behaviour (Ahmed, 2003).

Early sexual activity and low rates of contraceptive use combine to produce high rates of teenage pregnancy, particularly among those with little education and those living in rural areas. In the Dominican Republic, survey results indicated that among young women aged 15-19 years, 28 per cent in rural areas and 21 per cent in urban centres were mothers or were pregnant with their first child; of these teenagers, 60.7 per cent had no education, 34.2 per cent had a primary education, and 14.1 per cent had secondary schooling or higher (MEASURE DHS, 2007).

Fertility rates vary widely in the small island developing States (see table 5.5). The Seychelles have the lowest youth fertility rates, with 11.4 births per 1,000 women aged 15-19 years and 65.5 births per 1,000 women aged 20-24 years. The highest youth fertility rates are found in Sao Tome and Principe, with 118.4 and 273.5 births per 1,000 women in the age groups 15-19 and 20-24 respectively. The youth fertility rates of other small island developing States are somewhere in the middle and are comparable to fertility rates in the United States (58.1 and 114.2 births per 1,000 women aged 15-19 and 20-24 years respectively) (MEASURE DHS, 2007).

Table 5.5
Youth fertility in selected small island developing States

Region/Country	Births per 1,000 women	
	Age 15-19 (2007)	Age 20-24 (2007)
Africa		
Cape Verde	64.4	150.4
Comoros	62.5	191.1
Mauritius	26.8	104.0
Sao Tome & Principe	118.4	273.5
Seychelles	11.4	65.5
Caribbean		
Antigua & Barbuda	101.2	141.1
Dominica	20.0	80.6
Grenada	60.2	105.8
St. Kitts & Nevis	53.8	118.6
St. Lucia	35.5	92.4
St. Vincent & Grenadines	16.6	70.6
Trinidad and Tobago	11.9	66.1
Pacific		
Fiji	40.8	148.0
Kiribati	54.8	181.4
Marshall Islands	81.6	229.6
Micronesia, Federated States	33.0	133.4
Palau	61.8	114.1
Samoa	19.7	117.8
Solomon Islands	53.6	162.0
Tonga	35.5	139.2
Vanuatu	28.9	112.8
South Asia		
Maldives	85.8	204.1

Source: United States Census Bureau, International Data Base (2007) (available from www.census.gov/cgi-bin/ipc/idbsprd; accessed on 4 April 2007).

The prevalence of teenage pregnancies in small island developing States is a concern, especially given the limited support for child care. Early motherhood interferes with a young woman's ability to contribute to the economic and social development of her society, diminishes her opportunities in life, and poses certain health risks. Teenage pregnancy predisposes young girls to low educational attainment. Dropping out of school affects future job opportunities and earnings. Teen mothers are generally encouraged to continue with their education, but many choose not to, probably because schools are frequently not supportive.

HIV/AIDS

Related to early sexuality in small island developing States is the region's increasing vulnerability to HIV. The HIV prevalence rate in the Caribbean is the second highest in the world, and AIDS is the number one cause of death among adults in the subregion (Joint United Nations Programme on HIV/AIDS, 2006). Young women are particularly prone to HIV infection. In the Caribbean, HIV prevalence among female youth (1.6 per cent) is more than twice that registered for young males (0.7 per cent). In Trinidad and Tobago, females between the ages of 15 and 19 are six times more likely than males their age to be infected (Joint United Nations Programme on HIV/AIDS, 2006). HIV prevalence rates vary widely from one country to another, ranging from 0.1 per cent in Cuba to 2 per cent in Trinidad and Tobago and the Bahamas and 3.8 per cent in Haiti. Though Haiti has been making progress, prevention messages do not seem to be reaching young people. They are becoming sexually active at a younger age, and condom use appears to be declining (Joint United Nations Programme on HIV/AIDS, 2006). Cuba, with youth prevalence rates of 0.5 per cent among females and 0.9 per cent among males, has emerged as a model in its response to HIV/AIDS. Its programme to reduce mother-to-child HIV transmission and the accessibility of its antiretroviral treatment programme are unparalleled in the region (United Nations Population Fund, 2003; Joint United Nations Programme on HIV/AIDS, 2006).

Across the Caribbean subregion, the most common mode of HIV transmission is unprotected heterosexual intercourse. The rate of transmission among men who have sex with men is also significant, but this aspect of the epidemic is largely ignored. Societal norms have thus far precluded an open discussion on how to address this development. Continuing to treat this as a taboo topic will likely lead to increased HIV prevalence in the region (Joint United Nations Programme on HIV/AIDS, 2006).

In contrast to the situation in the Caribbean, the overall HIV/AIDS picture in the Pacific small island developing States is fairly positive, with relatively low rates of prevalence among youth. The exception is Papua New Guinea, where the incidence of HIV has been increasing at the alarming rate of 30 per cent annually since 1997. The country accounts for more than 90 per cent of all HIV infections reported in Oceania (excluding Australia and New Zealand). The growing epidemic is partly related to socio-cultural norms discriminating against women as well as high levels of violence against women (Joint United Nations Programme on HIV/AIDS, 2006). Some other Pacific small island developing States also exhibit increasing vulnerability to HIV. Low rates of contraceptive use prevail throughout the Pacific Islands, which could result in a future upsurge in the incidence of HIV/AIDS in the subregion. In Vanuatu, as well as in the Samoan capital of Apia, more than 40 per cent of pregnant women have tested positive for at least one sexually transmitted infection. In Dili, the capital of Timor-Leste, large proportions of sex workers, taxi drivers and men who have sex with men have tested positive for herpes simplex virus type 2 (Joint United Nations Programme on HIV/AIDS, 2006).

Among women living in the Pacific small island developing States, the prevalence of sexually transmitted infections is highest for those under the age of 25. This is believed to be partly attributable to the general lack of education among youth with regard to strategies for protection. The results of a survey published by the World Health Organization indicated that only 25.4 per cent of young respondents had correct beliefs about transmission and protection, and fewer than 1 in 10 young people involved in sex work consistently used condoms with commercial partners (World Health Organization, 2006).

Although studies indicate that reproductive health education leads to a lower probability of youth engaging in high-risk sexual behaviour, becoming pregnant, or contracting sexually transmitted infections such as HIV/AIDS, education about reproductive health is rarely provided in schools in Pacific small island developing States because of taboos regarding sexual matters and the belief that reproductive health education will encourage sexual experimentation among adolescents.

Factors contributing to young people's vulnerability to HIV/AIDS include unprotected sex (lack of condom use, which is sometimes related to lack of access to condoms); the high prevalence and rapid spread of other sexually transmitted infections (the pre-existence of one or more sexually transmitted infections increases the risk of HIV transmission upon exposure); the high mobility of people who are engaging in unprotected sex (for example, seafarers); the absence of discussion and education about reproductive health; promiscuity and high-risk sexual behaviour among young people; and poverty (United Nations Children's Fund, 2006). The mass movement of people in tourism is another major factor compounding the problem (CARICOM Secretariat, 2004).

Young people are important partners in the fight against HIV/AIDS. The Youth Ambassadors for Positive Living programme is part of a strategy to enable young people to realize their potential as active citizens through their participation in, contribution to, and engagement with development processes. Young people who have tested positive for HIV and those who have not contracted the disease work together to educate their peers on the dangers of HIV/AIDS. In Guyana and the Bahamas, 46 young men and women have been trained as peer educators. Their post-training activities have included conducting outreach activities such as live radio programmes aimed at providing other young people with the skills and information needed to encourage positive behaviour change. The programme is being replicated across the Caribbean.

Non-communicable diseases

The prevalence of non-communicable diseases is quite high in many small island developing States, especially in urban areas. The Pacific Islands have experienced a particularly sharp increase in non-communicable diseases, which is largely attributable to the growing incidence of obesity over the past several decades. Rates of obesity are rising rapidly among young people in particular, and unless this problem is addressed, chronic disease will become increasingly prevalent in the population as it ages. Some of the highest rates of obesity in the world are found in Oceania, particularly in American Samoa, the Cook Islands, French Polynesia, Nauru, Samoa and Tonga. In some cases, the rates are as high as 75 per cent (World Health Organization, 2003; Curtis, 2004).

One of the most common chronic diseases associated with obesity is diabetes—which in earlier times affected mainly older people. Today, however, increasing numbers of youth are developing early-onset diabetes (Secretariat of the Pacific Community/ Pacific Youth Bureau, 2005). Certain small island developing States in the Pacific, notably the Marshall Islands and Nauru, are among the countries with the highest rates of diabetes mellitus in the world (Williams, 2001). Obese youth are also at risk of developing hypertension, hyper-cholesterolemia (elevated blood cholesterol), and atherosclerosis—conditions that are predictive of coronary artery disease (Food and Agriculture Organization of the United Nations, 2002). This will have an enormous impact on the demand for health-care and support services and will place a tremendous strain on national economies.

In the Pacific Islands, the increase in the incidence of obesity is believed to be related to dietary changes, the relative lack of physical activity, and a possible genetic predisposition to the condition (Williams, 2001). Those whose diets once consisted of healthy staples such as fish and vegetables are now consuming foods that are higher in fat, sugar, and salt and lower in dietary fibre. The shift from employment in agriculture-based occupations to more sedentary office work has also contributed to the problem. To combat obesity, public health policies are needed to ensure the availability of nutritious low-fat, high-fibre foods, which are generally more costly and harder to find, and to create safe, accessible places that provide opportunities for physical activity (Curtis, 2004).

Suicide

In some small island developing States, suicide rates are alarmingly high. According to the most recent data available, suicide rates in the Pacific are among the highest in the world (Booth, 1998). Chuuk State, in the Federated States of Micronesia, has the highest male youth suicide rate in the world (182 per 100,000), followed by Samoa (64 per 100,000). These figures far exceed the top non-Pacific rate of 45 per 100,000 for Lithuania. Samoa has the highest female youth suicide rate (70 per 100,000), followed by Fiji (60 per 100,000 among young Fijian women of Indian descent), and rural China (37 per 100,000). Many theorists attribute female youth suicide in Fiji and other countries in Melanesia to the low status of women in these areas (Booth, 1999). Increased suicide rates among young males in Micronesia may be related to the weakening of extended family structures occurring as a result of socio-economic changes and the inability of nuclear families to both discipline and support young men (Hezel, 1989). The general transition in Pacific island societies from traditional to modern ways and the attendant intergenerational conflict and pressures on the younger generation are also believed to be contributing to the increasing rates of youth suicide (Booth, 1998).

Youth suicide is also a problem in small island developing States outside the Pacific. In Mauritius and in Trinidad and Tobago, suicide is the second leading cause of death among young people. In Belize, Cuba and Saint Lucia, it is the third most common cause of death for this age group (see the statistical annex).

Crime

A combination of factors including social alienation, lack of opportunity, and high unemployment among large numbers of youth in unstable, poorly managed urban settings can lead to gang violence and civil unrest (Ware, 2004). This was demonstrated in 2004 in towns in Timor-Leste and Solomon Islands, where gangs of male youths roamed the streets, looting shops and burning buildings. International military intervention was required to restore order. A similar situation prevailed during the civil war in Bougainville province in Papua New Guinea until order was restored in 1998. In all three instances, unemployed, frustrated young men were easily recruited into violent conflicts between opposing factions

(Chevalier, 2001). Volatile young men in such situations are often motivated by leaders who are pursuing political agendas and who use excuses of ethnic or interregional discrimination to incite violent unrest among male youth.

Among the Pacific small island developing States, Papua New Guinea has particularly severe law and order problems in its major towns, and youth gangs (referred to as raskols) are the main perpetrators of criminal acts. This may be attributable to a combination of the factors listed above (social alienation, lack of opportunity, and high unemployment among large numbers of youth in unstable, poorly managed urban settings) as well as to poor governance.

Escalating crime is also a significant challenge for Caribbean small island developing States (CARICOM Secretariat, 2004). Rates of violent crime are rising steadily in some countries, while problems such as drug trafficking and related activities are subject to "spikes". Regardless of the nature and prevalence of different types of crime, one consistent trend across the region is that the face of crime is getting younger (Bell, 2006).

Violent crime is usually concentrated in poor urban communities. Data for Jamaica show that most offences are committed by youth between the ages of 17 and 30. Young people constitute almost two thirds of those found guilty of crimes, with males four times more likely than females to be found guilty. It should be noted that 17- to 25-year-olds committed 56 per cent of all crimes, almost 50 per cent of murders, 44 per cent of manslaughters, 42 per cent of burglaries, and 39 per cent of sex offences. By and large, the perpetrators of major crime are males between the ages of 20 and 25. Young males are also usually the victims of homicides. Out-of-school male youth aged 13-19 years were found to be most at risk of substance abuse and drug dealing (Cunningham and Correia, 2003). Young people are also more inclined to be involved in criminal gangs. Gang violence is high in the Caribbean, with 12 per cent of female students and 20 per cent of male students having belonged to a gang at some point. In many cases, youth join criminal and drug-dealing gangs to compensate for the lack of formal employment opportunities or as a strategy for confronting violence in their communities (Cunningham and Correia, 2003).

THE SITUATION OF GIRLS AND YOUNG WOMEN

Poverty of opportunity and high unemployment have negatively affected young women. As noted previously, with few alternative forms of employment open to them, young unemployed women in small island developing States such as Papua New Guinea, Solomon Islands, and Vanuatu often resort to prostitution to survive. In Solomon Islands, for example, an unpublished study commissioned by UNICEF documented the sexual exploitation of girls as young as 12 years old, and of young women who visit the crews of freighters and fishing ships and the employees of logging companies. In some cases, based on a distorted form of the "bride price" tradition, young women have effectively been sold into a form of "sexual slavery" by their fathers (Christian Care Centre of the Church of Melanesia and the Regional Rights Resource Team, 2004; Callinan, 2006). Similar reports have come out of Vanuatu and Papua New Guinea (Wan Smol Bag and Regional Rights Resource Team, 2004; HELP Resources and United Nations Children's Fund, 2005)

Traditional views that a woman's role in society should be limited to that of wife and mother persist, though they are less strongly enforced, in many small island developing States today. In the light of high teenage pregnancy rates, families seek to protect their daughters' reputations and the family honour by restricting any activity that might expose girls to sexual risks. Consequently, adolescent girls are often denied the freedoms and choices allowed adolescent boys. In Tonga and Samoa, for example, families are often very strict with girls and limit their movements in an effort to prevent premarital sex. In some countries, preventing a girl from being "permanently spoiled" in terms of marriage prospects may include withdrawing her from school when she reaches puberty. While this certainly limits possibilities for early sexual contact among girls, it also interferes with their chances of completing their schooling and thus deprives them of opportunities for their future lives.

Although Pacific societies regard sexual contact between an adult and a minor as highly immoral, and while such interaction is illegal in all Pacific small island developing States, such crimes are only sporadically reported when they occur. Spreading knowledge publicly about such crimes is considered to bring great shame on families and to be highly destructive to small communities (United Nations Children's Fund, 2004a-c; 2005a-b; Government of the Republic of the Marshall Islands and United Nations Children's Fund, 2003; Government of the Cook Islands and United Nations Children's Fund, 2004). Silence, secrecy and the failure to report sexual abuse means that youth who are victimized by family members or others find little support or comfort. They face major difficulties dealing with the severe physical and mental consequences.

Girls in the Caribbean are also vulnerable to sexual violence, including abuse and exploitation. In Jamaica, for example, one in five girls aged 15-19 years reported being forced to have sex; for 16-year-olds, the proportion increased to one in four (Government of Jamaica and United Nations Children's Fund, 2004). The perpetrators are not always strangers, as young people are at risk of being violated by relatives, family friends, teachers, employers and others they may trust.

SUMMARY AND CONCLUSIONS

The geographic and natural resource characteristics of small island developing States translate into limited opportunities for industrial growth and a small formal labour market. At the same time, because of poor quality education, limited vocational training opportunities, and relatively little interest among youth in training for work outside the public sector, most young people in small island developing States do not have the skills required to secure formal sector employment. As a result, high-skill jobs often go to expatriates. With few formal sector jobs for young people, many youth in small island developing States see migration as the only means of finding employment. However, the current immigration policies of destination countries are skewed in favour of highly skilled migrants. This means that most youth from small island developing States cannot migrate. They must therefore join the ranks of the long-term unemployed or work in the informal sector or in subsistence agriculture, which is frequently seen as failure by society.

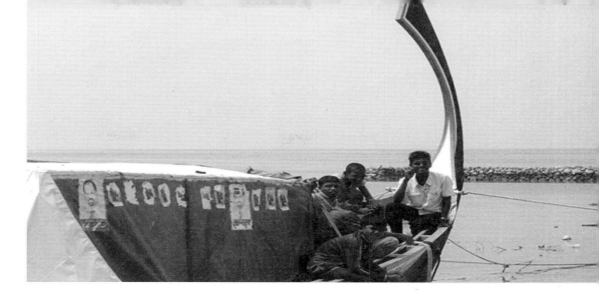

In small island developing States, particularly the Pacific Islands, the burden of lack of opportunity and the transition from small, kin-based societies to modern societies within a global economy falls heavily on youth, who develop expectations of employment in the modern economy that are seldom realized. The result is too often a situation in which unemployment, combined with rapid societal change and a clash of traditional cultures with modern ideas, leads to social alienation among youth. Such alienation expresses itself in a range of endemic social problems, including violence, risky sexual behaviour, and youth suicide.

With traditional gender and other social norms persisting and large portions of the population remaining economically vulnerable, the health and safety of youth in small island developing States remain seriously at risk. Youth, and young women in particular, continue to be at risk of contracting diseases such as HIV/AIDS and of abuse and exploitation in their homes and communities. In addition, the concentration of large numbers of dissatisfied youth in urban areas and their exposure to unscrupulous leaders ready to take advantage of them present risk factors for crime and violent conflict in small island developing States.

To address the poverty of opportunity faced by youth in small island developing States, urgent efforts are needed to improve the quality of education and employment prospects. In addition, there is a need for a variety of leisure activities that provide a positive outlet for young people's energies and frustrations as well as an opportunity to gain valuable knowledge, skills and attitudes. ▮▮▮▮▮▮▮▮▮▮▮▮

References

Abbot, David, and Steve Pollard (2004). Hardship and poverty in the Pacific: a summary. Manila: Asian Development Bank.

Ahmed, Aziza (2003). Gender and health in the Caribbean. Paper prepared for the ECLAC/CDCC/UNIFEM/CIDA/CARICOM Fourth Caribbean Ministerial Conference on Women: Review and Appraisal of the Beijing Platform for Action and the Outcome of the Twenty-Third Special Session of the General Assembly (2000), Saint Vincent and the Grenadines, 12-13 February 2003.

Appleyard, R.T., and Charles W. Stahl (1995). South Pacific Migration: New Zealand Experience an Implications for Australia. Canberra: Australian Agency for International Development (AusAID).

Asian Development Bank (2003). Poverty: Is it an issue in the Pacific? Manila.

_____ (2005). Project performance report on the Marshall Islands Community Health Project. Operations Evaluation Department. Manila.

_____ (2006). Country reports: Millennium Development Goals. Available from http://www.adb.org/papuanewguinea/png-mdgs.asp; http://www.adb.org/kiribati/mdg.asp; http://www.adb.org/MarshallIslands/mdgs.asp; and http://www.adb.org/Timor-Leste/ MDGs.asp (accessed on 27 July 2006).

Bell, Keith (2006). Youth crime and violence. Paper presented at the Sixth Commonwealth Youth Ministers Meeting, Nassau, 22-26 May 2006.

Booker, J. (2006). Calls for regional court to help tiny Pacific nations fight drugs. New Zealand Herald (21 August 2006). Available from http://subs.nzherald.co.nz/location/story.cfm?l_id=10&ObjectID=10397191.

Booth, Heather (1998). Pacific island suicide in comparative perspective. Working Papers in Demography, No 76. Demography and Sociology Program, Research School of Social Sciences. Canberra: Australian National University.

Callinan, Rory (2006). Generation exploited. Time Magazine, South Pacific edition (27 March 2006), pp. 19-25. Available from http://www.time.com/time/pacific/magazine/article/0,13673,503060327-1174745,00.html.

Caribbean Community (CARICOM) Secretariat (2004). The Ten Year Review of the Barbados Programme of Action: the Caribbean Process. Available from http://www.sidsnet.org/doc-share/other/20041124121539_Caribbean_Regional_Assessment_Rpt_as_of_Nov_24.pdf (accessed on 30 March 2007).

Chevalier, Christopher (2001). From chimera to chimaera: changing the realities for youth in Solomon Islands. Development Bulletin, vol. 56 (October), pp. 38-41. Special issue: Involving Young People in Development.

Christian Care Centre of the Church of Melanesia and Regional Rights Resource Team (2004). Commercial sexual exploitation of children and child sexual abuse in the Solomon Islands. Unpublished report. Suva, Fiji: United Nations Children's Fund, Pacific Office.

Connell, John (2003). Migration in Pacific island countries and territories. Migration Patterns and Policies in the Asian and Pacific Region. Asian Population Studies Series, No. 160. Bangkok: United Nations Economic and Social Commission for Asia and the Pacific.

Cunningham, Wendy, and Maria Correia (2003). Caribbean Youth Development: Issues and Policy Directions. World Bank Country Study. Washington, D.C.

Curtis, Michael (2004). The obesity epidemic in the Pacific Islands. Journal of Development and Social Transformation, vol. 1 (November).

Federation of St. Kitts and Nevis (2004). National assessment of the BPoA + 10, 1994-2003. Ministry of Finance, Development and Planning, October. Available from http://www.sidsnet.org/docshare/other/20041104160840_ST_KITTS_AND_NEVIS.pdf (accessed on 3 April 2007).

Food and Agriculture Organization of the United Nations (2002). The developing world's new burden: obesity. FOCUS. Available from http://www.fao.org/FOCUS/E/obesity/obes1.htm (accessed on 18 July 2007).

Gibson, John, and Scott Rozelle (2002). Poverty and access to infrastructure in Papua New Guinea. Department of Agricultural and Resource Economics, University of California, Davis. Working Paper No. 02-008.

Government of the Cook Islands and United Nations Children's Fund (2004). Cook Islands: A Situation Analysis of Children, Youth and Women. Suva: UNICEF Pacific Office, 2005.

Government of Jamaica and United Nations Children's Fund (2004). Mid-term review report: 2002 2006 Country Programme of Cooperation. Kingston: November. Available from http://www.unicef.org/jamaica/resources_2149.htm (accessed on 30 March 2007).

Government of the Republic of the Marshall Islands and United Nations Children's Fund (2003). Republic of the Marshall Islands: A Situation Analysis of Children, Youth and Women. Suva: UNICEF Pacific Office.

Gregory, A. (2006). Revolution warning for Pacific as "youth bulge" keeps growing. New Zealand Herald (1 July 2006). Available from http://subs.nzherald.co.nz/location/story.cfm?l_id=10&ObjectID=10389228.

HELP Resources and United Nations Children's Fund (Papua New Guinea) (2005). A situation analysis of child sexual abuse and the commercial sexual exploitation of children in Papua New Guinea. Unpublished report. Bangkok: United Nations Economic and Social Commission for Asia and the Pacific, January.

Hezel, Francis X. (1989). Suicide and the Micronesian family. The Contemporary Pacific, vol. 1, No. 1, pp. 43-74.

International Labour Office (2004). Key Indicators of the Labour Market. Third edition. Geneva.

_____ (2006). Global Employment Trends for Youth 2006. Geneva: International Labour Organization, August.

Joint United Nations Programme on HIV/AIDS (2006). 2006 Report on the Global AIDS Epidemic. Geneva.

McKenzie, David J. (2006). Remittances in the Pacific. Paper presented on 15 February 2006 at the Werner Sichel Lecture-Seminar Series 2005-2006: Immigrants and Their International Money Flows, held at Western Michigan University in Kalamazoo.

McMurray, Christine (2001). Youth employment in the Pacific. Working paper prepared for the ILO/Japan Tripartite Regional Meeting on Youth Employment in Asia and the Pacific, Bangkok, 27 February - 1 March 2002.

MEASURE DHS (2007). STATcompiler. Available from www.measuredhs.com (accessed on 4 April 2007).

Monsell-Davis, Michael (2000). Social change, contradictions, youth and violence in Fiji. In Reflections on Violence in Melanesia, Sinclair Dinnen and Alison Ley, editors. Annandale, Australia: Hawkins Press.

Pacific Islands Trade and Investment Commission and Asian Development Bank (2001). Business Information Guide to the Pacific Islands. Sydney.

Save the Children (Fiji) (2004). The commercial sexual exploitation and sexual abuse of children in Fiji: a situational analysis. Funded by the United Nations Economic and Social Commission for Asia and the Pacific.

Secretariat of the Pacific Community (2006). Football for Hope movement. Pacific Youth Festival Web page. Available from http://www.spc.int/Pacific_Youth_Festival_6.htm.

_____ Pacific Youth Bureau (2005). Component 3: Promoting healthy lifestyles. Pacific Youth Strategy 2010: Youth Empowerment for a Secure, Prosperous and Sustainable Future. Noumea, New Caledonia.

Statistics New Zealand (2002). Census snapshot: Pacific peoples. Available from http://www.stats.govt.nz/products-and-services/Articles/census-snpsht-pac-ppls-Jun02.htm.

United Nations (2006). International migration and development. Report of the Secretary-General (A/60/871).

United Nations Children's Fund (2004a). A Situation Analysis of Children, Youth and Women in the Federated States of Micronesia. Suva: UNICEF Pacific Office.

_____ (2004b). A Situation Analysis of Children, Youth and Women: Nauru. Suva: UNICEF Pacific Office.

_____ (2004c). A Situation Analysis of Children, Youth and Women: Niue. Suva: UNICEF Pacific Office.

_____ (2005a). A Situation Analysis of Children, Youth and Women: Kiribati. Suva: UNICEF Pacific Office.

_____ (2005b). Solomon Islands: A Situation Analysis of Children, Women and Youth. Suva: UNICEF Pacific Office.

_____ (2006). Pacific: Children and HIV/AIDS—A Call to Action. Bangkok: UNICEF East-Asia and Pacific Regional Office.

United Nations Development Programme (2006). Human Development Report 2006—Beyond Scarcity: Power, Poverty and the Global Water Crisis. New York.

United Nations Economic Commission for Latin America and the Caribbean (2006). Migration in the Caribbean—What do we know? (UN/POP/EGM-MIG/2005/09). Paper prepared for the Expert Group Meeting on International Migration and Development in Latin America and the Caribbean, Mexico City, 30 November - 2 December 2005.

United Nations Economic and Social Commission for Asia and the Pacific (2003). Migration patterns and policies in the Asian and Pacific region (ST/ESCAP/2277). Population and Poverty in Asia and the Pacific. Asian Population Studies Series, No. 160. Bangkok.

United Nations Educational, Scientific and Cultural Organization, Institute for Statistics (2006a). Global Education Digest 2006: Comparing Education Statistics Across the World (UIS/SD/06-01). Montreal.

_____ (2006b). Youth (15-24) literacy rates and illiterate population by region and gender for 2000-2004. Database September. Available from www.uis.unesco.org (accessed on 2 April 2007).

_____ (2007a). Assorted statistics. Database. Available from www.uis.unesco.org (accessed on 2 April 2007).

_____ (2007b). Statistical table 10. Database. Available from www.uis.unesco.org (accessed on 9 May 2007).

United Nations Population Fund (2003). Overview of adolescent life. State of World Population 2003—Making 1 Billion Count: Investing in Adolescents' Health and Rights. New York. Sales No. E.03.III.H.1.

_____ (2005). The unmapped journey: adolescents, poverty and gender. State of World Population 2005—The Promise of Equality: Gender Equity, Reproductive Health and the Millennium Development Goals. New York. Sales No. E.05.III.H.1.

United States Census Bureau (2007). International Data Base. Available from www.census.gov/ipc/www/idb/ (accessed on 4 April 2007).

Wan Smol Bag and Regional Rights Resource Team (2004). Commercial sexual exploitation of children and child sexual abuse in Vanuatu. Unpublished report. Suva: UNICEF Pacific Office.

Ware, Helen (2004). Pacific instability and youth bulges: the devil in the demography and the economy. Paper prepared for the Australian Population Association's 12th Biennial Conference—Population and Society: Issues, Research, Policy, Canberra, Australia, 15-17 September 2004.

Williams, D. (2001). Sweet temptations. Time Magazine, South Pacific edition, No. 33 (20-27 August 2001). Available from http://www.time.com/time/pacific/magazine/20010820/medicine.html.

World Bank (2006a). At Home and Away: Expanding Job Opportunities for Pacific Islanders through Labour Mobility. Washington, D.C. Available from http://web.worldbank.org/WBSITE/EXTER-NAL/COUNTRIES/EASTASIAPACIFICEXT/PACIFICISLANDSEXTN/0,,contentMDK:21020027~pagePK:141137~piPK:141127~theSitePK:441883,00.html.

_____ (2006b). World Development Report 2007: Development and the Next Generation. Washington, D.C.

World Health Organization (2003). Obesity and overweight. Fact sheet. Global Strategy on Diet, Physical Activity and Health. Available from http://www.who.int/hpr/NPH/docs/gs_obesity.pdf (accessed on 18 July 2007).

_____ (2006). Second generation surveillance surveys of HIV, other STIs and risk behaviours in 6 Pacific island countries (2004-2005), implemented by the ministries of health of Fiji, Kiribati, Samoa, Solomon Islands, Tonga and Vanuatu. Manila: WHO Regional Office for the Western Pacific.

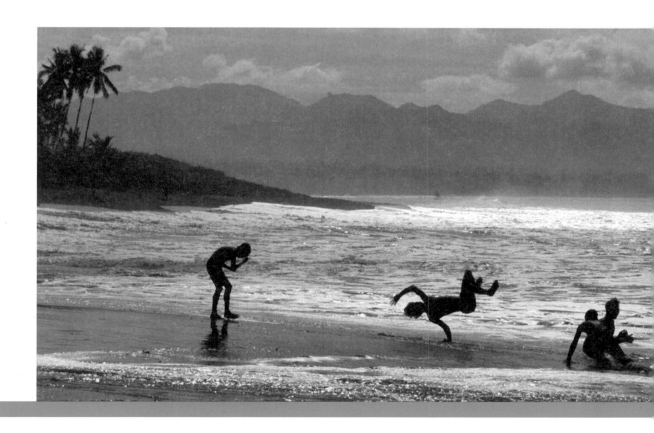

Chapter 6

Labour market challenges and new vulnerabilities for YOUTH in economies in transition

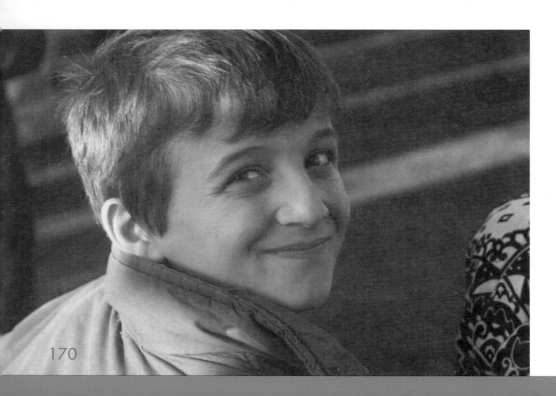

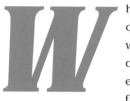**W**ho are the young people in Eastern Europe and the Commonwealth of Independent States (CIS)? What challenges are they facing? Those who are now between the ages of 15 and 24 were born in the last decade of the communist regimes. In the period 1980-1990, they experienced great changes in their immediate social environment, families and schools. The world around them became much less predictable, for better or for worse. Though youth typically feel confident that they will inherit a better world than their parents, within the countries in transition "the institutions, processes and social norms that facilitated a smooth passage from one generation to the next have weakened, been dismantled, are under construction or are in the process of fundamental transformation" (UNICEF Innocenti Research Centre, 2000). Young people in the region thus encounter a mix of difficulties, uncertainties and new possibilities.

The economies in transition continue to undergo substantial transformation and restructuring. Each country is different in terms of its socio-economic background, the pace at which the basic elements of centrally planned economies have been abandoned or the degree to which they have partially survived, and the speed of privatization. The severity of shocks following systemic change, as well as the level of success of the recovery process, has also differed widely. People's attitudes have been shaped by a lingering belief in the paternalism of higher authorities—whether at the State or the regional level—to solve pressing local issues and take care of local needs. Consequently, the conditions for active civic engagement and political participation in general differ greatly across the countries of the region. Equally different are the conditions for socio-economic participation. In many countries of the region, young people's access to economic and societal resources is limited, and very often youth are more vulnerable than older age groups. A lack of adequate education and employment opportunities, as well as exposure to violence and crime both as victims and as perpetrators, reinforces the social exclusion of young people and prevents them from participating in development and decision-making.

It is impossible to fully cover the wide range of youth-related challenges in this region in the present report. This chapter therefore focuses on exploring in depth two key impediments that prevent youth from developing and realizing their full potential: prevalent patterns of unemployment and other labour market disadvantages; and drug abuse and the spread of HIV/AIDS among young people in the region.

The first part of the chapter focuses on issues related to youth employment in the countries in transition in Eastern Europe and the CIS. It begins by reviewing changing expectations and experiences of youth in the context of the evolving socio-economic landscape. Next, key aspects of youth employment, such as unemployment, the informal economy and the quality of work, are considered. Finally, education and training issues, as well as barriers to and incentives for youth participation, along with their policy implications, are analysed. The second part of the chapter highlights the role of the growing HIV/AIDS epidemic in the region in further constraining the development of youth. It begins with an overview of HIV/AIDS prevalence and trends among youth, and the relationship to intravenous drug use in the region. It reviews the impact of HIV/AIDS on youth and society in the region. The summary and conclusions address policy measures at the national level geared towards improving the labour market situation for youth, as well as combating HIV/AIDS among youth and young drug users, focusing particularly on issues relating to prevention and treatment for both HIV/AIDS and drug addiction.

The intricacies of the challenges youth are facing often remain only partly understood at the national level. Information about labour market dynamics is limited; statistics often provide only a partial view, and the reliability of national data in the region leaves much room for improvement. Similar, if not larger, information gaps exist in the area of substance abuse and HIV/AIDS pandemics. There are also some inconsistencies among the age ranges used by statistical offices in defining the "youth" category. Such constraints inevitably limit the scope of analysis.

BETWEEN TWO WORLDS: YOUTH EMPLOYMENT AND THE LEGACY OF STATE SOCIALISM

To understand the challenges that young people face in the region, one has to understand the overall nature of the historic changes that have occurred. Under State socialism, stability in everyday life and work and the fulfilment of everyone's basic needs, including the provision of free education and health care, was ingrained in the system. The importance of this stability was consistently reinforced by official propaganda and echoed at school, in the workplace, and at official events. Political protest against the Government was strongly discouraged. Open discussion about the pros and cons of a market economy versus the existing system, not to mention the values of "liberal democracy" beyond the closed borders of the communist regimes, was taboo. Social participation existed in official forms and was highly regimented, while self-organization of any kind was discouraged.

In such a system, employment was provided for all by the State, and work was not just an option but a duty, while efficiency considerations and market demands were not taken into account. A young person of working age who did not have a job was an exceptional case and carried the stigma associated with challenging the basic tenets of society geared towards providing a job for everybody. Young people, when they completed high school, went through a regimented system of job placement with circumscribed opportunities and limited choice. However, a modicum of stability (even often on the verge of stagnation) provided young people with a feeling of security and assured a largely predictable path from school to work. Wage levels were largely compressed and modest but above a subsistence minimum. Low labour productivity was widespread. A guaranteed job gave access to all benefits and social services provided by State-owned enterprises. Guaranteed employment was a crucial part of the "social contract" and a precondition for access to a range of social services, including paid maternity leave and child-care benefits, nurseries and kindergartens, housing support, and holiday vouchers. Through various measures, the socialist State controlled young people's transition from school to work and continued to exercise open and covert control of an individual in society. In a certain sense, the system was designed to do without, or even to suppress, individual initiative and effort; the subordination of the individual to the collective was one of the pillars of communist ideology (Estrin, 1994).

The ideological aim of achieving full employment under the socialist system, through State intervention, irrespective of the degree of efficiency or effectiveness in the use of labour, contributed to a persistent oversupply of labour in the economy. Officially, levels of employment were consistently high and the participation rate was equal to the level of employment. However, many of those employed in socialist enterprises had to be on hand in case they were needed during peak work periods, so there was considerable "unemployment on the job" (Kornai, 1980; 2000). Young people hired for jobs were given limited responsibility, a low salary reflective of compressed wages, and little room for mobility. With the demise of State socialism and the elimination of artificial labour hoarding, employment rates for youth, as well as for the general population, decreased rapidly in all countries of the region starting at the beginning of the transition.

The socio-economic paradigm, and above all, the role of the State, changed considerably during the transition period. With the political and economic changes brought about by democratization and the end of the one-party monopoly on power, the role of the State diminished, and new expectations for young people's self-sufficiency and initiative emerged. Previously, the paternalistic State had provided various types of support for young people as a condition of their engagement in "socialist production", including financial support through budget transfers for start-ups, housing provision, and assistance to families with children. With the collapse of the system those types of financial subsidies were abolished, with some serious negative social consequences. For instance, increased financial hardship associated with unemployment or underemployment, coupled with difficulty in obtaining State-provided housing, had a negative impact on family formation. A combination of the above-mentioned factors may also have led to a decrease in fertility throughout the region. Overall, however, the family played, and continues to play, an important role in protecting its members against new risks and vulnerabilities. In this context, Gallup Organisation Hungary (2003) highlights some important factors explaining why youth in Eastern Europe are protracting their stay in the family home. Though similar patterns are seen in Western Europe, the reasons in Eastern Europe are somewhat different and include the lack of financial resources, the unavailability of suitable housing, and the need to save for the future (UNICEF Innocenti Research Centre, 2000).

With the rapid spread of democracy and free enterprise, the society in which the State played multiple roles—owner of the means of production, employer, and provider of social protection—ceased to exist. Although a new economy was created and social opportunities opened up, security and predictability were gone, and new sources of vulnerability emerged for society at large, including youth. Formative events in the lives of young people, such as joining the workforce, participating in training or education, and achieving professional fulfilment, took on new meaning in the climate of adjustment in the post-socialist era. New windows of opportunity opened up, particularly in business and entrepreneurship, though not everyone was able to take full advantage of these opportunities. The power of inertia and the difficulties of adjustment should not be underestimated. In many countries, after the fall of communism, there was still widespread failure to assume individual responsibility, and people tended to expect the State to solve their problems for them.

SOCIO-ECONOMIC TRANSITION

The overall economic situation in the region is perhaps best illustrated by trends in GDP over time. After the onset of the early phase of transition, in 1989, a serious economic recession affected the whole region. As a consequence, real GDP in 1995 was far below the 1989 level. Some countries in transition have experienced a relatively rapid economic recovery, while others are still facing prolonged recession with limited chances of improvement in the short term (see figure 6.1). Despite the considerable variation among the countries in the region in the level of GDP per capita, many of these economies, particularly in the CIS, remain interdependent. For example, economic upturns in the largest countries, including the Russian Federation, Ukraine and Kazakhstan, in 2003/04 benefited the whole region (Simai, 2006). Some countries in the region remain low-income agricultural economies, and many are characterized by a very high rate of primary exports (as a percentage of merchandise exports) against a low share of manufactured exports. In 2003, the primary export rate was particularly high in Azerbaijan (93 per cent) and Kazakhstan (82 per cent), ranged from 60 to 70 per cent in Moldova, Kyrgyzstan and the Russian Federation, and was over 30 per cent in most of the other CIS countries (United Nations Development Programme, 2005). In the absence of structural change and economic restructuring and diversification, including the expansion of the service sector, there are fewer opportunities for job creation. Whereas economic growth is a prerequisite for sustaining youth employment, the quality of that growth is equally crucial. For instance, the "jobless growth" that has been observed in several countries in the region by definition cannot alleviate the plight of young job seekers.

Figure 6.1

Per capita GDP and real GDP growth since 1989 in Eastern Europe and the CIS countries (1989 GDP level = 100)

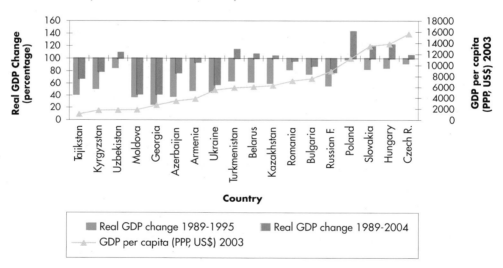

Source: United Nations Children's Fund, TransMONEE database (2005) (available from http://www.unicef-icdc.org/database).

Youth unemployment represents only one element of overall high aggregate unemployment and very low job creation, and it should be addressed holistically in the context of the wider "employment challenge" facing the entire economy and working population.

Although fluctuations in GDP levels reveal an important macroeconomic dimension, they do not tell the whole story of the transition. In many countries, the economic decline coincided with a substantial erosion of human capital as measured, for instance, by the Human Development Index (HDI) (United Nations Development Programme, 1998). As shown in figure 6.2, between 1985 and 2003, the position of countries in Eastern Europe and the CIS remained roughly the same or worsened, particularly in the early phase of the transition. Although certain social indicators remained quite strong in some countries, new challenges emerged. For example, obtaining a quality education became harder for many youth. This was primarily because education expenditures declined, falling by almost 20 per cent in Central Europe and by even more in some lower-income CIS countries. An inferior education creates a disadvantage for young people in the labour market, contributing to the difficulties in finding a decent first job. Health expenditures declined as well, falling by an average 30 per cent, and work-related benefits and social support systems were also scaled back (United Nations Development Programme, 2005; Simai, 2006). Difficulties in financing and maintaining social service delivery networks affected the quality and efficiency of the services provided, with a negative impact on health, education, and overall living conditions (Alam and others, 2005). Reduced access to and utilization of social services at the initial stage of the transition inevitably affected the well-being and development of young people.

Figure 6.2
Changes in the Human Development Index (HDI) in Eastern Europe and the CIS, 1985-2003

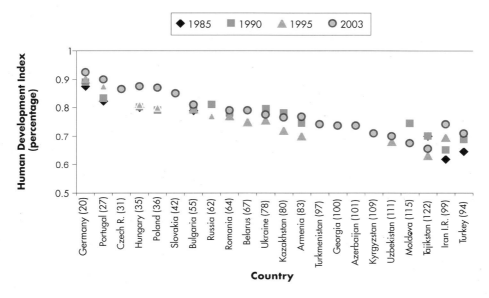

Source: United Nations Development Programme, *Human Development Report 2005—International Cooperation at a Crossroads: Aid, Trade and Security in an Unequal World* (New York).
Note: The HDI country ranking for 2003 is in parentheses.

Transitional labour markets are marked by the emergence of new opportunities, prospects and hopes, on the one hand, and by a decreasing demand for labour, higher levels of joblessness, and spells of long-term unemployment, on the other hand. These factors affect young people's transition to adulthood and represent a serious challenge for society and its stability. New windows of opportunity are important, and quite often new chances are seized by young people, but such opportunities are limited and may not compensate for the risks associated with substantially decreased social protection. The inability to find a job carries psychological costs, causes frustration and depression, and undermines motivation. Youth unemployment is also often associated with such social problems as violence, delinquency, alcohol and drug abuse, crime, and suicide (UNICEF Innocenti Research Centre, 2000).

In many cases, prolonged schooling has been used as a "safety valve" to cushion the negative impact of joblessness, effectively removing young people from the labour force, at least temporarily; others have withdrawn from the labour market after periods of unemployment, having given up hope of finding work in the formal economy. The inclusion among the officially unemployed of those young men and women who are no longer looking for a job would raise unemployment rates among youth considerably. The proportion of jobless youth who do not report looking for work is particularly high in those countries and regions in which the informal economy seems to be thriving (La Cava and others, 2004).

THE PERSISTENCE OF YOUTH UNEMPLOYMENT AND UNDEREMPLOYMENT

The emergence of youth unemployment as a persistent phenomenon is a new feature of the post-socialist era. The lack of jobs for young people figures prominently among the major social issues facing all economies in transition. As table 6.1 illustrates, the increase in youth unemployment from 1993 to 2003 in economies in transition surpassed the world average. The overall youth unemployment rate of 18.6 per cent for 2003 masks even higher rates for individual countries; in Bulgaria, the Czech Republic, Estonia, Latvia and Poland, for example, youth unemployment exceeded 20 per cent during the period 2002-2004 (European Foundation for the Improvement of Living and Working Conditions, 2007).

Table 6.1
Youth unemployment rates in economies in transition, 1993-2003

Region	Youth unemployment rate (percentage of labour force)		
	1993	2003	Change (percentage)
Economies in transition	14.9	18.6	+24.8
Developed market economies	15.4	13.4	-13.0
World average	11.7	14.4	+23.1

Source: International Labour Office, *Global Employment Trends for Youth 2004 (Geneva: International Labour Organization*, August 2004).

In the early stage of the transition, the youth unemployment rate was comparable to that of the developed market economies, but between 1993 and 2003 the situation changed drastically. During this period, the rate of youth unemployment declined by 13 per cent in the developed market economies but rose by almost 25 per cent in the economies in transition; by 2003, there was a differential of 5.2 percentage points between the two regions (see table 6.1).

The youth unemployment rate is an important indicator, but it does not reflect the complete set of employment challenges confronting young people. The duration of unemployment, for example, is a very important indicator as well, since longer spells of unemployment may be detrimental to a job search. A brief period without work may be considered a natural consequence of the desire to find an appropriate job, but the job-search period can be much longer when the labour market is not robust (International Labour Office, 2006). The interval of unemployment during the transition from school to work can be long in some countries, often exceeding six months (O'Higgins, 2003).

Data reliability is an extremely important factor in any analysis of the youth labour market in economies in transition. Data require careful interpretation; the standard and public statistics are based on definitions that are sensitive to irregularities. For example, under-employment is often disguised, translating into higher rates of employment and lower rates of unemployment (Brown and others, 2006; Godfrey, 2003; Kolev and Saget, 2005). In a number of countries, the (statistically) high level of employment reflects a failed or incomplete transition from a planned economy to a market economy, often masking serious underemployment.[1]

The ratio of youth to adult unemployment in the region generally ranges between 2 and 3. The fluctuations in this figure reveal a strong link between the youth labour market and general labour market situations. Though the overall ratio for the economies in transition may be similar to that for the developed market economies, the consistently higher overall unemployment rate in the former means that joblessness among youth sometimes reaches dramatic levels (Rutkowski and Scarpetta, 2005). Young people in economies in transition are disproportionately represented among new labour market entrants. Difficulties in effecting the transition from school to work reinforce the disadvantages faced by youth.

The incidence of poverty remains significantly higher among unemployed youth than among others of the same age. Children living in households with unemployed parents are more likely to experience unemployment themselves (Commander and Bornhorst, 2004), which vividly illustrates the negative impact of unemployment on the general population. Low family income often forces children to enter the labour market at a relatively young age, seeking any job they can get. Unemployed youth are often pushed to find work in the informal economy, where their situation may not improve significantly even though they are working (Godfrey, 2003; O'Higgins, 2003; Kolev and Saget, 2005). Poverty among youth who are working, whether in the formal or the informal economy, is widespread in the region and by implication is closely associated with social exclusion. In the economic and social domains, many youth in the region have become marginalized. Unemployment is contributing to risky behaviour among youth, including unsafe sex and drug abuse. The socio-economic implications of these conditions are serious, including potentially costly health crises and the transmission of poverty to the next generation.

The challenges of finding a new job

Job prospects for young people are strongly connected to the general labour market situation and a country's overall economic prospects. In spite of the economic recovery that occurred in most economies in transition following the initial transitional recession, employment prospects have been quite dim. Those who have been able to adjust to the new demands of the labour market have benefited from new opportunities, though many have floundered, even in those countries that are more advanced in their market-driven restructuring. As the total number of jobs has decreased, finding a first job and entering the labour market has become increasingly difficult across the board. Between 1996 and 2005, the youth employment rate decreased in most Eastern European countries (see figure 6.3). Job prospects for youth largely depend on the stage of economic reform, and then on the structure of the labour market. Youth in countries that have experienced a protracted recession remain particularly disadvantaged, as they have few chances for a solid start and are likely to face serious difficulties in obtaining a decent job and a steady legal income.

Figure 6.3
Employment rate for youth in Eastern Europe (as a percentage of the population aged 15-24 years), 1996-2005

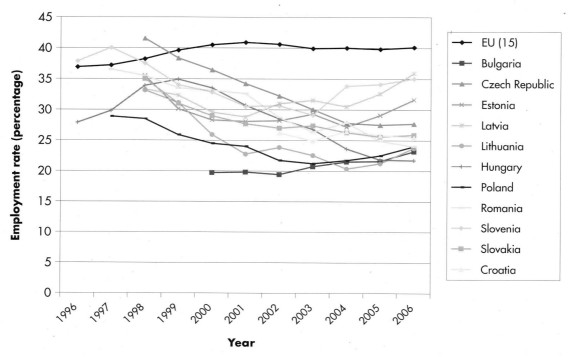

Source: Compiled from Eurostat online data, based on labour market surveys (available from http://epp.eurostat.ec.europa.eu; accessed on 16 August 2007).

Note: Employment rates represent employed persons as a percentage of the same-age total population. Employed persons are those aged 15 years and over who, during the reference week, performed work, even if just one hour per week, for pay, profit or family gain, or were not at work but had a job or business from which they were temporarily absent because of illness, a holiday, an industrial dispute, education/training, or other such reasons.

Serious job losses accompanied economic restructuring, which included widespread privatization and the closing of unprofitable enterprises in most countries of the region. New jobs were created at a much slower rate and within a different structure, in information and communication technology and other high-tech industries, and in services, trade and the banking sector (Kőrösi, 2005). A large share of the people who lost their jobs remained unemployed for an extended period, sometimes with little hope of ever finding a new job. Most of the unemployed workers had a low level of education or had attended vocational schools, a prevalent form of education all over the region, where training was narrow in focus and limited to fit the demands of the centrally planned economies. A large proportion of these people dropped out of the labour market, retired early, or lived on various kinds of social benefits, while others engaged in various informal economic activities.

Where there are insufficient employment opportunities, young people may also give up hope of ever finding a job and drop out of the labour force altogether. According to the International Labour Office, the most worrisome increase in the proportion of young people who are not in employment, education or training (also known as the NEET rate) has occurred in Central and Eastern Europe. The high prevalence (33.6 per cent) of youth who are not in school and not employed is a good indicator of the non-utilized potential of the young labour force and of the level of discouragement among youth in the region. The International Labour Office considers discouragement the most "damaging" reason for inactivity. In countries recovering from conflict, such as Croatia and Bosnia and Herzegovina, youth are likely to experience frustration that may lead to destructive behaviour (International Labour Office, 2006).

During the post-communist transition (1993-1999) in Hungary, capital investment in new sectors largely displaced unskilled labour, but for younger and older skilled workers job prospects were somewhat better, with young people often enjoying an advantage (Kertesi and Köllő, 2002). Youth with qualifications similar to those of older workers were expected to do well in training programmes, take part in on-the-job training, and become valued employees, especially in large foreign-based companies. Transnational companies and banks, large retailers, and fast-food chains often preferred to hire youth. In some of the other economies in transition, such as the Czech Republic and Poland, the replacement of older workers with younger workers was less vigorous but still significant.

Forms of employment

Eastern Europe and the CIS experienced the process of transition and adjustment to various economic shocks very differently. In the former, economic shocks led to a decline in employment, while in the latter, by and large, wages fell sharply in conjunction with a dramatic increase in underemployment. At the beginning of the transition the contribution of services to GDP was relatively low across the region, but the situation changed over time. As the process of restructuring unfolded in Central and Eastern Europe, new jobs were created in the service sector, and the sectoral distribution of employment shifted, sometimes providing additional opportunities for youth. Between 1990 and 2001, the share of the service sector in GDP grew significantly (by over 10 percentage points) in Azerbaijan, Bulgaria, the Czech Republic, Kazakhstan, Poland and the Russian Federation (International Labour Office, 2004). In some countries in the region, however, labour shifted back to subsistence agriculture, with little room for the creation of decent jobs for youth. Employment in the large informal economy, which is mainly driven by insufficient job opportunities in the formal economy, constitutes a last resort in the survival strategy of the population, including youth. Young people living in depressed regions have been at a disadvantage. In many rural areas, new investment has been rare, and in small settlements the only jobs available have been in local government and public services, and these are usually taken by older workers.

Self-employment has emerged as an important alternative for young people. Though new ventures may sometimes be developed as a response to prolonged unemployment, they can survive and even be transformed into prosperous businesses. In many countries of the region, successful new ventures have been undertaken in the service sector, including software development and design and other ICT-based activities. Establishing such enterprises in the larger metropolitan areas has facilitated their success and further growth. However, not all types of self-employment are equally prosperous. In the Central Asian CIS countries and in the Caucasus, many are "own-account" workers, functioning as independent contractors with no long-term employees; such self-employment often demands long hours, produces a relatively small income, and is carried out partly or mostly in the informal sector. Young people often participate in family-based economic activities, engaging in various forms of street trading or small-scale agriculture, running small shops, or providing personal services. Sometimes, self-employment is de facto confined to the informal economy owing to a lack of legal employment opportunities elsewhere. Small-scale entrepreneurs often feel that they need to succeed quickly, fearing that the development of their enterprises will be adversely affected by changes in the political and economic environment. Self-employed youth are in a vulnerable position in the labour market, as they are typically ineligible for unemployment insurance or social assistance.

Owing to insufficient formal employment opportunities, youth are disproportionately represented in the informal economy (Rutkowski and Scarpetta, 2005; Godfrey, 2003), where they may be compelled to accept inferior working conditions. Estimates on the size and importance of the informal economy in the region indicate that the share of the working-age population engaged in informal employment is quite high. Such activity is particularly prevalent in the Caucasus; in Georgia and Azerbaijan, around half of the working-age population participates in the informal economy, compared with about 40 per cent in most of the remaining CIS countries. In the Asian CIS countries, a third of the working-age population is involved in informal activities. There is also a sizeable informal economy in the new European Union member countries. In Romania almost one fourth, in Bulgaria one third, and in Poland and Hungary around one fifth of the working-age population is engaged in informal work (Schneider, 2002; Schneider and Klinglmair, 2004).

The main reasons for young people's participation in the informal economy include the dearth of formal sector jobs, the increased competition for a limited number of vacancies, and the lack of social networks and skills for marketing oneself to potential employers (International Labour Office, 2006). In countries without adequate unemployment benefits and social protection systems, youth are willing to accept poor-quality jobs that offer little or no security. Participation in the informal economy represents an employment option of last resort in the CIS countries. Conversely, in Eastern Europe, formal employment is less attractive because of the high tax burden and the relative lack of employment opportunities. Informal activities offer some relief but do not constitute a permanent solution; they often mitigate, but do not necessarily prevent, income poverty.

Underemployment

Underemployment is difficult to document, as it is often linked to part-time work, and survey results do not indicate whether individuals in such circumstances hold part-time jobs or have been forced to work less, with lower pay, because of employers' economic difficulties (Cazes and Nesporova, 2004). In some cases, the decision to work part-time is voluntary, but when it is not, it can jeopardize a person's income, social protection coverage, and overall well-being. Forced breaks in work and administrative leaves have been common, especially in the CIS, and a similar situation prevailed in the Eastern European economies during the first years of the transition.

Most of the labour market reforms in the economies in transition have centered around liberalizing temporary contracts by extending the maximum duration of fixed-term contracts or by legalizing temporary work agencies. Many of the Eastern European economies in transition have made their labour markets more flexible by reducing restrictions on temporary employment, with more modest reductions in the protection of permanent workers (Rutkowski and Scarpetta, 2005). In many of the economies in transition, the growing acceptance of "alternative" arrangements such as temporary and part-time work derives from the inability of job-seekers to find permanent full-time employment. Research undertaken during the early part of the present decade indicated that while the proportion of employees in flexible positions in the economies in transition was below that prevailing in the European Union, the reverse was true with respect to involuntary part-time work. The share of employees with involuntary fixed-term (limited as opposed to permanent) contracts was even higher in the economies in transition (Employment in Europe, 2002).

Another type of underemployment is linked to the mismatch of skills. Because jobs in their fields of study or specialization are unavailable, young people often accept positions in which they are unable to make full use of their capabilities (International Labour Office, 2006). Though it is often said that skill or knowledge deficits make it more difficult to find a job, this is not always the case. In Eastern European and CIS countries, young people may be overqualified for certain positions. However, because they do not wish to endure long periods of unemployment, they accept work that does not correspond to their educational and skill levels; this constitutes one form of underemployment. Education can be a "boon or a hindrance" depending on the economic status of the country (International Labour Office, 2006).

Disadvantaged youth in search of livelihoods

Labour market disadvantages are not distributed evenly among all young people. Rates of unemployment are higher among youth with disabilities and ethnic minorities living in geographically or economically disadvantaged regions than among the general youth population. Youth unemployment rates are dramatically higher for those with low levels of educational attainment; in most cases, young people with less than an upper secondary education are more likely to be unemployed than those with upper secondary or higher educational qualifications. Young people who have an upper secondary education but lack vocational skills, however, are in a similarly disadvantaged situation.

Socio-economic background is an important factor in determining the likelihood of a young person remaining in school or dropping out early, though relevant indicators vary widely from one country to another. Eurostat surveys for the European Union (15) show that young people leaving education at an early stage usually have parents with low levels of education, and the corresponding share of early drop-outs is even higher in Eastern Europe (similar to Southern Europe) (Iannelli, 2003). In Hungary, one in three (and in Romania, one in two) young people who leave school early have parents with low levels of education. The probability of unqualified youth becoming unemployed is high, and the likelihood of their breaking the intergenerational cycle of low educational attainment is low.

The relationship between parental education and the occupational standing of young people in their first significant job was analysed using the PISA International Socio-Economic Index of Occupational Status indicator. Throughout Europe, a young person's social background is a strong predictor of his or her occupational status: the higher the parents' educational attainment, the higher the children's occupational status (Iannelli, 2003). In Hungary, the situation of the Roma is a case in point. Roma youth suffer from multiple disadvantages owing to low levels of education and discrimination in both schooling and employment. These children may grow up in a family or a community setting where regular patterns of employment are not prevalent, since most or all of the local working-age population live on welfare benefits and/or engage in informal activities. These young people do not have a chance to observe a routine associated with regular work in the formal economy and often do not feel the need to have a regular job (Kertesi, 2004; Kertesi and Kézdi, 2005).

Changing patterns of education and labour market prospects

The share of young people attending school and the number of years they stay in school have an impact on the labour force participation rate of youth. Before the transition, primary and secondary school enrolment was very high, with literacy rates of 99 per cent in every country. During the transition there was an alarmingly sharp drop in primary school enrolment, particularly in the poorer CIS countries and those experiencing civil conflict. Primary school enrolment decreased significantly in Moldova, Tajikistan, Armenia, Georgia and Turkmenistan (World Bank, 2003). The primary school drop-out rate was also high in Bulgaria and Romania. In Central Europe enrolment generally remained high, though in some countries children belonging to ethnic minorities (such as the Roma) often dropped out of school, left school early, or avoided it altogether (Kertesi, 2004). The effective exclusion of these groups made it more difficult for them to enter the labour market, increasing their prospects for long-term unemployment.

The changes occurring in secondary enrolment during the transition are shown in figure 6.4. Before the transition, many of the secondary schools were vocational schools training young people to meet the needs of the socialist economy. Many young people between the ages of 15 and 18 acquired skills that were not marketable in the new demand-driven economy. Because of the restructuring of the education system and shifts in enrolment patterns, the proportion of children in school declined in some parts of the region, especially in the age group 15-18 (see figure 6.4). Although a number of changes have been introduced in secondary education, the old system of vocational training (with its various inefficiencies) still exists.

Figure 6.4
Economies in transition: Gross secondary and vocational/technical school enrolment in selected countries, 1989-2003

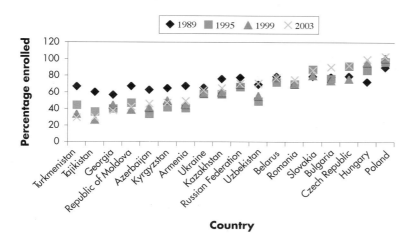

Source: United Nations Children's Fund, TransMONEE database (2005) (available from http://www.unicef-icdc.org/database).
Note: The data reflect all enrolments in the given year.

In contrast to secondary school enrolment, there has been no drop in higher-education enrolment in most of the economies in transition. At the beginning of the transition, 10 to 20 per cent of 19- to 24-year-olds were enrolled in higher education throughout the region. In Eastern Europe and most of the CIS countries, enrolment in higher education has increased—somewhat slowly at the beginning of the transition and more rapidly in recent years. In Poland and Hungary, gross enrolment ratios have increased to more than 50 per cent. In other countries, between 30 and 40 per cent of the young adult population are pursuing higher studies (see figure 6.5). The only countries in which the share of the youth population enrolled in higher education has dropped are Armenia, Tajikistan, Turkmenistan and Uzbekistan.

Figure 6.5

Economies in transition: gross higher education enrolment in selected countries, 1989-2003

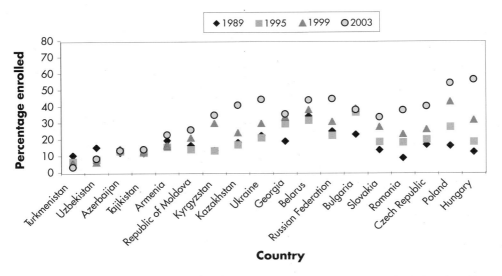

Source: United Nations Children's Fund, TransMONEE database (2005) (available from http://www.unicef-icdc.org/database).
Note: The data reflect all enrolments in the given year as a percentage of the population aged 19-24.

The share of young women in tertiary education has increased in many countries of the region and now exceeds that of young men. The gross enrolment ratio for female youth in tertiary education has almost doubled in the past five years. This increase may reflect the fact that some youth, especially young women, tend to "wait" in the education system, postponing the school-to-work transition in the hope that eventually the economy will improve to a point where decent jobs become more available (International Labour Office, 2006).

Substantial problems exist in the education and training systems across the region. A mismatch between labour market needs and graduate qualifications is evident in many of the economies in transition. Those leaving school without marketable skills may have a relatively hard time securing their first job; those hoping to improve their chances of finding employment may have to take retraining courses. Many vocational schools have not changed significantly since the socialist era, and youth coming out of these institutions tend to have limited opportunities in the emerging labour markets. In the short run, the new system of social support for the unemployed may help young people.

Higher-education enrolment effectively removes young people from the labour market, at least temporarily, decreasing the share of unemployed youth. Returns on investments in education have been improving in general, though many graduates face an uncertain job market. For some, higher education enhances job prospects in the long run; however, the influx of large numbers of highly qualified young people into the labour market may translate into high rates of unemployment and/or underemployment, particularly during periods of slow growth and limited job creation. In Hungary, the sharp increase in the proportion of youth in higher education led to a heated debate on the capacity of the market to absorb qualified young people and the possible need to forecast the flows of such youth into the labour market.

Wages

Another important policy issue in the economies in transition is minimum wage, including a sub-minimum wage for youth. The effect of minimum wage regulations on youth employment is a major concern in the region, even though the question is not new and there is no clear empirical evidence relating to the subject. Some researchers contend that minimum wages have stronger disemployment effects (disincentive effects on employment) in disadvantaged poor areas and among the low-skilled. They refer to international evidence showing that high national minimum wages negatively affect employment prospects for low-productivity workers, youth with little labour market experience, and workers with low skills and in remote regions (Rutkowsky and Scarpetta, 2005).

The above notwithstanding, country-specific evidence and equity considerations cannot be disregarded when taking policy decisions. In Poland, a sub-minimum wage for young people has been introduced as a means to expand youth employment. By offering wage incentives for young workers in economically depressed regions, authorities in Poland hope to promote job creation for those youth who are hardest hit by unemployment. So far, the country's sub-minimum wage (80 per cent of the regular minimum wage) has proved effective in reducing youth unemployment. Further reform efforts in this area may be desirable. One important consideration is that social benefit programmes are often tied to the minimum wage (that is, they are relatively high when the minimum wage is relatively high), which creates disincentives to work (Rutkowsky and Scarpetta, 2005).

NEW VULNERABILITIES: SUBSTANCE ABUSE AND THE SPREAD OF HIV/AIDS AMONG YOUTH

Further complicating the development of youth in Eastern Europe and the CIS is the fact that the region has the fastest-growing HIV/AIDS epidemic in the world, with young people accounting for over half of all new infections (Joint United Nations Programme on HIV/AIDS, 2005).[2] Existing data on HIV/AIDS prevalence among youth are incomplete. In particular, prevalence estimates for youth aged 15-24 years are often not provided on a country-by-country basis for Eastern Europe and the CIS, and descriptive statistics tend to refer to different age groups, such as "people under 30" (Joint United Nations Programme on HIV/AIDS, 2006b).

Though not comprehensive, the statistics that are available strongly indicate that the overwhelming majority (more than 80 per cent) of people living with HIV/AIDS in Eastern Europe and the CIS countries are under the age of age 30 (United Nations Children's Fund, 2004). In Ukraine, 25 per cent of those diagnosed with HIV are under 20 years of age. In Belarus, 60 per cent of those diagnosed are aged 15-24 years, and in both Kazakhstan and Kyrgyzstan approximately 70 per cent are under 30 (Joint United Nations Programme on

HIV/AIDS, 2005). In the Russian Federation, there were more than 50,000 new HIV infections among young people 15-24 years old in 2001, compared with close to zero in 1995 (Joint United Nations Programme on HIV/AIDS, Inter-agency Task Team on Young People, 2004). Table 6.2 provides estimates of the numbers of people living with HIV in Eastern European and CIS countries. In some of the countries with relatively low prevalence rates, the incidence of HIV infection has been extremely high during the past few years. In Azerbaijan and Tajikistan, the numbers of people living with HIV almost quadrupled between 2003 and 2005, rising from 1,400 to 5,400 in the former and from 1,300 to 4,900 in the latter. During the same period, the number doubled in Georgia (from 2,800 to 5,600) and almost tripled in Uzbekistan (from 11,000 to 31,000) (Joint United Nations Programme on HIV/AIDS, 2006b).

Table 6.2
Estimated numbers and proportions of people living with HIV in Eastern Europe and the CIS

Country	Number of Adults 15 years and older (2003)		Percentage of Adults 15-49 years (2003)		Number of Adults 15 years and older (2005)		Percentage of Adults 15-49 years (2005)	
	Estimate	Low-high estimates	Estimate	Low-high estimates	Estimate	Low-high estimates	Estimate	Low-high estimates
Albania	..	..	..	..	..	..	..	<0.2
Armenia	2 600	1 700–3 900	0.1	0.1 - 0.2	2 900	1 800–5 800	0.1	0.1 – 0.6
Azerbaijan	1 400	680–4 600	<0.1	<0.2	5 400	2 600–17 000	0.1	0.1 – 0.4
Belarus	18 000	9 700–44 000	0.3	0.2 – 0.8	20 000	11 000–47 000	0.3	0.2 – 0.8
Bosnia and Herzegovina	..	..	..	..	..	..	<0.1	<0.2
Bulgaria	..	..	..	..	..	..	<0.1	<0.2
Croatia	..	..	..	..	..	..	<0.1	<0.2
Czech Republic	1 500	900–2 500	<0.1	<0.2	1 500	900–2 500	0.1	<0.2
Estonia	8 600	4 100–28 000	1.1	0.5 – 3.7	10 000	4 800–32 000	1.3	0.6 – 4.3
Georgia	2 800	1 500–4 800	0.1	0.1 – 0.2	5 600	2 700–18 000	0.2	0.1 – 2.7
Hungary	3 000	1 800 – 5 000	0.1	<0.2	3 200	1 900–5 300	0.1	<0.2
Kazakhstan	10 000	9 000–33 000	0.1	0.1 – 0.4	12 000	11 000 – 76 000	0.1	0.1. – 3.2
Kyrgyzstan	1 100	<2 000	<0.1	<0.2	4 000	1 900 – 13 000	0.1	0.1. – 1.7
Latvia	7 400	4 500–12 000	0.6	0.3 – 1.0	10 000	6 100 – 17 000	0.8	0.5 – 1.3
Lithuania	1 300	640–4 300	0.1	<0.1–0.2	3 300	1 600 – 11 000	0.2	0.1. – 0.6
Moldova	23 000	12 000–56 000	0.9	0.5 – 2.2	28 000	15 000 – 69 000	1.1	0.6 - 2.6

Country	Number of Adults 15 years and older (2003)		Percentage of Adults 15-49 years (2003)		Number of Adults 15 years and older (2005)		Percentage of Adults 15-49 years (2005)	
	Estimate	Low-high estimates	Estimate	Low-high estimates	Estimate	Low-high estimates	Estimate	Low-high estimates
Poland	25 000	15 000–42 000	0.1	0.1 – 0.2	25 000	15 000–42 000	0.1	0.1– 0.2
Romania	..	..	..	..	..	..	<0.1	<0.2
Russian Federation	760 000	450 000–1 300 000	0.9	0.5 – 1.5	940 000	560 000–1 600 000	1.1	0.7 - 1.8
Serbia and Montenegro	9 000	5 400–15 000	0.2	0.1 – 0.3	10 000	6 000–17 000	0.2	0.1 - 0.3
Slovakia	<500	<1 000	<0.1	<0.2	<500	<1 000	<0.1	<0.2
Tajikistan	1 300	700–2 300	<0.1	<0.2	4 900	2 300–16 000	0.1	0.1. - 1.7
Turkmenistan	..	..	..	..	<500	<1 000	<0.1	<0.2
Ukraine	380 000	240 000–540 000	1.3	0.8 – 1.9	410 000	250 000–680 000	1.4	0.8 - 4.3
Uzbekistan	11 000	5 400–36 000	0.1	<0.1– 0.3	31 000	15 000–100 000	0.2	0.1 - 0.7
The former Yugoslav Republic of Macedonia	<500	<1 000	<0.1	<0.1– 0.3	<500	<1 000	<0.1	<0.2

Source: Joint United Nations Programme on HIV/AIDS, *2006 Report on the Global AIDS Epidemic* (Geneva: 2006), annex 2: HIV and AIDS estimates and data, 2003 and 2005.

Notes: Two dots (..) indicate that an item is not available or is not separately reported. The low and high estimates reflect the range in which the correct estimate is expected to fall.

Injecting opiates such as heroin from contaminated needles, syringes or other drug injection paraphernalia is the chief mode of HIV transmission in the countries of Eastern Europe and the CIS; injecting drug users account for more than 70 per cent of HIV cases in the region. Young people under the age of 20 are believed to comprise up to 25 per cent of those who inject drugs in the economies in transition (Joint United Nations Programme on HIV/AIDS, Inter-agency Task Team on Young People, 2004). In some countries, such as Latvia and the Russian Federation, youth appear to constitute the majority of injecting drug users (Aceijas and others, 2006). In the Russian Federation, young people under 30 years of age account for 80 per cent of HIV cases deriving from injecting drug use (Joint United Nations Programme on HIV/AIDS, 2004).

Injecting drug use is a relatively new phenomenon in the countries of Eastern Europe and the CIS, and youth are being exposed to trafficked drugs. Drug use began escalating in the region during the severe socio-economic crisis immediately following the collapse of communism and the break-up of the Soviet Union. It has continued to increase within the context of profound social changes and economic hardships, including the transition to a market economy, high unemployment (especially among youth), widening inequalities, and increased insecurity. The economic hardships highlighted in the first part of this chapter have been especially difficult for young people, many of whom are failing to complete secondary school and/or are among the growing ranks of the poor and jobless. These circum-

stances, along with other factors such as the breakdown of the family, emotional distur-
bances, and peer pressure or adherence to group norms (such as drug use) make youth
more vulnerable to injecting drug use, placing them at a higher risk of becoming infected
with HIV.

There has also been a consolidation of transnational drug trafficking as the region has
been integrated into international drug trafficking routes and inundated with opium-based
drugs such as heroin. Several of the Central Asian republics (Azerbaijan, Kazakhstan,
Kyrgyzstan, Tajikistan, Turkmenistan and Uzbekistan) are in close proximity to Afghanistan,
which, during the period of profound transformation in the economies in transition,
emerged as the world's largest grower of opium poppies, accounting for three quarters of
global production (World Bank, 2005a; International Harm Reduction Development
Program, 2006). These countries straddle major drug trafficking routes into the Russian
Federation and Europe; in some parts of this area, heroin is believed to be cheaper than
alcohol (Joint United Nations Programme on HIV/AIDS, 2004a).

The transmission of HIV/AIDS among young injecting drug users

The sharing of needles and syringes, which is the norm among injecting drug users in
Eastern Europe and CIS countries, is the cause of much of the HIV transmission within this
group. The practice is particularly common in prisons throughout the region. Research in
the Russian Federation indicates that many young people are incarcerated for drug use and
continue sharing needles in jail, spreading HIV (World Bank, 2005a).

The burgeoning sex trade in the region is also a matter of concern within the present
context. Risky sexual behaviour often accompanies injecting drug use, greatly increasing
the risk of HIV infection. The prevalence of sexually transmitted infections is generally high
among drug users, reflecting a strong tendency to engage in risky sexual behaviour. Young
women having unprotected sex with injecting drug users account for an increasing share of
those newly diagnosed with HIV. Young women may also contract HIV from casual or regular male sexual partners who are infected as a result of injecting drug use.

Although condoms offer protection from sexually transmitted HIV infection, rates of
use are generally low among youth in the region. In the Russian Federation, one survey
found that fewer than half of young people between the ages of 16 and 20 used condoms
when having sex with casual partners. Among injecting drug users, consistent condom use
averages less than 20 per cent (Joint United Nations Programme on HIV/AIDS, 2004).

In several countries, including Kazakhstan, Ukraine and Uzbekistan, the significant
overlap between injecting drug use and sex work is fuelling the heterosexual transmission
of HIV and contributing substantially to the countries' growing HIV epidemics. Most who
enter sex work do so in their teens or early twenties. It is estimated that in Eastern Europe
and Central Asia, 80 per cent of sex workers are under the age of 25. There are also indications that sex workers who inject drugs may be younger than those who do not. A study
in St. Petersburg, Russian Federation, found that 33 per cent of sex workers under 19 years
of age tested positive for HIV (Joint United Nations Programme on HIV/AIDS, 2006b).
Condom use among sex workers in the region is seldom reported to be higher than 50 per
cent (Joint United Nations Programme on HIV/AIDS, 2004).

Another factor affecting heterosexual transmission, particularly the rising incidence of HIV infection among young women, is the increase in labour migration. A sizeable and largely female mobile workforce has emerged in the informal economy; growing numbers of women are migrating in search of work. In addition, while the prevalence of injecting drug use among women is still relatively low, the numbers have risen significantly during the past decade. Young women are included in the increasing feminization of the epidemic in some countries; in the Russian Federation, among the newly reported HIV cases in 2004, there were more young women between the ages of 15 and 20 who had become infected than young men of the same age group (Joint United Nations Programme on HIV/AIDS and World Health Organization, 2005).

It should also be noted that the data on HIV prevalence only reflect the situation of those people and groups (such as injecting drug users) that have been tested. It is possible that there are "hidden" epidemics among persons or groups that are not regularly tested, such as men who have sex with men. Such sexual activity is severely stigmatized across the region and is not commonly talked about or acknowledged. Consequently, there are not much data or information about HIV prevalence rates among this group. Very limited data indicate, however, that there is cause for concern. In Odessa, Ukraine, 7 of 25 men who had had sex with men and were tested were found to be HIV-positive, as were 2 of the 22 men tested in Mykolaiv, Ukraine (Joint United Nations Programme on HIV/AIDS and World Health Organization, 2005).

Consequences for the lives of young people

The HIV/AIDS epidemic has had a broad impact on youth and society in Eastern Europe and the CIS. At the individual level, young people experience deep trauma when they are infected with HIV early on in their lives. HIV diagnosis and AIDS-related illness also has an enormous impact on the family and household.

The rapid spread of HIV/AIDS in Eastern Europe and the CIS, particularly among young people, also has important implications for the labour force and for society as a whole. The epidemic, which now affects mainly young injecting drug users, might become generalized among the population in several countries or across the region. The personal emotional and financial burden and the collective social and economic costs of such an epidemic would be quite high (United Nations Office on Drugs and Crime, 2003). Clearly, the stakes are high in the struggle to combat HIV/AIDS and injecting drug use among youth in the region.

Social exclusion is a major negative social consequence of HIV/AIDS—and perhaps a contributor as well. In Eastern Europe and the CIS, those with the highest likelihood of exposure—young injecting drug users, sex workers (including youth), prison inmates and, possibly, men who have sex with men—are often at the margins of society and are vulnerable to stigmatization, discrimination and social exclusion, which may include limited access to health services. It is asserted that one factor undermining efforts to prevent HIV/AIDS in the region is the overall state of denial and complacency with regard to HIV and drug abuse at all levels and the general stigmatization and marginalization of drug users and their families (United Nations Office for Drug Control and Crime Prevention, 2001). Fear, stigma and discrimination discourage those affected by HIV/AIDS from seeking treatment and assistance, and contribute to further social exclusion.

There is evidence that Governments and civil society institutions in Eastern Europe and the CIS are becoming more strongly committed to combating the growing HIV/AIDS epidemic (Piot, 2006). Effective political leadership is essential within this context, and efforts to address the crisis are being intensified at the highest levels, particularly in the Russian Federation and Ukraine, the two largest and most severely affected countries in the region. The Russian Federation has significantly increased its financial commitment to AIDS programmes and has indicated that it will embark on an urgent programme to fight the epidemic. In the Ukraine, the President has taken personal responsibility for the national response to AIDS, and the Ukrainian National Coordination Council on HIV and AIDS has been touted as a model for the engagement of all government sectors and civil society in the fight against this major threat (Kallings, 2006).

COMBATING THE SPREAD OF HIV/AIDS AND CONFRONTING INJECTING DRUG USE AMONG YOUTH: PREVENTION AND TREATMENT

Since youth are at the centre of the HIV/AIDS epidemic in Eastern Europe and the CIS and make up a significant portion of the injecting drug user population, they must be a major focus of prevention and treatment policies, programmes and activities.

Prevention efforts among youth are essential for containing and reversing the current HIV/AIDS trends in Eastern Europe and the CIS. Information and education on the risks of HIV and how it is transmitted must be provided to young people, particularly those in high-risk groups. Knowledge is the starting point for reducing the incidence of HIV. Youth who are or will be sexually active need accurate information on how to prevent the sexual transmission of HIV, and youth who are or will be injecting drugs need to understand the importance of using clean needles and know how to obtain sterile injecting equipment. This and other relevant information is often not available to young people in the region; those materials that are available are seldom written specifically for a younger audience, rendering them less effective in educating youth.

Targeted school-based programmes can play a critical role in HIV prevention. School attendance enables students to benefit from integrated HIV/AIDS awareness and sexuality education. Higher levels of educational attainment are associated with safer sexual behaviour and delayed first sexual intercourse. A general finding from outside Eastern Europe and CIS is that young people's risk of HIV infection is closely correlated with the age of sexual initiation. The percentage of young women and young men who have had sex before the age of 15 is one of five new core indicators for generalized epidemics (Joint United Nations Programme on HIV/AIDS, 2006b). Abstinence and delayed sexual initiation are among the central strategies for preventing HIV infection among young people (Joint United Nations Programme on HIV/AIDS, 2006b). The limited information available within the region indicates that 29 per cent of all youth in Moldova, 13 per cent of all youth in the

Russian Federation, and 1 per cent of female youth aged 15-19 years in Azerbaijan reported having had sex before the age of 15 (Joint United Nations Programme on HIV/AIDS 2006b). It should be noted that because the prevalence of HIV in the region is strongly linked to injecting drug use, school-based HIV prevention programmes must include a strong focus on education about injecting drug use and its link to HIV transmission.

In Eastern Europe and the CIS, 40 per cent of in-school youth have access to HIV prevention education, but the same is true for only 3 per cent of out-of-school youth (United Nations Population Fund, 2006). Statistics from 2003 revealed wide intraregional disparities in the prevalence of schools with teachers who had been trained in life-skills-based HIV education and who had taught it during the previous year at the secondary level; individual country rates were 15 per cent for Armenia, 55 per cent for Kazakhstan, 13 per cent for Kyrgyzstan, 100 per cent for the Russian Federation, and 3 per cent for Tajikistan (Joint United Nations Programme on HIV/AIDS, 2006b). These figures indicate that school-based HIV prevention programmes are available in some countries and areas of the region, but that such programmes are not numerous or widespread enough to cover even half of the in school youth. Clearly, school-based HIV prevention programmes do little for youth who are not in school. Of particular concern is the fact that many youth who are injecting drugs and would benefit from such programmes do not attend school.

Research undertaken in the CIS indicated that only 7 per cent of young men and women aged 15-24 years were equipped with comprehensive and correct knowledge about HIV/AIDS. Those countries in Eastern Europe and CIS in which young women between the ages of 15 and 24 had virtually no comprehensive or correct knowledge of HIV/AIDS included Albania (0 per cent), Tajikistan (1 per cent), Azerbaijan (2 per cent), Turkmenistan (3 per cent), and Uzbekistan (8 per cent). The corresponding figure was 19 per cent in Moldova, and male and female youth in the Russian Federation appeared relatively well-informed, with 48 per cent possessing comprehensive and correct knowledge about HIV/AIDS (United Nations Population Fund, 2006; Joint United Nations Programme on HIV/AIDS, 2006b).

Research has shown that one-time exposure to relevant information is not enough to induce people to adopt safer behaviours or to effect long-term behavioural change; HIV/AIDS prevention messages that are reinforced over time have proved more effective. Experience indicates that peers are often the most effective deliverers of HIV prevention messages and services, and that celebrity role models such as sports figures can sometimes catch the attention of young people and help them understand the risks of HIV in ways that schoolteachers and even parents cannot (Kallings, 2006).

Peer involvement should constitute at least part of the HIV prevention strategy targeting youth in Eastern Europe and the CIS—particularly young injecting drug users. The topics covered within such a context should include raising knowledge about HIV and HIV transmission, condoms and negotiating condom use, safer drug injection practices, reducing the risks surrounding sexually transmitted diseases, and decreasing high-risk sexual behaviour.

For those most at risk in Eastern Europe and the CIS, including young, unemployed and marginalized injecting drug users and sex workers, there are several layers of stigma to overcome. It is therefore important to create an environment that encourages members of these groups to come forward and be tested for HIV, to seek and receive treatment, and to help prevent the further spread of the disease. An accommodating political and social environment is especially important for marginalized teenagers and youth, who may already be dealing with issues of exclusion or ostracism.

Confidential voluntary counselling and testing are essential for both the prevention and treatment of HIV/AIDS among young people. Fear of stigma and discrimination often prevents young people from accessing health services; they also have confidentiality concerns and do not wish to expose themselves to disapproval or criticism from health-care providers. Confidential voluntary counselling and testing services are especially important for youth, as many do not know how or where to access preventive health services, and young people in general are less likely to seek treatment for sexually transmitted infections. Within Eastern Europe and the CIS, youth access to and knowledge of voluntary counselling and testing services vary considerably from one country to another. Available data indicate that the proportions of young women aged 15-19 years who know where to get an HIV test are 6 per cent in Tajikistan, 24 per cent in Albania, 36 per cent in Armenia, 56 per cent in Moldova, and 73 per cent in the Ukraine (Joint United Nations Programme on HIV/AIDS, 2004).

Messages and programmes for youth must address issues such as access to condoms, treatment for sexually transmitted diseases, and strategies for preventing mother-to-child transmission; more targeted efforts should include harm reduction programmes for injecting drug users to decrease their risks of transmitting HIV among themselves.

In order to successfully combat the growing regional HIV/AIDS epidemic and prevent the transmission of HIV, there is a clear need to address the issues of HIV/AIDS and injecting drug use as youth issues, taking into account the context in which youth live and the pressures they may face. Reaching young people with HIV/AIDS education and prevention programmes is of particular importance in overall efforts to halt the transmission of HIV. There is also a need to focus specifically on youth who are drug users or at risk of drug use, as young people make up a significant proportion of this subpopulation, whose members currently face the highest risk of HIV transmission.

Reaching young injecting drug users with HIV/AIDS prevention information and HIV/AIDS and drug abuse treatment programmes is a major challenge. Since the sale, purchase, and use of illicit drugs are illegal, young injecting drug users attempt to remain underground and hidden, making it difficult to communicate or establish a working relationship with these individuals. As mentioned above, there are also problems relating to stigma, discrimination, social exclusion, and limited or conditional access to medical treatment. One major factor affecting the availability of treatment is the political issue of using public funds for programmes targeting young injecting drug users; both policy makers and members of the general public may be unsympathetic to the plight of this group, viewing drug use primarily as a law enforcement issue. Programmes that might benefit such youth could focus on HIV prevention (through the provision of financing for free needle exchanges), on HIV prevention combined with drug treatment (including the medical administration of oral replacement drugs so drug users no longer rely on needle injection), and on the treatment of injecting drug users who have contracted HIV and/or developed AIDS. It is important that a balance be struck in such programmes so that drug use is sufficiently destigmatized to facilitate the prevention of HIV transmission and the rehabilitation of injecting drug users, but without unintentionally encouraging or promoting illegal drug use.

SUMMARY AND CONCLUSIONS

Facilitating youth employment and ensuring that young people have access to decent and productive work are among the most important ways to foster their participation in the economy while also promoting development. Unfortunately, economic participation among young people in Eastern Europe and the Commonwealth of Independent States has been negatively affected by the major transitions occurring in the region; youth have been particularly hard hit by the lack of jobs, evidenced by the fact that the rate of youth unemployment in most economies in transition is more than double the overall unemployment rate. These circumstances have deepened young people's social exclusion. This has undoubtedly facilitated the spread of the HIV/AIDS pandemic in the region, as social exclusion, vulnerability and poverty among youth often lead to certain types of risky behaviour, including substance abuse and unsafe sex. Economies in transition are struggling to establish appropriate policy mechanisms and frameworks to address this new major threat, in part by challenging entrenched stigmas and widespread prejudice.

Youth participation through wage employment, self-employment and entrepreneurship plays an important role in the socio-economic engagement of youth. While conditions shaping participation differ substantially from one country to another, democratization opens up new possibilities and meaningful targets for social and political participation.

During the transition period, the Governments of most countries in Eastern Europe and the CIS, in cooperation with their social development partners, placed the associated goals of fighting youth unemployment and expanding youth employment high on their agendas. The results have been mixed, at best, in part because the process of shifting from centrally planned to market-driven development has not been completed in many respects. Countries are still in the process of identifying and eliminating inefficiencies in labour and capital use and reallocating resources.

Although the level of insecurity in the region has increased, young people generally appear to be more optimistic than their elders. They are often perceived as the natural beneficiaries of the transformation that is taking place, as they are being given new political opportunities associated with democracy-oriented reforms and are typically more receptive to new ideas and better able to adjust to market-oriented economic changes. According to the results of opinion polls conducted in the countries of the region, young people support political and economic change more strongly than do members of the older generation. In the central part of Eastern Europe and in the Baltic States, for example, more than 50 per cent of those between the ages of 18 and 34 think that the economic situation is better today than in 1989. This belief declines across age groups, with only about 35 per cent of those aged 65 and over agreeing with this assertion (European Bank for Reconstruction and Development, 2007).

Youth policies at the national level cannot be truly effective if young people are not regarded as assets of society, important agents of change, and critical stakeholders. Youth participation and representation at various levels of governance are crucial. The needs of young people must be addressed in a comprehensive manner using a multi-sector approach that places youth empowerment at the epicentre of national programmes and policies. Whether focused on education, health or the labour market, youth policies should reflect the input of young people; youth should be given a say in matters that affect them directly or indirectly.

Policy measures implemented at the national level have been geared towards offering young job-seekers employment or helping them increase their chances of finding work (through advisory services, training or retraining, and other measures). The experiences of several countries have shown that retraining and improving qualifications to better meet the demands of the market help young people up to the age of 25 secure employment (Nekolová and Hála, 2007). Governments have tried to enhance the employability of youth in general, and of certain vulnerable groups in particular, to give them better access to the labour market. Social protection policies have been geared towards creating skills and competencies.

Policies that are preventive in nature have been implemented in the areas of (formal and non-formal) education, health, and employment and have proved to be more cost-effective than remedial policies. Reviews of international programmes addressing youth employment confirm that the most effective programmes are those that integrate youth employment policy into an integrated package of services tailored to youth needs (La Cava and others, 2004).

With respect to the HIV/AIDS epidemic in Eastern Europe and the CIS, the main issue for the region, especially in the context of youth development, is how to reduce the transmission of HIV through injecting drug use. This issue has broad relevance for everyone in the region but is of particular relevance to youth and young injecting drug users. It is vitally important not only to disseminate information about HIV prevention and ensure access to quality health care, but also to find effective ways to help drug users stop injecting drugs and overcome drug abuse, or at the very least to reduce and minimize the HIV transmission risks associated with injecting drug use. Such efforts are also of value for the more general reasons of public health, social inclusion and human compassion.

Since youth are at the centre of the HIV/AIDS epidemic in Eastern Europe, they also represent a large part of the solution. In order to successfully combat the growing HIV/AIDS epidemic in the region, there is a clear need to address the issues of HIV/AIDS and injecting drug use as youth issues. There is an urgent need to focus specifically on youth who are injecting drugs or are at risk of becoming drug users, as young people make up a significant proportion of this subpopulation in the region and therefore face the highest risk of HIV transmission. Youth sex workers also need to be given priority and focused attention.

Young people need to be provided with information on HIV prevention and substance abuse and encouraged to take advantage of youth-friendly health services such as voluntary counselling, testing and treatment in a safe and supportive environment free from stigma, discrimination and disapproval. They need to be armed with information about reducing risky behaviour and provided with the training and life skills (such as negotiating abstinence and condom use) that will allow them to do so. They also need to be given access to condoms. For those youth who inject drugs, appropriate drug dependence treatment options must be made available, and drug users must have access to clean needles and syringes to reduce the risk of HIV transmission through the injection of drugs.

In order for the region to avoid a generalized HIV/AIDS epidemic and the attendant burdens and human and financial costs, strong political leadership and a serious commitment at the highest level of government are necessary. Relevant education, prevention and health-care measures must be scaled up to slow the increasing incidence of HIV infection, and care must be provided for those who are already infected. The countries of the region must vigorously combat HIV/AIDS and prevent its spread among youth in general and among young injecting drug users in particular.

[1] Underemployment is difficult to measure. The most commonly used method, a survey question (included in labour force surveys) covering those who are working fewer hours, that is, less than 35 hours per week, yields extremely high estimates of underemployment (especially when examining the youth situation). When the indicator includes those who are "looking for work", the picture becomes more reliable, and the rate is considerably lower. Nevertheless, it is difficult to determine the number of underemployed youth (as a subset of employed youth) owing to their relatively disadvantaged position in the labour market. For example, youth in rural areas may work longer hours, though their work may be cyclical and fluctuate from season to season. In the case of rural youth, and also the self-employed, accurate statistical data are scarce. In addition to hours of work, low labour returns are of concern (Godfrey, 2003).

[2] Not all sources (including Joint United Nations Programme on HIV/AIDS, 2005) specify the age group they are referring to when they use the term "young people" (also see, for example, Piot, 2006). Some UNAIDS sources also refer to "young people under 30". However, even without the age group specified in detail, the information from these sources is inclusive of youth aged 15-24 when the term "young people" is used.

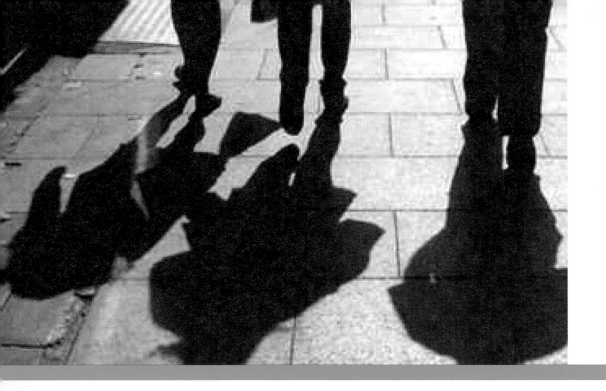

References

Aceijas, C., and others (2006). Estimates of injecting drug users at the national and local level in developing and transitional countries, and gender and age distribution. *Sexually Transmitted Infections*, vol. 82 (supplement 3), pp. 10-17.

Alam, Asad, and others (2005). Affordable access to quality services. *Growth, Poverty, and Inequality: Eastern Europe and the Former Soviet Union*. Washington, D.C.: World Bank.

Brown, David J., and others (2006). Nonstandard forms and measures of employment and unemployment in transition: a comparative study of Estonia, Romania, and Russia. IZA Discussion Paper No. 1961. Budapest: February.

Cazes, Sandrine, and Alena Nesporova (2003). Labour Markets in Transition: Balancing Flexibility and Security in Central and Eastern Europe. Geneva: International Labour Office.

_____ (2004). Labour markets in transition: balancing flexibility and security in Central and Eastern Europe. *OFCE Revue*, special issue (April).

Commander, Simon, and Fabian Bornhorst (2004). Integration and the well-being of children in the transition economies. Innocenti Working Papers, No. 98. Florence: UNICEF/Innocenti Research Centre, October.

Estrin, Saul (1994). The inheritance. In *Labor Markets and Social Policy in Central and Eastern Europe: The Transition and Beyond*, Nicholas Barr, editor. London: Oxford University Press.

European Bank for Reconstruction and Development (2007). *Life in Transition: A Survey of People's Experiences and Attitudes*. London.

European Commission. Directorate-General for Employment and Social Affairs (2002). *Employment in Europe 2002: Recent Trends and Prospects*. Luxembourg: Office for Official Publications of the European Communities.

European Foundation for the Improvement of Living and Working Conditions (2007). Youth and work. Dublin.

Freeman, David H. (2005) Youth employment promotion: a review of ILO work and the lessons learned. Geneva: International Labour Organization.

Gallup Organisation Hungary (2003). *Youth in New Europe.* Candidate Countries Eurobarometer 2003.1. European Commission.

Godfrey, Martin (2003). *Youth Employment Policy in Developing and Transition Countries: Prevention as well as Cure. Social Protection* Discussion Paper No. 0320. Washington, D.C.: World Bank.

Iannelli, Cristina (2003). Young people's social origin, educational attainment and labour market outcomes in Europe: youth transitions from education to working life in Europe, part III. *Statistics in Focus* (Population and Social Conditions: Theme 3-6/2003). Luxembourg.

International Harm Reduction Development Program (2006). *Harm Reduction Developments 2005: Countries with Injection-Driven HIV Epidemics.* New York: International Harm Reduction Development Program of the Open Society Institute.

International Labour Office (2004). *Global Employment Trends for Youth 2004.* Geneva: International Labour Organization, August.

_____ (2006). *Global Employment Trends for Youth 2006.* Geneva: International Labour Organization, August.

Joint United Nations Programme on HIV/AIDS (2004). *The Changing HIV/AIDS Epidemic in Europe and Central Asia* (UNAIDS/04.18E). Geneva: April.

_____ (2005). At great risk of HIV/AIDS: young people in Eastern Europe and Central Asia. Ministerial Meeting: Urgent Response to the HIV/AIDS Epidemics in the Commonwealth of Independent States, Moscow, 31 March - 1 April 2005. Available from http://www.unodc.org/pdf/event_2005-03-31_young_people.pdf (accessed on 7 July 2006).

_____ (2006a). Eastern Europe and Central Asia. Fact sheet. Available from http://www.unaids.org/en/Coordination/Regions/EasternEuropeandCentralAsia.asp (accessed on 7 July 2006).

_____ (2006b). *2006 Report on the Global AIDS Epidemic.* Geneva.

_____ UNAIDS Inter-agency Task Team on Young People (2004). *At the Crossroads: Accelerating Youth Access to HIV/AIDS Interventions.* New York.

Joint United Nations Programme on HIV/AIDS and World Health Organization (2005). Eastern Europe and Central Asia. AIDS Epidemic Update: December 2005. Geneva.

Kallings, Lars O. (2006). Can we halt the epidemic in Eastern Europe and Central Asia? Facing the prevention challenge. Speech given at the first Eastern European and Central Asian AIDS Conference, Moscow, 16 May 2006. Available from http:///www.unaids.org/en/Coordination/Regions/EasternEuropeandCentralAsia.asp (accessed on 7 July 2006).

Kertesi, Gábor (2004). The employment of the Roma: evidence from Hungary. Budapest Working Papers on the Labour Market (BWP), No. 2004/1. Budapest: Institute of Economics, Hungarian Academy of Sciences.

_____ and Gabor Kézdi (2005). Roma children in the transformational recession: widening ethnic schooling gap and Roma poverty in post-communist Hungary. Budapest: Central European University.

Kertesi, Gábor, and János Köllő (2002). Labour demand with heterogeneous labour inputs after the transition in Hungary, 1992-1999—and the potential consequences of the increase of minimum wage in 2001 and 2002. Budapest Working Papers on the Labour Market (BWP), No. 2002/5. Budapest: Institute of Economics, Hungarian Academy of Sciences.

_____ (2003). Fighting "low equilibria" by doubling the minimum wage? Hungary's experiment. IZA Discussion Paper No. 970. Bonn: Institute for the Study of Labor, December.

Kolev, Alexandre, and Catherine Saget (2005). Towards a better understanding of the nature, causes and consequences of youth labor market disadvantage: evidence for South-East Europe. Social Protection Discussion Series, Paper No. 0502. Washington, D.C.: World Bank, March.

Kornai, János (1980). *Economics of Shortage.* Amsterdam: North-Holland.

_____ (2000). What the change of system from socialism to capitalism does and does not mean. *Journal of Economic Perspectives*, vol. 14, No. 1 (winter), pp. 27-42.

Kőrösi, Gábor (2005). Framework 5 Project on Competitive Pressures and Its Social Consequences in EU Member States and in Associated Countries (COMPPRESS) HPSE-CT-2002-00149; WP3 Competition-driven labour market developments: their institutional and policy implications; (and) Deliverable 23: Labour market adjustment of Bulgarian, Hungarian and Romanian enterprises. Comparative study. Budapest: December.

La Cava, Gloria, and others (2004). Young people in South Eastern Europe: from risk to empowerment—final report. Washington, D.C.: World Bank, June.

Nekolová, Markéta, and Jaroslov Hála (2007). Contribution to EIRO thematic feature on youth and work: case of the Czech Republic. Available from http://www.eurofound.europa.eu/eiro/2005/12/tfeature/cz0512101t.html.

O'Higgins, Niall (2003). *Trends in the Youth Labour Market in Developing and Transition Countries.* Social Protection Discussion Series, Paper No. 0321. Washington, D.C.: World Bank.

Piot, Peter (2006). Facing the challenge. Keynote speech to the First Eastern European and Central Asian AIDS Conference, Moscow, 15 May 2006. Available from http://www.unaids.org/en/Coordination/Regions/EasternEuropeandCentralAsia.asp (accessed on 7 July 2006).

Rutkowski, Jan, and Stefano Scarpetta, editors (2005). *Enhancing Job Opportunities: Eastern Europe and the Former Soviet Union.* Washington, D.C.: World Bank.

Schneider, Friedrich (2002). The size and development of the shadow economies of 22 transition and 21 OECD countries. IZA Discussion Paper No. 514. Bonn: Institute for the Study of Labor, June.

_____ and Robert Klinglmair (2004). Shadow economies around the world: What do we know? IZA Discussion Paper No. 1043. Bonn: Institute for the Study of Labor, March.

Simai, Mihaly (2006). Poverty and inequality in Eastern Europe and the CIS transition economies (ST/ESA/2006/DWP/17). DESA Working Paper No. 17. February.

United Nations Children's Fund. CEE/CIS and Baltics Regional Office (2004). HIV/AIDS in Europe and Central Asia. Press release (22 February).

United Nations Children's Fund. UNICEF Innocenti Research Centre (2000). *Young People in Changing Societies.* Regional Monitoring Report No. 00/13. Florence, Italy.

_____ (2004). *Innocenti Social Monitor for 2004: Economic Growth and Child Poverty in the CEE/CIS and the Baltic States.* Florence, Italy.

_____ (2006). Children in CEE/CIS. TransMONEE database. Available from http://www.unicef-icdc.org/databases/.

United Nations Development Programme. Regional Bureau for Europe and the CIS (1998). *Poverty in Transition?* New York.

_____ (2004). *HIV/AIDS in Eastern Europe and the Commonwealth of Independent States— Reversing the Epidemic: Facts and Policy Options.* Bratislava.

_____ (2005). *Human Development Report 2005—International Cooperation at a Crossroads: Aid, Trade and Security in an Unequal World.* New York.

United Nations Office for Drug Control and Crime Prevention (2001). Interview with Dr. Peter Piot, Executive Director of UNAIDS. ODCCP Update. Vienna, June 2001. Available from http://www.unodc.org/unodc/newsletter_2001-06-30_1_page005.html (accessed on 26 July 2006).

United Nations Office on Drugs and Crime (2003). *Global Illicit Drug Trends 2003.* Sales No. E.03.XI.5.

_____ (2004). *HIV Prevention among Young Injecting Drug Users.* Sales No. E.04.XI.20.

United Nations Population Fund (2006). Youth and HIV/AIDS fact sheet. Available from http://www.junfpa.org/swp/2005/presskit/factsheets/facts_youth.htm (accessed on 7 July 2006).

World Bank (2003). *Averting AIDS Crises in Eastern Europe and Central Asia: A Regional Support Strategy.* Washington, D.C.

_____ (2005a). *Combating HIV/AIDS in Europe and Central Asia.* Global HIV/AIDS Program, Europe and Central Asia Human Development Department, Europe and Central Asia Region. Washington, D.C.

_____ (2005b). Young and at risk: living with HIV. News and Broadcast Web page (28 March 2005). Available from http://go.worldbank.org/34mamb8aj0

World Health Organization. Child and Adolescent Health and Development (2004). Steady...ready...go! Information brief. Geneva. Available from http://www.who.int/child-adolescent-health/New_Publications/ADH/IB_SRG.pdf (accessed on 30 October 2006).

World Health Organization, Joint United Nations Programme on HIV/AIDS, and United Nations Office on Drugs and Crime (2004). Reduction of HIV transmission through drug-dependence treatment (WHO/HIV/2004/04). Policy brief. Geneva: World Health Organization.

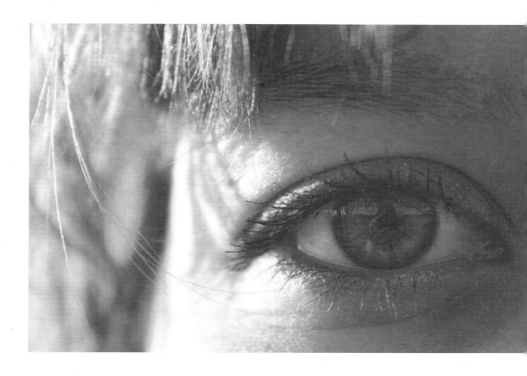

Chapter 7

Opportunities for **YOUTH** development in developed market economies: an unequal playing field

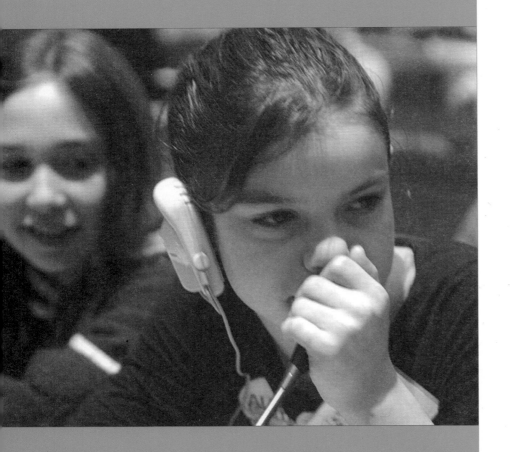

The developed market economies have made considerable progress over the years in addressing a number of issues that affect youth development. For example, coverage of primary schooling is universal, and gender access to primary and secondary education is almost equal, with girls being slightly overrepresented at tertiary levels. Ninety-eight per cent of boys and girls complete primary education, compared with 84 per cent for the developing regions. Youth in developed market economies are more likely than those living in other regions to obtain high educational qualifications, increasing their chances of securing a satisfactory position in the labour market. With respect to health, under-five, infant and maternal mortality rates are low, and most young children are immunized against killer childhood diseases before they reach adolescence. Although the period of youth tends to be among the healthiest periods of life, those young people in developed countries who need health care are, on average, more likely than youth in developing regions to have access to advanced health care.

The positive environment for youth development is supported by the buoyant economies of most countries in the region. Per capita income in developed countries is the highest in the world, and the economies of many countries in the region continue to grow at healthy rates. The vast economic resources available in these countries, in addition to the high level of infrastructure development, provide opportunities that are unmatched in other parts of the world. These factors have helped to create environments that are, in many respects, conducive to youth development and participation in society. As a result of these factors, young people in developed market economies are particularly well-positioned to access the opportunities brought about by globalization. Access to these opportunities is also facilitated by the availability of information and communication technologies, whose benefits have been more fully realized in this region than in any other, equipping young people with the skills to thrive in knowledge-based information societies.

Though notable progress has been achieved, there are still major differentials in youth development opportunities within and between the developed market economies. There remain large numbers of young people who are unable to access the benefits of national growth and development and participate fully in society. Inequalities in youth development are apparent in all countries for which data are available, including those in which social welfare systems are well established. Inequalities are often linked to factors such as class, ethnicity, race, gender and migrant status.

This chapter examines the nature and extent of inequalities in youth development in developed countries, focusing on education, employment and health—three core areas of the World Programme of Action for Youth in which developed countries have made considerable progress at the aggregate level but exhibit considerable inequalities of opportunity across population groups. It is argued in the chapter that the elimination of these disparities requires the implementation of policies that facilitate the inclusion of young people and help alleviate economic disadvantages. Such policies have become particularly important in the context of increased international migration to developed countries, a trend that, on its own, can contribute to social exclusion.

EDUCATION: OPPORTUNITIES AND PERFORMANCE ARE UNEQUAL WITHIN AND BETWEEN COUNTRIES

A good education is an essential building block for youth development. It is of enormous importance in enabling young people to contribute to development and to reap the full benefits and opportunities offered by their environments. Education also provides knowledge and empowerment for overcoming various negative factors arising from the environment. It can provide a link to well-remunerated jobs that can help young people break out of poverty. Individuals with low educational qualifications are at greater risk of marginalization because they are less likely to secure a satisfactory position in the labour market.

The majority of young people in developed countries achieve the basic compulsory levels of education, and many proceed to higher levels. The completion rate for upper secondary education has risen to above 8 in 10. More than half of the young people in the region will enter tertiary programmes that offer degree-level qualifications, and the rate of completion of tertiary education to the level of a traditional degree is now above one third (Organization for Economic Cooperation and Development, 2007). More than 40 per cent of young people in Australia, Denmark, Finland, Iceland, Italy, the Netherlands, New Zealand and Norway now complete university studies, with graduation rates tending to be highest in countries where programmes are of short duration; in Germany and Austria, where programmes are longer, only around 20 per cent of young people receive degrees (Organization for Economic Cooperation and Development, 2007). Major differentials in educational outcomes within and between countries are common, however. Social affiliation also has a significant effect on educational attainment (Hatcher, 1998). In many countries, these differentials persist despite policy measures to foster greater integration.

Young people in Canada, the United Kingdom of Great Britain and Northern Ireland, and the United States of America generally attain much higher levels of education than do those in France and Sweden, but "low" levels of education among youth are least likely in Sweden and the United Kingdom. Disparities in performance are also evident elsewhere and in specific subject areas of study. Data from the Organization for Economic Cooperation and Development (2006) indicate that in Greece, Italy, Portugal and the United States, at least a quarter of the students exhibit a very low level of mathematics proficiency (level 1 or below) within the six-level Programme for International Student Assessment (PISA) framework. In Finland, however, more than 93 per cent of students range between the second and sixth levels of proficiency (see table 7.1). At the tertiary level, rates of graduation vary widely from one country to another, ranging from around 20 per cent in Austria and Germany to just over 50 per cent in the United States and 80 per cent in Japan (Organization for Economic Cooperation and Development, 2006).

Table 7.1
Mathematics proficiency among students in developed countries according to Programme for International Student Assessment standards

Country	Level of proficiency in mathematics						
	Below Level 1 (under 358 points)	Level 1 (358-420 points)	Level 2 (421-482 points)	Level 3 (483-544 points)	Level 4 (545-606 points)	Level 5 (607-668 points)	Level 6 (above 668 points)
Finland	1.5	5.3	16.0	27.7	26.1	16.7	6.7
Canada	2.4	7.7	18.3	26.2	25.1	14.8	5.5
Netherlands	2.6	8.4	18.0	23.0	22.6	18.2	7.3
Australia	4.3	10.0	18.6	24.0	23.3	14.0	5.8
Iceland	4.5	10.5	20.2	26.1	23.2	11.7	3.7
Denmark	4.7	10.7	20.6	26.2	21.9	11.8	4.1
Ireland	4.7	12.1	23.6	28.0	20.2	9.1	2.2
Japan	4.7	8.6	16.3	22.4	23.6	16.1	8.2
New Zealand	4.9	10.1	19.2	23.2	21.9	14.1	6.6
Switzerland	4.9	9.6	17.5	24.3	22.5	14.2	7.0
Austria	5.6	13.2	21.6	24.9	20.5	10.5	3.7
France	5.6	11.0	20.2	25.9	22.1	11.6	3.5
Sweden	5.6	11.7	21.7	25.5	19.8	11.6	4.1
Norway	6.9	13.9	23.7	25.2	18.9	8.7	2.7
Belgium	7.2	9.3	15.9	20.1	21.0	17.5	9.0
Luxembourg	7.4	14.3	22.9	25.9	18.7	8.5	2.4
Spain	8.1	14.9	24.7	26.7	17.7	6.5	1.4
Germany	9.2	12.4	19.0	22.6	20.6	12.2	4.1
United States	10.2	15.5	23.9	23.8	16.6	8.0	2.0
Portugal	11.3	18.8	27.1	24.0	13.4	4.6	0.8
Italy	13.2	18.7	24.7	22.9	13.4	5.5	1.5
Greece	17.8	21.2	26.3	20.2	10.6	3.4	0.6
OECD total	11.0	14.6	21.2	22.4	17.6	9.6	3.5
OECD average	8.2	13.2	21.1	23.7	19.1	10.6	4.0

Source: Organization for Economic Cooperation and Development, *Education at a Glance 2006: OECD Indicators* (Paris: 2006) (available from www.sourceoecd.org/education).

Note: Countries are in ascending order based on the percentage of students who failed to achieve the lowest level of proficiency.

In Canada and the United States, literacy skills among youth aged 16-25 years have been found to be strongly associated with the educational background and social status of the parents (Willms, 1999). Youth from advantaged families fare better than those from families with lower social status and low levels of parental educational attainment. Even in Sweden, a welfare State known for its strong orientation towards social equity and equality, major differentials exist between social classes with respect to educational access. For example, whereas 90 per cent of Swedish children who have university-educated parents attend upper secondary school, only 70 per cent of those born to unskilled workers are enrolled at this level. Further, those with university-educated parents are much more likely to be enrolled in three- or four-year academic institutions rather than in vocational programmes. Although Sweden saw declines in educational inequality in the past, there has been no further reduction in inequality since 1970 (Hatcher, 1998).

Tertiary education opportunities, in particular, are strongly linked to socio-economic status. Though often hidden in the complex systems of tertiary education in many countries, inequality in access (owing to costs and other factors) is considerable in the developed market economies. In the United States, the varied tracks that exist for young people to enter tertiary education ostensibly provide opportunities even for those who have had a less-than-successful experience in secondary school (Karen, 2002). Nevertheless, those from low socio-economic backgrounds are less likely than those from higher socio-economic backgrounds to enrol in tertiary studies.

The differences in young people's educational performance across countries undoubtedly reflect various underlying individual and societal factors as well as demographic and socio-economic factors. A recent study reveals that low-income students appear to perform significantly better on standardized tests when they attend schools where fewer than 50 per cent of the students are poor than when they attend schools with a higher percentage of poor students (Association for Supervision and Curriculum Development, 2007). The factors underlying this relationship are not entirely clear. Educational attainment differentials in developed countries also reflect choices that are made by poorer students and their families at difficult transition points in the education system. Whereas those from poorer backgrounds are more likely to drop out of school if they fail a grade or face difficulties in performance (see box 7.1), those from wealthier backgrounds are more likely to find the resources to take remedial action to ensure success.

Box 7.1

Each year in the United States, hundreds of thousands of students drop out of school. It is estimated that approximately one in eight children (12.5 per cent) never graduate from high school, though there are significant variations by State. The proportions of eighth-grade students who graduate from high school five years later range from 55 per cent in Florida to 87 per cent in New Jersey.

An important indicator of the likelihood of school completion is socio-economic background. The dropout rate for students from low-income households is 10 per cent, compared with 5.2 per cent for those from middle-income households and 1.6 per cent for students from high-income households. High school dropouts are more likely to come from single-parent families or from families in which one or both parents are unemployed. Young people (aged 18-24) of Hispanic descent are less likely to complete school (64 per cent) than African American youth (84 per cent) or white youth (92 per cent). Native American youth also have a relatively high likelihood of dropping out.

High school dropouts tend to be older than their grade-level peers, and they are more likely to be males than females. Females who drop out often do so because of pregnancy. The probability of students living in urban areas completing school is lower than that of suburban or non-metropolitan residents. The risk of dropping out of school is especially high for youth with disabilities; during the 1999-2000 school year, only 57 per cent of youth with disabilities graduated with regular diplomas. Of youth with disabilities who do not complete school, the highest proportions are students with learning disabilities (32 per cent) and students with emotional/behavioural disabilities (50 per cent).

Dropping out of school perpetuates inequalities by interfering with the ability of youth to participate in society and in the labour market. Unemployment and underemployment are widespread among those who have not completed high school. High school dropouts are 72 per cent more likely than high school graduates to be unemployed, and job opportunities available to those without a high school diploma often do not pay a living wage. A high school graduate earns an average of US$ 9,245 more per year than someone who did not complete school. Incarceration is also more likely among high school dropouts. Almost 80 per cent of individuals in prison do not have a high school diploma. Those who fail to complete high school suffer losses on many levels, but society also loses. Besides crime prevention and prosecution, other costs to society include welfare and unemployment benefits as well as billions of dollars in lost tax revenues.

Various efforts have been made to reduce the dropout rate. The 2001 No Child Left Behind Act is aimed at holding schools accountable for student progress using indicators of adequate yearly progress, including measures of academic performance and rates of school completion. Pressure is increasing on schools to improve rates of school completion and the acquisition of academic and social skills necessary to participate in society and the economy. Since it is difficult to change the "status variables" associated with dropping out (such as socio-economic standing, disability or ability level, and family structure), interventions have focused on the variables that can be influenced by students, parents, educators and community members to increase school completion (such as attendance, poor academic performance, identification with school, and support services). Focusing on these variables also addresses the various "push factors" that students often cite as reasons for dropping out of school.

Source: Camilla A. Lehr and others, *Essential Tools—Increasing Rates of School Completion: Moving from Policy and Research to Practice; A Manual for Policymakers, Administrators, and Educators* (Minneapolis: Institute on Community Integration Publications Office, 2004).

The persistent, and in some cases widening, racial gap in educational performance can largely be attributed to significant and increasing social and economic inequalities across society, particularly in the inner cities, where large concentrations of ethnic minorities reside. It is apparent that metropolitan areas often present many challenges and disadvantages for poorer individuals and families. In the United States, opportunities in these areas "are considerably greater for non-Hispanic white children than for blacks and Hispanics, with Asian children tending to fall in the middle. Black and Hispanic children are more likely to live in poor families than other children." Additionally, the disadvantaged groups tend to be relegated by poverty to "neighborhoods and schools with unfavorable socio-economic environments—a kind of double, or triple, jeopardy" (Acevedo-Garcia and others, 2007, p. 33).

It should also be mentioned that there are still large intercountry differentials in the educational "readiness" of young people even before they begin the transition to adulthood. According to the rankings of UNICEF (2007) in a major study of child well-being in rich countries, the reading, mathematical and scientific literacy of 15-year-olds varies widely across developed countries, with 15-year-olds from Canada and Finland being most prepared and those from Greece and Portugal among the least prepared. This means that youth begin their transition to adulthood with different capacities to navigate the challenges and harness the opportunities offered in a changing global economy.

There are a number of common consequences of these differentials, among the most important of which are diminished opportunity (resulting in higher unemployment and underemployment, especially among youth), domestic poverty, disparagement by the rest of the population, and the emergence of groups that may encourage youth delinquency and conflict. There is evidence that some of the education differentials across groups in developed market economies have not remained stagnant. Improvements are apparent in some areas; in particular, some racial convergence in schooling in the United States has been observed. Kalmijn and Kraaykamp (1996) attribute this to the influence of legal and institutional changes, including such factors as school desegregation, bussing, scholarships for black students, and affirmative action. Much remains to be done, however; as long as inequalities in education exist in developed market economies, they translate into differentials in young people's preparedness and capacity to access the full benefits afforded by these buoyant economies.

INFORMATION AND COMMUNICATION TECHNOLOGIES: AN IMPORTANT COMPLEMENT TO EDUCATION BUT ONE WITH UNIQUE CHALLENGES

Information and communication technologies (ICT) play a major role in education and in the social and economic lives of youth in the developed market economies. Schools are increasingly using the Internet to access the wide range of materials it offers to supplement instruction materials and to interact with students. Many young people use the Internet as the primary source of information on subjects ranging from leisure activities and health to politics and employment. In Europe, use of career resource sites jumped 21 per cent to involve 9.5 million youth between 2005 and 2006. This jump outpaced the total increase in youth Internet use in Europe, which grew by about 10 per cent to 36.4 million youth during the same period (comScore Europe, 2006). In areas of high Internet penetration, these services may facilitate matches between young people and specific areas of the job market.

Youth are prolific users of social networking sites such as Facebook, MySpace and MyYearbook, which allow users to post a personal profile with photos and descriptions of interests and hobbies. Internet technologies are also increasingly serving as hubs for communication, identity formation and social networking among youth in the region and are embedded into the lives of more and more young people every day. In addition to using the new technology as an information source, youth also have made an impact on the landscape of the Internet. A range of features such as discussion boards, live chats, news feeds, online polling and social networking tools allow youth to engage in different forms of civic participation, which may involve supporting or criticizing a political candidate, organizing around an issue of concern, or forming a community reflecting common interests.

Access, opportunities and the actual use of ICT resources and other digital media differ within and between developed market economies. While computers are becoming more widely available in schools, their accessibility remains variable. Some countries have more than one computer for every five students, but the ratio is less than 1 to 10 in Germany, Greece, Portugal and Spain (Organization for Economic Cooperation and Development, 2006). The overall rate of personal computer use among youth is lowest in Greece and Ireland, at 59 per cent, while in Austria, Denmark, Finland, Iceland, Luxembourg, the Netherlands, Norway and Sweden, rates of youth computer use are above 95 per cent (International Telecommunication Union, 2006).

As opportunities to benefit from ICT continue to increase and differ within and across countries, so do the risks. Youth are vulnerable to risks such as exploitation, abuse, fraud and online pornography. These risks multiply as access to the Internet becomes easier and more widespread for users of all ages. Youth, as well as adults, can be the perpetrators as well as the victims of ICT-engineered crime, but youth are more exposed to risk since they are avid users of digital media both socially and in schools. In order to address these risks, various mechanisms have been established in collaboration with Governments to ensure appropriate regulation of ICT and the digital pathway. However, young people from poorer socio-economic backgrounds may have less access to these resources and protection and may be more vulnerable to scams and misrepresentations, yielding to fraudulent offers of jobs or a better life that the Internet may appear to offer.

EMPLOYMENT: WITH DIMINISHING OPPORTUNITIES FOR WORK, YOUTH STAY IN SCHOOL LONGER OR ENGAGE IN VOLUNTEERISM

Employment is an important avenue for social, economic and civic integration, allowing people to earn an income and become contributing members of society on multiple levels. In the specific context of employment, those who have work can join professional and labour organizations and interact with colleagues. People who have decent jobs are more invested in society and, through their connection to economic life, are likely to develop an interest in the political context in which they work, which can also lead to increased community and political participation. The economic security provided by stable work gives people the opportunity to engage fully in domestic, social and political activities. Employment income also enables individuals and their families to gain access to basic social services, including education and health care, which are essential for staying out of poverty. Given the central role that employment plays in providing incomes and basic livelihoods for individuals and families, social exclusion in employment can have consequences that extend well beyond the workplace.

Overall, young people in the developed market economies have better labour market prospects than do youth in other world regions. Many youth seek a degree of economic independence by entering the labour market even before they have completed their education and may work part-time throughout their schooling. The varied options provided by education systems in these regions, including distance learning, combined with opportunities for part-time work, enable many young people to hold a job while pursuing an education. Youth unemployment rates for the region as a whole decreased from 15.4 per cent in 1993 to 13.4 per cent in 2003 (International Labour Office, 2004). Between 1995 and 2005, the size of the youth labour force in the region declined by 5 per cent (see table 7.2). This may have contributed to the overall decline in unemployment, as the number of unemployed youth fell from 10.2 million in 1995 to 8.5 million in 2005. Female and male youth are almost equally likely to participate in the labour market, the gap between male and female labour force participation rates having narrowed between 1995 and 2005.

Table 7.2
Indicators of youth participation in the labour force: developed economies and the European Union

Indicator	1995	2005	Percentage change
Size of the youth labour force (thousands)	67 740	64 501	-5.0
Youth share of total working age population (percentage)	17.2	15.7	-9.6
Number of employed youth (thousands)	57 459	56 020	-2.6
Number of unemployed youth (thousands)	10 281	8 481	-21.2
Youth labour force participation rate			
Males	56.9	54.0	-5.4
Females	50.1	49.6	-1.0
Total	53.6	51.8	-3.5
Youth employment to population ratio	45.4	45.0	-0.9
Ratio of youth to adult unemployment	2.3	2.3	—

Source: Compiled from International Labour Office, *Global Employment Trends for Youth 2006* (Geneva: International Labour Organization, August 2006).
Note: A dash (—) indicates that the amount is nil or negligible.

Despite strong positive overall labour market features at the aggregate level, many youth in developed economies have difficulty obtaining decent, stable long-term employment and may experience sequences of short-term jobs, be forced to take jobs below their skill level, or move frequently between sectors and industries. As table 7.2 indicates, a smaller proportion of both males and females were in the labour force in 2005 than in 1995. This decline in the proportion of youth in the labour force is small, but it reflects a growing tendency for youth to remain in education for longer periods or to enter into internships or other volunteer positions in order to improve their employability. There is a growing tendency among young people to delay the age at which they enter the labour force in order to complete additional years of schooling. The labour force participation rate of youth aged 15-19 years has been dropping in recent years in a number of countries, including Belgium, France, Greece, Italy and Luxembourg (International Labour Office, 2005).

The complex role of education

It has been demonstrated that better-educated young workers have higher earnings, greater job stability and greater upward mobility over time (Lloyd, 2006). Tertiary education, in particular, is generally perceived as a guarantor of decent and well-paid work in developed market economies. Graduates of tertiary institutions earn considerably more than those who have completed only upper secondary or post-secondary education. While the earnings differentials between men and women remain substantial, the financial rewards from tertiary education tend to be greater for women in Australia, Canada, Ireland, the Netherlands, Norway, Spain, Switzerland and the United Kingdom (Organization for Economic Cooperation and Development, 2006).

While a higher level of education clearly offers certain advantages, even university graduates are increasingly experiencing insecurity and uncertainty in their employment prospects. Although they may be qualified in terms of having met school requirements, many do not receive specific job training. The amount of non-formal job-related training in which adults engage over their lifetime varies both by country and according to previous qualifications. In countries such as Greece, Italy and the Netherlands, adults that have completed their tertiary studies spend an average of around 300 hours or less in such training over their lives; this compares with over 1,000 hours in Denmark, Finland, France and Switzerland (Organization for Economic Cooperation and Development, 2006). Because young people's lack of experience is often a reason for their failure to secure employment, there has been a recent increase in internships and other volunteer work. In Germany, for example, a discussion has emerged around the so-called "internship generation", which is likely to be of relevance to other developed market economies. It is a common perception that university graduates must do at least one internship before being able to find employment.

Two recent studies in Germany, one conducted by Grühn and Hecht (2007) and the other by Briedis and Minks (2007), have tried to shed light on this phenomenon; the former study was commissioned by the German trade-union federation and polled graduates of two large German universities, while the latter was conducted at the request of the Ministry of Education and was based on a survey of almost 12,000 graduates nationwide. Both studies found that internships were far more common for some areas of study (social sciences, art and culture studies, and media-related studies) than for others (technical or science-related studies). Both studies also found that young women were more likely than young men to pursue an internship after their studies (even within the same area of study). Briedis and Minks (2007) found that one out of eight graduates of technical colleges and one out of seven university graduates had done one or more internships after completing their formal studies. Twenty per cent of the university graduates had done two or more internships. A total of 37 per cent of the graduates studied by Grühn and Hecht (2007) had done at least one internship after finishing university.

Although the above data relate to Germany, the situation is likely to be similar in other developed economies. Internships in developed countries appear to have become a waiting stage for those who are unable to find suitable immediate employment or for those who seek to improve their chances of finding a good job. Internships may open doors to future employment with businesses or offices where the interns served. In the two German studies, the main reasons respondents gave for doing an internship was to obtain work experience, to facilitate the search for employment, and to meet the desire for practical qualifications in an area of specialization. Unemployment was also given as a reason for participating in internships. The fact that internships may pay little or no money did not seem to matter. Indeed, 17 per cent of technical college graduates and 34 per cent of university graduates did not receive any remuneration. Of those university graduates who were paid, 22 perceived their remuneration to be good or satisfactory, while 29 per cent perceived it to be bad or unsatisfactory (Briedis and Minks, 2007). Among interns, females tend to be paid less than males. Since remuneration is often insufficient to cover living expenses, two thirds of interns rely on their parents to help them financially during their internships, while 40 per cent have a second job (Grühn and Hecht, 2007). This implies that students who are able to afford this form of volunteerism, while also positioning themselves for good jobs later, are mainly those from higher socio-economic groups whose families or other sponsors are able to support them during their internships.

A particularly instructive source of data for examining these and related aspects of youth labour force participation in developed market economies is the Luxembourg Income Study, a cooperative research project involving 30 countries in Europe, North America, Asia and Oceania. The project, which began in 1983, provides time series data on areas such as employment characteristics, occupations, and education, and suggests that the transition of youth to independent adulthood has slowed in industrialized countries. Based on these data, Bell and others (2007) note that a major reason for this delayed transition is that labour market conditions have made it harder for young people to secure well-paid employment; they also note that in countries other than the United States, it appears that well-compensated jobs now require more schooling. They argue, therefore, that there has been a "failure to launch" among youth in these countries.

There are various indications of this failure. Although developed countries have successfully churned out increasing numbers of youth with secondary and tertiary qualifications, these countries are changing fast with globalization, and labour markets have not been able to accommodate this large group of skilled young graduates (United Nations, 2005). Job prospects are even worse for unskilled workers. In the absence of full-time opportunities in the formal economy early in their careers, young people are turning to entrepreneurship, internship and self-employment, often in the informal economy. Those in the informal economy often work for low pay and have few prospects for the future. When youth do work, their patterns of work vary by age, sex, and across countries (see figure 7.1). Data on young people who work full-time and for the full year in Germany, Italy, the United Kingdom and the United States suggest that, during the mid-1990s, such employment was highest among male youth aged 18-25 years in the United Kingdom and the United States. This may suggest that, in addition to differences in factors such as the length of the educational cycle and military service, there are differences across developed countries in young people's perception of the need to work. It may also suggest that, despite the difficulty many young people have in making the transition to full-time work, in some countries youth are still able to secure long-term, full-time jobs with relative ease.

Figure 7.1
Percentage of young adults working full-time for the full year, by age and sex, selected countries

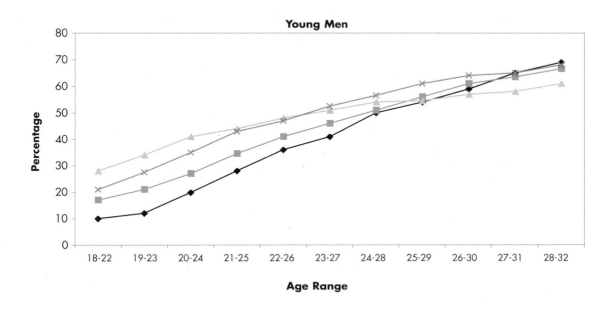

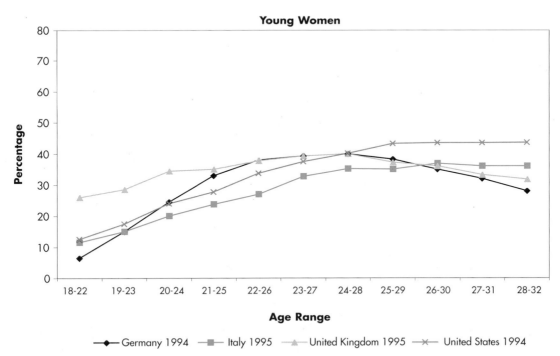

Source: Timothy M. Smeeding and Katherin Ross Phillips, "Cross-national differences in employment and economic sufficiency", *Annals of the American Academy of Political and Social Science*, vol. 580, No. 103 (2002), p. 108.

Note: The figures estimate the level of economic independence (measured by full-year, full-time work) at a point in time averaged over 11 overlapping, five-year age ranges.

Table 7.3 suggests that the chances of youth being unemployed vary by gender, though the direction and size of this relationship varies across countries. In most of the countries for which data are presented in table 7.3, young women enjoy a slightly better employment situation, but in a few countries they are at a disadvantage. In Greece and, to a lesser extent, Spain, young women are much more likely than young men to be unemployed. In both countries, this differential narrowed between 2003 and 2005. The tendency for young women to fare slightly better than young men in the labour market is possibly due to the higher average educational attainment of women in the region (International Labour Office, 2004). Nevertheless, women tend to earn less than young men, even with the same qualifications. The trend in unemployment between 2003 and 2005 for each sex was mixed, but rates for both sexes increased the most in Sweden.

Table 7.3
Share of youth who are unemployed in selected developed countries, by sex

Country	2003			2005		
	Females	Males	Female minus male unemploy-ment rate	Females	Males	Female minus male unemploy-ment rate
Austria	8.9	7.3	1.6	10.3	10.4	-0.1
Belgium	21.3	22.2	-0.9	22.1	21.0	1.1
Canada	11.8	15.3	-3.5	10.6	14.2	-3.6
Denmark	9.2	9.2	—	8.6	8.6	—
Finland	21.6	21.9	-0.3	19.5	20.6	-1.1
France	21.9	20.4	1.5	25.4	21.9	3.5
Germany	14.4	14.9	-0.5	14.3	15.6	-1.3
Greece	36.6	18.9	17.7	34.8	18.7	16.1
Iceland	7.0	9.5	-2.5	6	8.5	-2.5
Ireland	8.4	9.7	-1.3	8	9.1	-1.1
Italy	27.6	20.5	7.1	27.4	21.5	5.9
Luxembourg	12.7	9.7	3.0	16.4	11.8	4.6
Netherlands	6.3	6.3	—	8.4	8.0	0.4
Norway	10.7	12.4	-1.7	11	12.2	-1.2
Portugal	17.0	12.4	4.6	19.1	13.6	5.5
Spain	30.8	20.2	10.6	23.5	16.7	6.8
Sweden	13.7	13.0	0.7	22.1	23.0	-0.9
United Kingdom	10.5	13.8	-3.3	11.3	14.5	-3.2
United States	11.4	13.4	-2.0	10.1	12.4	-2.3

Source: United Nations Economic Commission for Europe; data accessed from www.unece.org on 14 May 2007.
Note: A dash (—) indicates that the amount is nil or negligible.

Unemployment, underemployment and poor earning capacities have a variety of consequences for youth. Apart from compelling them to remain in education, these factors can be linked to dependency on parents, family problems, alcohol and drug consumption, and delinquency. Youth who end up in the informal economy and are subjected to working conditions that compromise their health and well-being (owing to long hours, repetitive functions, and inadequate health and other social protections) are likely to suffer further economic, health and social consequences in the future. Youth unemployment and underemployment also have serious societal implications. One of the most far-reaching consequences is that unemployment can lead to the exclusion of young people by spawning or deepening poverty. Such consequences are detrimental to youth themselves and can also extend across generations.

Implications for youth poverty

There appear to be direct linkages between access to educational and employment opportunities and youth poverty. Although developed market economies have the highest per capita incomes in the world, a number of countries in the region have recorded high and increasing levels of economic inequality (Förster and Mira d'Ercole, 2005), with large pockets of young people in these countries living in poverty.

Reliable estimates of youth poverty are difficult to find in both developing and developed countries. However, since poverty is a household-level rather than an individual-level indicator, its rate of prevalence among youth is probably reflected in the prevalence rates for adults. This would imply that, as with adults, wide differentials exist within and between developed countries in the levels of youth poverty. Poverty is likely to be more severe among youth than among adults because young people often lack the knowledge and the means to manoeuvre around difficult economic circumstances. A study based on the 1999 Poverty and Social Exclusion Survey of Britain (PSE) found that a substantial proportion of young people (aged 16-25 years) reported incomes that were significantly below those reported by the population as a whole (Fahmy, 1999). The study also found a lack of correspondence between income and deprivation measures of poverty. While income poverty was higher among youth than in the general population, deprivation indicators of poverty (the inability to afford three or more socially perceived necessities) were lower among youth as a group.

Youth poverty has contributed to the large increases in economic inequality that have been observed in the United States over the past four decades (Smeeding, 2005). The country has both the highest and the most rapidly rising overall rate of inequality among OECD countries. The tendency for youth to be consigned to low-skill employment, their vulnerability to unemployment, and the absence of social safety nets leave them more vulnerable to poverty than adults. Not surprisingly, data from the Luxembourg Income Study in the developed market economies suggest that between 1985 and 2000 there was a decline in young adults' ability to form independent households (Bell and others, 2007). Bell and others (2007) add that "there has been an actual postponement in establishing independent households" (p. 16).

The degree of difficulty experienced in making the transition to independent adult-hood varies across countries and by sex. As shown in figure 7.2, young people in the United Kingdom are most likely to complete the transition early; almost 60 per cent of females and about 35 per cent of males aged 20-24 years are heads of household, or their partners or spouses are. Young men and women in Italy are least likely to make an early transition to independent adulthood. Bell and others (2007) note that the earlier transition for young people in the United Kingdom could be because of the availability of subsidized or affordable housing in the United Kingdom, and that cultural factors or the high cost of home ownership may discourage youth in Italy from living independently at a relatively young age. Cultural factors are also likely to be important in the United Kingdom. Furthermore, many young households tend to live in private rented homes and do not benefit from subsidized housing.

Figure 7.2

Percentage of young adults in selected developed countries who are heads of household or their spouses, by age and sex, 1995-2000

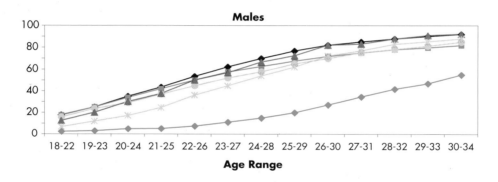

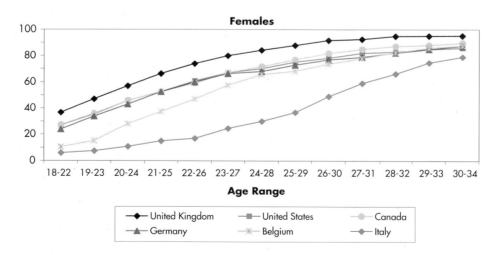

Source: Lisa Bell and others, "Failure to launch: cross-national trends in the transition to economic independence", Luxembourg Income Study Working Paper Series, No. 456 (2007), figure 1.

Young adults who live independently of their parents are more likely to live in poverty. A study on the situation in the United Kingdom found that youth who lived independently of parents, and therefore did not have access to parent-paid or subsidized housing, were much more likely to be poor; in fact, 48 per cent of these youth were found to be poor (Fahmy, 1999). This tendency for poverty to be more severe among youth who live independently is apparent, to varying degrees, in other countries in the region, cutting across Belgium, Germany, Italy, Canada and the United Kingdom, and there are indications that the extent of poverty typically worsens over time (Bell and others, 2007).

Clearly, evidence of the economic and financial growth of developed market economies conceals a more complex and uncertain situation for young people. Youth poverty and vulnerability in this region may be hidden because of protection and social insurance through income and other support from parents and other family members. Youth who are unable to benefit from the resources of kin often face a more uncertain future.

HEALTH: MANY OLD HEALTH CHALLENGES EASE, BUT NEW RISKS THREATEN THE WELFARE OF YOUTH

Youth in developed countries generally experience some of the best health conditions in which to mature into healthy and independent adulthood. Advances in medical technology, environmental controls, an abundant food supply, and good access to basic and emergency health care mean that most young people can stay healthy and, when unwell, can receive care. These benefits, however, are not equally available or affordable to all. Health-related inequalities have been found to exist everywhere, though they vary considerably in intensity from country to country (Feinstein, 1993). Unhealthy lifestyles compromise the physical and mental health of youth and leave many at risk of ill health or death; some are unable to make an independent transition to adulthood even if they survive. High-quality, affordable health care may be inaccessible to youth owing to poverty, the lack of health insurance coverage, a lack of relevant knowledge, and/or inefficiencies in health-care delivery.

Although better knowledge about health and access to a comprehensive array of health services would play a major role in reducing disparities in health outcomes in developed countries, access to care and correct information about health issues also varies greatly across the region. These variations arise from factors such as parental background, residence, education, race, and income. Pervasive gaps in quality health care have been reported for various ethnic minorities and those of lower socio-economic status, placing youth within these groups at increased risk of suffering from poor health (Wagstaff, 2002; Agency for Healthcare Research and Quality, 2005).

Lifestyle: accidents and alcohol affect the lives and well-being of young people

According to a recent report from the World Health Organization (Toroyan and Peden, 2007), road traffic accidents are the leading cause of injury and death among youth, with the risks differing across demographic and socio-economic groups. A recent study covering Australia, Canada, New Zealand, Sweden, the United Kingdom and the United States has also noted that rates of death due to injury are two to three times higher among those from lower socio-economic groups than among the members of groups with higher socio-economic status (Hjern and Bremberg, 2002). In Canada, more than one third of all deaths among 15- to 19-year-olds, and just under a third of all deaths among those aged 20-24 years, were caused by road vehicle accidents in 2006, and an estimated 29,000 teenagers and 30,000 young adults were injured (Canadian Council on Social Development, 2006). In the United States, approximately 75 per cent of all deaths among children and youth between the ages of 10 and 24 resulted from motor-vehicle crashes, other unintentional injuries, homicide and suicide (Grunbaum and others, 2001).

It is essential to ensure that adequate protections are in place for working youth, especially those involved in manual labour. Because young people may be less experienced at using equipment in manual jobs, they face higher risks of accidental dismemberment and death related to their occupations. A United States study of young people aged 14-17 years engaged in non-farm work found that common hazards included ladders, scaffolding, forklifts, tractors, riding mowers, and working around loud noises. More than half of the youth surveyed had been injured at least once while working (Dunn and others, 1998). Occupational accidents among youth are related to lack of experience as well as to inadequate safety measures to protect young people in the workplace.

Injuries and death from motor vehicle and other accidents are often the result of behavioural choices young people make, especially regarding drinking and the use of illicit drugs and other illegal substances. Alcohol and drug use can compromise the ability of youth to make rational decisions when operating machinery or motor vehicles. Data from a national survey of high school students in the United States in 2003 indicate that during the 30 days preceding the survey, 30 per cent of students had ridden with a driver who had been drinking alcohol; 45 per cent had drunk alcohol themselves; 17 per cent had carried a weapon; and 22.4 per cent had used marijuana. In addition, during the 12 months preceding the survey, 33 per cent of high school students had been in a physical fight, and 8.5 per cent had attempted suicide (Grunbaum and others, 2003). Some 31 per cent of young Americans aged 18-25 years who were interviewed by the Pew Research Center (2007) reported that they smoked cigarettes, and 9 per cent admitted to having taken illegal drugs. The age at which these activities are initiated is becoming progressively younger. In the Netherlands, 47 per cent of male youth and 49 per cent of female youth had their first cigarette at or before the age of 13, and in the United States, 36.1 per cent of current smokers aged 18-24 years started smoking before the age of 16 (Hibell and others, 2000; Centers for Disease Control and Prevention, 2004). It is estimated that 30 per cent of 15-year-olds in Finland and 33 per cent of 15-year-old Germans use tobacco at least once per week (Wilkinson and Marmot, 2003).

Poor youth health outcomes linked to lifestyle factors in developed countries are often a result of choice, but the outcomes also reflect the consequences of youth alienation from opportunities for their healthy self-development. Poverty and a lack of access to education and opportunities for structured and constructive leisure activities may leave young people vulnerable to negative peer pressure. Policies to address the growing lifestyle-related health challenges of youth in developed countries therefore require a more holistic approach. Reducing these risks involves changing personal behaviour, but it also requires changes in social and economic structures that exclude youth, especially those with disadvantaged socio-economic backgrounds. Changes in broader socio-environmental conditions are essential, for example, in achieving long-term reductions in youth drinking and associated problems (Wagenaar and Perry, 1994). It is also necessary to explore opportunities for youth development that arise through intergenerational programmes and other opportunities for exchange between young people and older persons. Perhaps most important is that programmes fostering youth development should build on the strengths of young people rather than trying to "fix" them by addressing particular problems such as dropping out of school, substance abuse, or early pregnancy (Quinn, 1999).

Sexuality, pregnancy and reproductive health

Risky sexual behaviour and early sexual experience among young people in developed market economies are critical concerns because these factors contribute greatly to the increasing incidence of sexually transmitted diseases, including HIV. Sexually transmitted diseases are recognized as a major public health problem among young people in most of the industrialized world (Singh, Darroch and Frost, 2001). It is estimated that in the United States, those aged 15-24 years represent 25 per cent of the sexually active population but acquire nearly one half of all new sexually transmitted diseases. Teenagers and young adults are likely to be at greater risk of contracting such diseases than are older adults because they are more likely to have multiple partners and to have unprotected sex with high-risk partners. In Canada, women who had acquired a sex partner recently or who had had two or more sex partners in the previous 12 months were found to be at increased risk of infection (Public Health Agency of Canada, 2004).

Young women are particularly vulnerable to the consequences of risky sexual behaviour. Chlamydia is the most commonly reported sexually transmitted disease in many parts of the developed world, with the highest rates usually found among adolescent females and young women. In Canada, between 1997 and 2002, infection rates increased by 60 per cent in the general population but by much more among youth (Canadian Council on Social Development, 2006). In the United Kingdom, chlamydia rates are highest among women aged 16-19 years and among men between the ages of 20 and 24. The incidence of chlamydia is often highest among economically disadvantaged young women (Centers for Disease Control and Prevention, 1998). Similar patterns apply to the incidence of gonorrhoea.

In general, young people tend to have poorer access to reliable information on sexually transmitted diseases than do adults (Panchaud and others, 2000). Those who are from poorer socio-economic backgrounds are particularly less likely to have access to quality care and accurate information. Other barriers to the prevention and treatment of sexually transmitted diseases include the lack of insurance, the unavailability of transportation, and the prevalence of facilities and services that are designed for adults and may intimidate youth or compromise confidentiality (Centers for Disease Control and Prevention, 1998).

Beyond the risk of contracting sexually transmitted diseases, precocious and risky sexual behaviour exposes many young people, especially those from poorer socio-economic backgrounds, to the risk of becoming parents before they complete their education. Young parents are often forced to find opportunities to earn an income to support their new families, but this often occurs before they have acquired the skills necessary to succeed in the labour market. Differences linked to socio-economic status exist within countries. In the United Kingdom, for example, the risk of becoming a teenage mother is almost 10 times higher among women whose families are in the lowest socio-economic class than among those from higher social and economic classes. In Sweden, teenagers from broken homes are far more likely to become pregnant. These differentials exist within a context in which adolescent pregnancy rates over the past 25 years have dropped significantly (Guttmacher Institute, 2002). A comprehensive study of socio-economic disadvantage and adolescent women's sexual behaviour across five developed countries—Canada, France, Sweden, the United Kingdom and the United States—illustrates that early pregnancy and childbearing in the developed world are much more likely to occur among youth with low levels of education and income. The authors note that "being disadvantaged is associated with an early age at first intercourse, less reliance on or poor use of contraceptives, and lower motivations to avoid, or ambivalence about, having a child" (Singh, Darroch and Frost, 2001, p. 251).

Obesity and related chronic diseases

Obesity is a growing problem among youth in developed countries and is associated with a number of other health risks. In some parts of the region, obesity has become a serious public health crisis. The percentage of obese and overweight youth has increased dramatically in many of the developed market economies, especially in urban areas (World Health Organization, 2007; Food and Agriculture Organization of the United Nations, 2005). In the United States, it is estimated that over two thirds of adults and one third of children and adolescents are overweight or obese, and obesity has become the second leading cause of preventable disease and death (Ogden and others, 2002; 2006). In Canada, the proportion of young people who are overweight or obese has increased from 15 to 26 per cent in the past 25 years. Sedentary lifestyles with long hours spent in front of the television or the computer contribute to these trends (Canadian Council on Social Development, 2006).

Overweight children and adolescents are likely to remain obese as adults. Obesity is associated with increased risk of the occurrence among young people of chronic diseases that were once prevalent only in adulthood, including diabetes, hypertension, and high cholesterol. There is evidence that the incidence of diabetes is rising in many parts of the world, but especially in the developed market economies (World Health Organization, 2007). In the United States, type 2 diabetes is occurring more often among youth aged 15-19 years. Those most likely to be affected are obese, sedentary females between the ages of 10 and 18 who have a strong family history of type 2 diabetes (Fagot-Campagna, Ros Burrows and Williamson, 1999). Over the long term, treatment costs for obesity-related conditions such as diabetes and heart disease have been pushing up health spending in the United States, amid increasing fears that obesity might slow or stop longevity gains and promote disability (Graham, 2007).

The association between socio-economic status and obesity is complex and varies by country, age, gender and ethnicity. Although a variety of physiological factors may act in combination to produce clinical obesity (Power, Miller and Alpert, 2007), various studies suggest that those of lower socio-economic status are more likely to be obese (Ball and Crawford, 2005; Drewnowski and Specter, 2004; Sobal and Stunkard, 1989; Wang, 2001; Wang and Zhang, 2006). This may be the result of cost considerations in choosing food since unhealthy food is generally cheaper than healthy alternatives; food with a higher nutritional content tends to be priced much higher than "cheaper calories", making a better diet less accessible to youth from poorer households. At the same time, poorer people have fewer exercise and health-care options (Kleinfield, 2006). Recent studies suggest that the association between socio-economic status and obesity is weakening, though patterns and trends differ across age, gender and ethnic groups (Wang and Zhang, 2006; Zhang and Wang, 2004).

A focus on nutrition—including better information on the nutrients in foods typically consumed by youth, as well as regulatory measures aimed at establishments involved in food processing and distribution—can have a positive effect on alleviating the burden of obesity among youth. A recent study of a group of schools in Sweden that banned sweets and sodas found that the number of overweight children dropped from 22 to 16 per cent, while over the same time span, another group of schools that did not make such changes saw the proportion of overweight students rise from 18 to 21 per cent (Graham, 2007). The best results seem to be achieved when the Government, business and civil society organizations, and health-care groups work together to prevent or reduce obesity by ensuring a supply of healthier foods, the availability of after-school activities, and better management of chronic disease, and when young people and their families make a commitment to pursue a healthier lifestyle.

MIGRANT YOUTH IN DEVELOPED COUNTRIES: THE BOTTOM OF THE INEQUALITY LADDER?

Precise age-disaggregated data on migrants are scant; however, it is believed that young people constitute a significant share of the world's 175 million migrants (United Nations, 2005). The developed market economies are a favourite destination; in 1990, 53 per cent of all migrants resided in the region, and by 2005 the proportion had grown to 61 per cent (United Nations, 2006). Migrants now constitute 9.5 per cent of the population in developed countries, compared with 1.4 per cent in less developed regions (United Nations, 2005). The average age of migrants tends to be much lower than the median age of the population in host countries (Kupiszewska and Kupiszewski, 2006).

Youth from developing countries comprise about one third of the overall migrant flow and one fourth of the total number of migrants worldwide. If the definition of youth were extended to include those aged 25 to 29, young people would account for half of the migrant flow and one third of the total stock of migrants (United Nations Population Fund, 2006).

With the influx of young migrants, youth populations in developed countries are becoming increasingly diverse. They represent a range of nationalities and a wide array of abilities, attitudes, cultures and ethnicities. Migrant youth may exhibit patterns of transition to adulthood that are different from those of native-born youth in their host countries. In the Netherlands, for example, cohabitation and family formation are approached very differently by migrant youth and Dutch youth (see box 7.2). There are also differences and similarities between each of the migrant groups. This may have long-term implications for youth transitions to independent living. The diversity of youth populations in developed countries presents opportunities for strengthening international and intercultural solidarity among young people and for promoting more "globalized" youth participation in development. However, it also presents critical challenges and the threat of exclusion for those who are not able to compete or who are viewed as different.

Box 7.2

THE TRANSITION TO ADULTHOOD AMONG MIGRANT AND NON-MIGRANT YOUTH IN THE NETHERLANDS: PARENTAL BACKGROUND PLAYS AN IMPORTANT ROLE

A recent study on family life transitions among migrant and Dutch youth in the Netherlands revealed the importance of the parental family in the transition to adulthood. Today, 25 per cent of people between the ages of 15 and 30 in the Netherlands have at least one foreign-born parent (Statistics Netherlands, 2007). This high proportion of young people with migrant backgrounds has important implications for society.

In a study that included young adults from the four largest migrant groups (Turks, Moroccans, Surinamese and Antilleans) and those of Dutch origin, no major differences were found in the preferred timing of a transition to independent living, or in the actual patterns of leaving home. Although no clear distinctions could be made between the preferences and choices of Dutch and migrant youth in the family life domain, some differences were apparent in the areas of union formation and the timing of marriage and childbearing. In comparison with migrant youth, Dutch youth had a stronger preference for premarital cohabitation and postponing marriage and parenthood.

For young adults of Dutch and migrant origin alike, the socio-structural position of the parents was found to be an important factor in preferences and choices regarding family life transitions. The educational attainment of parents, parental religiousness, and the family structure in which the young adult grew up were found to be related to preferences regarding union formation, childbearing, gender role perspectives, and co-residence. Children of more highly educated parents had a greater preference for cohabitation before marriage, a tendency to postpone major family life transitions, and a more egalitarian outlook on gender roles. Growing up in a family in which kinship ties were strong and parent-child relationships were good resulted in more traditional attitudes and behaviour regarding family life transitions. These findings suggest that it is important to take into account the socio-structural position of, as well as the nature and quality of relationships within, the parental family when studying the transition to adulthood among both migrant and Dutch youth.

Source: H.A.G. de Valk, "Pathways into adulthood: a comparative study on family life transitions among migrant and Dutch youth" (Utrecht University/ICS dissertation series, Thela Thesis, 2006).

Migrant diversity in developed market economies has increased, with a widening array of countries of origin represented. Migrant flows often reflect historical political or economic ties. For example, in 1999, 43.5 per cent of foreigners in France were of African extraction (Organization for Economic Cooperation and Development, 2003), a reflection of France's long colonial history in Africa. Such ties have become less influential, however, as today's migrants tend to move wherever opportunities are perceived to be greatest and barriers to entry weakest. In the past few years, foreigners from Eastern Europe (especially Poland) have become increasingly prevalent in the migrant population of Ireland. Thirty-eight per cent of migrants entering Ireland in 2004/05 were from the 10 accession countries of the European Union, with 17 per cent of total immigrants coming from Poland (Central Statistics Office of Ireland, 2005). This sudden rise in immigration is partly attributable to the fact that Ireland, Denmark and the United Kingdom were the only EU-15 countries that did not impose migration restrictions on new accession members after the expansion of the European Union in May 2004. The strong performance of the Irish economy through the 1990s was another pull factor for migrant labour.

Youth are driven to migrate by a combination of factors that may include domestic political and economic difficulties and foreign demand for specific skills. The Governments of host countries recognize the need to address the shrinkage of the labour force arising from population ageing, and young people (local or foreign) constitute a ready and relatively cheap supply of labour for this purpose. Migrants work in many different fields, but an increasing number are being recruited into the service industry, especially within the health sector, to meet the care needs of an ageing population. Individuals also migrate for the purpose of family reunification, which explains why migration trends have remained strong in spite of economic downturns in parts of the developed world. Family reunification constitutes the major reason for migration in many of the OECD countries (Organization for Economic Cooperation and Development, 2003). The need for asylum represents another important reason for migration; in 2005, 2.6 million refugees lived in the developed market economies and comprised 2.3 per cent of international migrants worldwide (United Nations, 2006).

Large numbers of young people migrate to developed countries to take advantage of educational opportunities. Australia, New Zealand and the United States are the most popular destinations for educational migrants from Asia. Migrant students or young people who are the children of migrants often find better study opportunities in their host countries, but they are also faced with a number of unique challenges.

Many of the Governments of developed countries appreciate and benefit from the skills of migrant populations but also face major challenges in integrating migrants fully into their national populations. Migrant integration and incorporation have long constituted an important concern for social scientists. The discourse on migration in the United States goes back a long way and reflects the crucial role of migration in American history. Migration history loomed less centrally in studies of European history until roughly the 1980s, but the work carried out since that time now provides for similar discussions in Europe. It must be noted, however, that it is difficult to characterize the gist of the burgeoning social science literature concerned with the integration of migrant youth in Europe; integration processes are complex, and scholars use diverse approaches, so the evidence appears mixed and variable from one country to another.

Insight into the process of migrant youth integration can be gleaned from a study comparing second-generation migrant populations in Austria, Belgium, France, Germany, the Netherlands and Sweden (Crul and Vermeulen, 2003). The study found quite disparate outcomes, which appeared to be linked to the diverse institutional settings in which second-generation migrant youth lived. Turkish-background youth in Germany and Austria suffered far less unemployment than Turkish-background youth in France, Belgium and, to a lesser extent, the Netherlands. This is because of the apprentice system linked to vocational school education in Austria and Germany. In Belgium, France and the Netherlands, a significant number of Turkish-background youth held professional or white-collar jobs, but many highly qualified and unqualified second-generation Turkish members of the labour force were unemployed owing to the difficult transition from school to employment.

More recent research suggests a worsening state of affairs. Unemployment among youth in general, and among Turkish-background youth in particular, is increasing in Austria and Germany, largely because the apprenticeship systems that for decades successfully linked schooling to employment are collapsing as many of the firms that participated in and benefited from the programmes have relocated (Tamas and Münz, 2006).

Whether migrant youth are better off or worse off than native youth with respect to participation in education appears to depend on their country of residence and country of origin. It also depends on the factor(s) precipitating their migration. Ethnic disparities in educational attainment, with some immigrants doing brilliantly in schools and others doing poorly, were evident in the United States as early as a century ago (Suarez-Orozco, 1991). In New Zealand, in 1996, people born overseas were more likely than those born locally to have degree-level qualifications, and the proportion of Asian-born youth who were studying full-time was much higher than the corresponding rate for New Zealand-born youth (Fabian, 1999). The brilliant performance of some immigrant minorities in the education system may relate to the fact that certain migrant youth, depending on their family and cultural background, are under considerable pressure to succeed.

A primary problem relates to how migrants with varied backgrounds are assimilated into new education systems. A study carried out for the Australian Bureau of Immigration, Multicultural and Population Research and the New South Wales Ministry of Education found that although most newly arrived immigrants of secondary school age are placed in intensive English programmes before being transferred into mainstream education, almost half of the secondary students in New South Wales government schools who are in need of specialized English as a second language (ESL) instruction do not receive such assistance (Iredale and Fox, 1997). A consequence of the lack of preparedness for participation in education is that a large number of students underperform and drop out of school; they may be caught between two cultures and become marginalized. In the United States, approximately 54 per cent of illegal immigrants aged 18-24 years do not have a high school diploma or General Educational Development credential; the corresponding rates for legal immigrants and nationals are 27 and 15 per cent respectively (Van Hook, Bean and Passel, 2005).

In many developed countries, migrant youth are underrepresented in advanced studies. In Sweden, for example, many second-generation youth, especially those of Turkish origin, end up in vocationally oriented programmes, probably because of language barriers. Westin (2003), who tracked the progress of second-generation migrants in schooling and the labour market, found that despite participation in established remedial language programmes, up to one third of second-generation youth dropped out of the education system—a much higher rate than for Swedish youth in general (Westin, 2003). A second-chance system of adult education programmes run by municipal councils has become increasingly important to second-generation youth; in the long run, these young people may do better educationally than earlier migrant generations (Westin, 2003).

Though pockets of youth with migrant backgrounds have been successfully integrated in their communities, the social inclusion of migrants remains a challenge. Many migrant youth and those with migrant backgrounds do not benefit fully from the basic services and human development opportunities that are available in the host country. This is especially true for undocumented migrants, who, in line with national policies, may be excluded from programmes and services. Paradoxically, these migrants are often those most in need of such services, including health, education and unemployment benefits. Even where such services are available, undocumented migrants are likely to refrain from using them out of fear of prosecution.

Migrants of all ages are particularly vulnerable to exploitation. During the period of actual migration, they may be victimized by traffickers. Desperate to find a job, many will be compelled to accept work from unscrupulous employers and will become the victims of ineffective labour law enforcement (Porter, 2006). Large numbers of immigrants endure unhealthy or physically arduous working conditions and receive no employment benefits. In the absence of effective integration policies, migrant workers are likely to be concentrated in low-wage employment, where their income is more subject to stagnation.

One way in which migrants have adjusted to the challenges in their destination countries is by settling in areas in which others of similar national, ethnic or immigration backgrounds reside. Although this may be an effective way of obtaining social support, it can also deepen a young migrant's alienation from the host country. Socially marginalized migrant youth may become involved in criminal activities or exhibit other forms of antisocial behaviour.

IMPLICATIONS FOR SOCIAL INTEGRATION AND YOUTH PARTICIPATION

As youth in the developed market economies increasingly encounter challenges during their transition to adulthood, they are taking a firmer and more visible stance against what they perceive to be the sources of these difficulties. They are also increasingly involved in advocating for community, national and international development. Though their participation in formal political processes is frequently limited, many engage in a variety of community and development activities on a voluntary basis. Young people in many developed countries are becoming increasingly involved in voluntary associations, community groups and private associations that form social networks which may not target political power directly but nonetheless encourage political participation. A study examining youth political participation in 22 countries found evidence of a growing global civil society. The study noted an enormous upsurge in organized voluntary activity through global associations (Kovacheva, 2005). The Internet has facilitated this participation by providing citizens with an online opportunity structure. Digital communication technologies have proved a useful tool for motivating young people to address issues that are important to them. Studies surrounding the 2004 European Parliament elections and the 2002 elections in the United States have shown that online initiatives were successful in motivating young people to become more involved in public affairs (Ward, 2005). To encourage the political engagement of youth, the environment should be designed to appeal to their affinity for networks and communities of interest (Bennet, 2003). Many youth also engage in protests and other forms of civil disobedience to present their positions and defend their right to employment, health services, fair wages and social protection.

It is apparent that youth in developed countries are not disinterested in political processes, as is argued, for example, by Youniss and others (2002). Studies reflecting, for example, that 60 per cent of Japanese youth express little or no interest in national politics and that fewer than half say they want to do anything for Japan (Stevenson and Zusho, 2002), and those that suggest similar disinterest in the formal political systems throughout Europe and in the United States (Kovacheva, 2005; O'Toole and others, 2003; Hooghe and Stolle, 2005; Blanch, 2005; Pirie and Worcester, 2000), may be overlooking the emergence and entrenchment of a new form of political activism among youth. While young people in developed countries appear to be relatively uninterested in traditional forms of political participation, many are actively engaged in new forms of expression and civic involvement that address their concerns and interests directly. Perhaps this is in response to the fact that opportunities for political participation in the developed market economies tend to be highly structured and institutionalized. Youth may perceive these structures as too formalized and restricted and believe that they are inadequate to meet their needs (Forbrig, 2005; O'Toole and others, 2003; Pirie and Worcester, 2000).

It may therefore be argued that a cultural shift in political participation has occurred in many developed countries. Young people today may not be active in formal political circles, but they are passionate and proactive when it comes to advocating for environmental protection, human rights, gender equality and self-expression, for example (Inglehart, cited in Kovacheva, 2005). In the changing political context, young people should not necessarily be expected to embrace the same political institutions and values as those of previous generations.

Unconventional forms of political and social participation need to become more fully integrated into the conceptualization of democracy to allow youth more opportunities to be engaged. The Council of Europe's Steering Committee for Intergovernmental Cooperation in the Youth Field has developed a proactive understanding of youth participation, recognizing that "participation is not an aim in itself but an approach to becoming (an active citizen that involves) taking an active role both in the development of one's own environment and in European cooperation" (CDEJ, 1997, p. 7, cited in Kovecheva, 2005). Youth should be allowed and encouraged to participate in the political sphere on their own terms. While it is important to transmit to youth the value of conventional participation, even when the immediate effects may appear negligible, the political system can only remain viable if citizens are active, both conventionally and unconventionally (Blanch, 2005).

SUMMARY AND CONCLUSIONS

The opportunities available to youth living in developed market economies are unmatched in other parts of the world. Nevertheless, inequalities in youth development persist, particularly in the areas of education, ICT access, employment and health. Unequal opportunities in these areas are largely the result of socio-economic differences, but inequalities linked to ethnicity, race, sex, and migrant status also play an important role.

Throughout the region, enrolment and completion rates are high at all levels of education, but there are still major intercountry and intracountry differentials in educational outcomes. Disparities in educational performance reflect not only socio-economic differences among students, but also differences in educational systems. Educational inequalities create an uneven playing field in terms of opportunities for youth to make a smooth transition to adulthood. The disadvantaged face unemployment, underemployment, poverty, social isolation, and the risk of being drawn into antisocial groups. Evidence that some of the education differentials across groups have diminished in the region offers a reason for hope, however.

Information and communication technologies are taking on an increasingly important role in the lives of youth. They are used not only as a source of education and information, but also as a means to find employment and to interact with peers. While gender differentials in computer and Internet use are small, there seem to be variations across and within countries in terms of opportunities for youth to use these technologies. At a time when the ability to use the Internet is becoming a prerequisite for participation in the global economy, Governments need to ensure that all youth have ICT access. However, additional steps need to be taken to minimize the potential risks to youth that are associated with Internet use, including exploitation and abuse.

It is a matter of concern that, despite fairly good labour market conditions, many young people in developed economies have difficulty obtaining stable, decent long-term employment corresponding to their skill levels. The resulting tendency for youth to remain in education for longer periods of time, or to enter into internships or other volunteer positions in order to improve their employability, has had an unequalizing effect on labour market opportunities for youth. The increasing importance employers are placing on previous work experience represents an advantage for those youth whose families can afford to support them during internships, which are frequently poorly remunerated. This situation calls for increased corporate responsibility in ensuring that internships are sufficiently remunerated or that part-time internship options are available, so that youth from all backgrounds are able to gain work experience. Public or private stipends for volunteers and interns from disadvantaged backgrounds would ensure greater equality in entry-level labour markets. Finally, increased opportunities for apprenticeships and entry-level jobs that require little or no prior job experience are needed.

The health and well-being of youth in developed market economies are being compromised by inequalities in access to health care and by the behavioural choices young people make, particularly with respect to drinking, drugs and sexual encounters. Among youth from disadvantaged backgrounds, poor choices are to a large extent the result of alienation from opportunities and the lack of constructive leisure activities to which their better-off peers have access. Increasing levels of obesity among youth are beginning to have consequences for health systems in the more developed economies. Governments, businesses, parents and health-care professionals need to form partnerships and address the problem by improving nutrition, food distribution mechanisms, and leisure activities.

With the influx of young migrants into the developed market economies, youth populations in these countries are becoming increasingly diverse. To foster social cohesion, inequalities linked to migrant status need to be reduced, and efforts to facilitate social integration need to be stepped up. This can be achieved through greater efforts to promote migrant youth integration into the educational system, and by improving employment opportunities for youth with migrant backgrounds. Active labour market policies can be instrumental in this regard.

Civic involvement among youth in the developed market economies has shifted from political engagement to high levels of community volunteer and development activity. Such types of civic engagement constitute an important form of non-formal education for youth and also provide tangible benefits to the community. The energy and creativity of youth are powerful resources from which societies should draw in the interest of social and political development. In order to broaden the political landscape and make it more inclusive, youth must be allowed to express how they themselves conceive politics and to become politically active in ways that may be non-traditional but offer greater personal fulfilment. To avoid inequalities in participation and non-formal learning, practical strategies must be developed to encourage the involvement of youth from disadvantaged socio-economic backgrounds in volunteer activities.

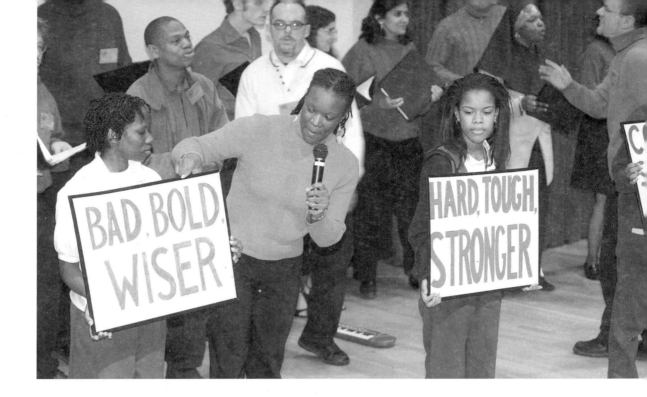

References

Acevedo-Garcia, Dolores, and others (2007). Children left behind: how metropolitan areas are failing America's children. Report from *diversitydata.org*, Harvard School of Public Health and Center for the Advancement of Health. January. Available from http://diversitydata.sph.harvard.edu/children_left_behind_final_report.pdf.

Agency for Healthcare Research and Quality (2005). Women's health care in the United States: selected findings from the 2004 National Healthcare Quality and Disparities Report. Fact sheet. AHRQ publication No. 05-P021. May.

Association for Supervision and Curriculum Development (2007). Watching out for our poorest schools. *Is It Good for the Kids?* Web column by ASCD Executive Director Gene Carter. Available from http://www.ascd.org/portal/site/ascd/index.jsp/.

Ball, Kylie, and David Crawford (2005). Socioeconomic status and weight change in adults: a review. *Social Science and Medicine*, vol. 60, No. 9 (May), pp. 1987-2010.

Bell, Lisa, and others (2007). Failure to launch: cross-national trends in the transition to economic independence. Luxembourg Income Study Working Paper Series, No. 456.

Bennett, W. Lance (2003). Civic learning in changing democracies: challenges for citizenship and education. Center for Communication and Civic Engagement, Working Paper No. 4.

Blanch, Daniel (2005). Between the traditional and the post modern: political disaffection and youth participation in Galicia. In *Revisiting Youth Political Participation*, Joerg Forbrig, editor. Strasbourg: Council of Europe Publishing.

Briedis, Kolja, and Karl-Heinz Minks (2007). Generation Praktikum—Mythos oder Massenphänomen? HIS: Projektbericht. April.

Brubaker, Rogers (1992). *Citizenship and Nationhood in France and Germany*. Cambridge, Massachusetts: Harvard University Press

Canadian Council on Social Development (2006). *The Progress of Canada's Children and Youth 2006*. Available from http://www.ccsd.ca/pccy/2006/tools.htm.

Centers for Disease Control and Prevention (1998). Special focus profiles: section 8—STDs in adolescents and young adults. In *1998 Sexually Transmitted Disease Surveillance Report*. Available from http://0-www.cdc.gov.mill1.sjlibrary.org/nchstp/dstd/Stats_Trends/1998Surveillance/98PDF/Section8.pdf (accessed on 28 May 2007).

_____ (2004). Health behaviors of adults: United States, 1999-2001. Data from the National Health Interview Survey, 2004.

Central Statistics Office, Ireland (2005). Population and migration estimates, April 2005. Available from http://www.cso.ie/releasespublications/documents/population/current/popmig.pdf.

comScore Europe (2006). March European traffic to career resources, job search and training/education sites increases 27 percent versus year ago. Press release (25 April 2006). Available from http://www.comscore.com/press/release.asp?press=844.

Crul, M., and H. Vermeulen, editors (2003). *The Future of the Second Generation: The Integration of Migrant Youth in Six European Countries.* Special issue of International Migration Review, vol. 37, No. 4 (winter).

Drewnowski, Adam, and S.E. Specter (2004). Poverty and obesity: the role of energy density and energy costs. *American Journal of Clinical Nutrition*, vol. 79, No. 1 (January), pp. 6-16.

Dunn K.A., and others (1998). Teens at work: a statewide study of jobs, hazards, and injuries. *Journal of Adolescent Health*, vol. 22, No. 1, pp. 19-25.

Eitzen, D. Stanley (1992). Problem students: the sociocultural roots. *Phi Delta Kappan*, vol. 73, No. 8 (April).

Fabian, Angela (1999). People born overseas. Statistics New Zealand. Available from http://www.stats.govt.nz.

Fagot-Campagna, Anne, M.T. Ros Burrows and P.D. Williamson (1999). The public health epidemiology of type 2 diabetes in children and adolescents: a case study of American Indian adolescents in the Southwestern United States. *Clinica Chimica Acta*, vol. 286, No. 1 (August), pp. 81-95.

Fahmy, Eldin (1999). Youth, poverty and social exclusion. Working Paper No. 27. Poverty and Social Exclusion Survey of Britain/University of Bristol, Townsend Centre for International Poverty Research. Available from http://www.bris.ac.uk/poverty/pse/99PSE-WP27.pdf (accessed on 13 July 2007).

Feinstein, Jonathan S. (1993). The relationship between socioeconomic status and health: a review of the literature. *The Milbank Quarterly*, vol. 71, No. 2, pp. 279-322.

Food and Agriculture Organization of the United Nations (2005). *The State of Food Insecurity in the World 2004: Monitoring Progress towards the World Food Summit and Millennium Development Goals.* United Nations publication, Sales No. E.05.LI.4.

Forbrig, Joerg (2005). Democratic politics, legitimacy and youth participation. In *Revisiting Youth Political Participation*, Joerg Forbrig, editor. Strasbourg: Council of Europe Publishing.

Förster, Michael, and Marco Mira d'Ercole (2005). Income distribution and poverty in OECD countries in the second half of the 1990s. Social, Employment and Migration Working Papers, No. 22. Paris: Organization for Economic Cooperation and Development.

Graham, Jed (2007). Overweight Americans to weigh on nation's future health costs. *Investor's Business Daily* (30 May 2007).

Grühn, Von Dieter, and Heidemarie Hecht (2007). *Generation Praktikum?* Studie des Arbeitsbereichs Absolventenforschung der FU Berlin im Auftrag der DGB-Jugend und der Hans-Böckler-Stiftung. February.

Grunbaum, Jo Anne, and others (2001). Youth risk behaviour surveillance—United States, 2001. Morbidity and Mortality Weekly Report, surveillance summaries (28 June 2001). Centers for Disease Control and Prevention. Available from http://www.cdc.gov/mmwr/preview/mmwrhtml/ss5104a1.htm.

Guttmacher Institute (2002). Teenagers' sexual and reproductive health: developed countries. *Facts in Brief.*

Hatcher, Richard (1998). Class differentiation in education: rational choices? *British Journal of Sociology of Education*, vol. 19, No. 1, pp. 5-24.

Hibell, Bjorn, and others (2000). *The 1999 ESPAD Report: Alcohol and Other Drug Use among Students in 30 European Countries.* Stockholm: Swedish Council for Information on Alcohol and Other Drugs.

Hjern, A., and S. Bremberg (2002). Social aetiology of violent deaths in Swedish children and youth. *Journal of Epidemiology and Community Health*, vol. 56, No. 9, pp. 688-692.

Hooghe, Marc, and Dietlind Stolle (2005). Youth organisations within political parties: political recruitment and the transformation of party systems. In Revisiting Youth Political Participation, Joerg Forbrig, editor. Strasbourg: Council of Europe Publishing.

International Labour Office (2004). Global Employment Trends for Youth 2004. Geneva: International Labour Organization, August.

_____ (2005). *Key Indicators of the Labour Market*. Fourth edition. Geneva.

International Telecommunication Union (2006). Data on youth computer use for the years 2004 and 2005. With Eurostat (2006).

Iredale, Robyn, and Christine Fox (1997). The impact of immigration on school education in New South Wales, Australia. *International Migration Review*, vol. 31, No. 3 (fall), pp. 655-669.

Kalmijn, Matthis, and Gerbert Kraaykamp (1996). Race, cultural capital, and schooling: an analysis of trends in the United States. *Sociology of Education*, vol. 69, No. 1, pp. 22-34.

Karen, David (2002). Changes in access to higher education in the United States: 1980-1992. *Sociology of Education*, vol. 75, No. 3, pp. 191-210.

Kleinfield, N.R. (2006). Modern ways open India's doors to diabetes. *The New York Times* (13 September 2006).

Kovacheva, Siyka (2005). Will youth rejuvenate the patterns of political participation? In *Revisiting Youth Political Participation*. Joerg Forbrig, editor. Strasbourg: Council of Europe Publishing.

Kupiszewska, D., and M. Kupiszewski (2006). Non-national populations in the EU member States. *Statistics in Focus* (August). Luxembourg: Eurostat.

Lloyd, Cynthia B., editor (2006). *Growing Up Global: The Changing Transitions to Adulthood in Developing Countries*. National Research Council and Institute of Medicine of the National Academies. Washington, D.C.: National Academies Press.

Ogden, Cynthia L., and others (2002). Prevalence and trends in overweight among US children and adolescents, 1999-2000. *Journal of the American Medical Association*, vol. 288, No. 14, pp. 1728-1732.

_____ (2006). Prevalence of overweight and obesity in the United States, 1999-2004. *Journal of the American Medical Association*, vol. 295, No. 13, pp. 1549-1555.

Organization for Economic Cooperation and Development (2003). T*rends in International Migration 2003*. Paris: SOPEMI.

_____ (2005). *Education at a Glance 2005: OECD Indicators*. Paris. Available from www.sourceoecd.org/education.

_____ (2006). *Education at a Glance 2006: OECD Indicators*. Paris. Available from www.sourceoecd.org/education.

_____ (2007). *Education at a Glance 2007: OECD Indicators*. Paris. Available from www.sourceoecd.org/education.

O'Toole, Therese, and others (2003). Tuning out or left out? Participation and non-participation among young people. *Contemporary Politics*, vol. 9, No. 1 (March), pp. 45-61.

Paunchaud, Christine, and others (2000). Sexually transmitted diseases among adolescents in developed countries. *Family Planning Perspectives*, vol. 32, No. 1, pp. 24-32 and 45.

Pew Research Center for the People and the Press (2007). *How Young People View Their Lives, Futures and Politics: A Portrait of "Generation Next"*. Available from http://people-press.org/reports/pdf/300.pdf (accessed on 15 March 2007).

Pfaff, Nicolle (2005). Adolescent ways of political learning: results from Eastern Germany. In *Revisiting Youth Political Participation*, Joerg Forbrig, editor. Strasbourg: Council of Europe Publishing.

Phillpots, Greg, and Peggy Causer, editors (2006). *Regional Trends*, No. 39, 2006 edition. Basingstoke: Palgrave Macmillan for the Office for National Statistics, United Kingdom. Available from http://www.statistics.gov.uk/RegionalTrends39/.

Pirie, Madsen, and Robert Worcester (2000). *The Big Turn-Off: Attitudes of Young People to Government, Citizenship and Community*. London: Adam Smith Institute.

Porter, Edwards (2006). Here illegally, working hard and paying taxes. *The New York Times* (19 June 2006).

Power, Carrie, Sally K. Miller and Patricia T. Alpert (2007). Promising new causal explanations for obesity and obesity-related diseases. *Biological Research for Nursing*, vol. 8, No. 3, pp. 223-233.

Public Health Agency of Canada (2004). E.coli 0157: Alberta (update). *Infectious Diseases News Brief* (5 November 2004). Available from http://www.phac-aspc.gc.ca/bid-bmi/dsd-dsm/nb-ab/2004/nb4504_e.html.

Quinn, Jane (1999). Where need meets opportunity: Youth development programmes for early teens. *The Future of Children*, vol. 9, No. 2, When School Is Out (fall), pp. 96-116.

Singh, Susheela, Jacqueline E. Darroch and Jennifer J. Frost (2001). Socioeconomic disadvantage and adolescent women's sexual and reproductive behavior: the case of five developed countries. *Family Planning Perspectives*, vol. 33, No. 6 (November/December), pp. 251-258 and 289.

Smeeding, Timothy M. (2005). Public policy, economic inequality, and poverty: the United States in comparative perspective. *Social Science Quarterly*, vol. 86 (supplement), pp. 955-983.

Sobal, J., and A.J. Stunkard (1989). Socio-economic status and obesity: a review of the literature. *Psychological Bulletin*, vol. 105, No. 2 (March), pp. 260-275.

Stevenson, Harold W., and Akane Zusho (2002). Adolescence in China and Japan: adapting to a changing environment. In *The World's Youth: Adolescence in Eight Regions of the Globe*, B. Bradford Brown, Reed W. Larson and T.S. Saraswathi, editors. Cambridge: Cambridge University Press.

Suárez-Orozco, Marcelo M., editor (1991). *Migration, Minority Status and Education: European Dilemmas and Responses in the 1990s*. Theme issue of *Anthropology and Education Quarterly*, vol. 22, No. 2, pp. 99-120.

Tamas, Kristof, and Rainer Münz (2006). *Labour Migrants Unbound? EU Enlargement, Transitional Measures and Labour Market Effects*. Stockholm: Institute for Futures Studies.

Toroyan, T., and M. Peden, editors (2007). *Youth and Road Safety*. Geneva: World Health Organization.

United Nations (2005). *World Population Prospects: The 2004 Revision*. New York.

_____ (2006). World population monitoring, focusing on international migration and development. Report of the Secretary-General (E/CN 9/2006/3).

United Nations Children's Fund (2007). *Child Poverty in Perspective: An Overview of Child Well-being in Rich Countries*. Report Card No. 7. Florence, Italy: UNICEF Innocenti Research Centre.

United Nations Population Fund (2006). *Moving Young—State of World Population 2006: Youth Supplement*. Sales No. E.06.III.H.2. Available from http://www.unfpa.org/swp/2006/moving_young_eng/introduction.html.

Van Hook, Jennifer, Frank D. Bean and Jeffrey Passel (2005). Unauthorized migrants living in the United States: a mid-decade portrait. Feature story, *Migration Information Source* (September). Migration Policy Institute. Available from http://www.migrationinformation.org/Feature/display.cfm?id=329 (accessed on 15 May 2007).

Wagenaar, A.C., and C.L. Perry (1994). Community strategies for the reduction of youth drinking: theory and application. *Journal of Research on Adolescence*, vol. 4, No. 2, pp. 319-345.

Wagstaff, Adam (2002). Poverty and health sector inequalities. *Bulletin of the World Health Organization*, vol. 80, No. 2, pp. 97-105.

Wang, Y. (2001). Cross-national comparison of childhood obesity: the epidemic and the relationship between obesity and socioeconomic status. *International Journal of Epidemiology*, vol. 30, No. 5, pp. 1129-1136.

_____ and Q. Zhang (2006). Are low socioeconomic status American children and adolescents at increased risk of obesity? Trends in the association between overweight and family income between 1971 and 2002. *American Journal of Clinical Nutrition*, vol. 84, pp. 707-716.

Ward, Janelle (2005). An opportunity for engagement in cyberspace: political youth Web sites during the 2004 European Parliament election campaign. *Information Polity*, vol. 10, No. 3-4, pp. 233-246. Special issue: *The World Wide Web and the 2004 European Parliament Election*, Wainer Lusoli and Nicholas W. Jankowski, editors.

Westin, C. (2003). Young people of migrant origin in Sweden. *International Migration Review*, vol. 37, No. 4 (winter), pp. 987-1010. Special issue: The Future of the Second Generation: The Integration of Migrant Youth in Six European Countries.

Wilkinson, Richard, and Michael Marmot, editors (2003). *Social Determinants of Health: The Solid Facts*. Second edition. Copenhagen: WHO Regional Office for Europe.

Willms, J. Douglas (1999). *Inequalities in Literacy Skills among Youth in Canada and the United States*. International Adult Literacy Survey. Ottawa: Statistics Canada.

World Health Organization (2007). Obesity and overweight. Chronic disease information sheet. Global Strategy on Diet, Physical Activity and Health. Available from http://www.who.int/dietphysicalactivity/publications/facts/obesity/en/.

Youniss J., and others (2002). Youth civic engagement in the twenty-first century. *Journal of Research on Adolescence*, vol. 12, No. 1, pp. 121-148.

Zhang, Qi, and Youfa Wang (2004). Trends in the association between obesity and socioeconomic status is U.S. adults: 1971 to 2000. *Obesity Research*, vol. 12, pp. 1622-1632.

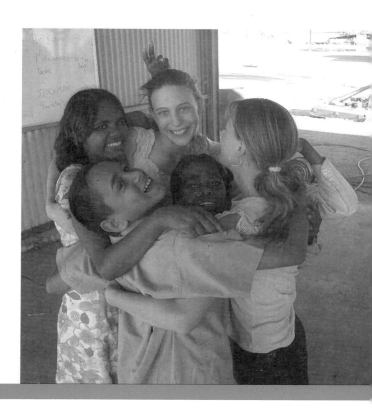

Chapter 8

Ensuring *YOUTH* development
around the world:
the way **forward**

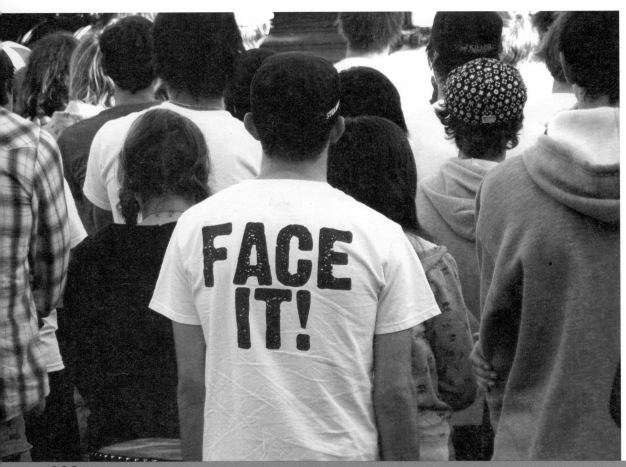

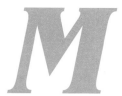ore than 10 years after the adoption of the World Programme of Action for Youth to the Year 2000 and Beyond, many youth continue to have limited access to opportunities for self- development, which reduces the contribution they can make to national development.

The preceding chapters paint a mixed picture of contemporary youth development, highlighting visible progress in some areas but persistent challenges and obstacles in many others. Youth have a vital role to play in shaping present and future societies, and their transition to independent adulthood is crucial in this regard. More than 10 years have passed since the adoption of the World Programme of Action for Youth, which emphasizes that "every State should provide its young people with opportunities for obtaining education, for acquiring skills and for participating fully in all aspects of society, with a view to, inter alia, acquiring productive employment and leading self-sufficient lives" (United Nations, 1996, paragraph 8(a)). Notable progress has been made in many areas; however, much remains to be done at all levels to translate this goal into reality.

The review of regional experiences suggests that young people the world over are in a better position than past generations of youth to contribute to development. However, there are still far too many who face barriers and constraints arising from their backgrounds or from the social environment in which they live. Regardless of their place of birth or current residence, young people continue to experience similar sets of difficulties that impinge on their healthy and timely transition to adulthood. Apart from health, education and employment issues, such areas as poverty reduction and the availability of opportunities for volunteer work and for the advancement of young women and girls continue to present a challenge. There are differences in the severity of the challenges and opportunities for youth in each of these areas of development. For example, developing regions have made considerable progress in education, but access has not expanded equally within or between countries. In sub-Saharan Africa and parts of Asia, access to quality education, especially at the secondary and tertiary levels, is still a major problem for many youth.

Regional differences in the ability of young people to make the transition to adulthood are undoubtedly related to overall levels of economic development as well as the extent to which countries have invested in key areas of youth development. In both developed and developing countries, young people are increasingly finding mechanisms to overcome the challenges, but there are often costs involved. For example, many well-educated and well-qualified youth spend years "waiting" in further education, internships, or volunteer positions for job opportunities to open up. In developing regions, young people often migrate in search of better opportunities. Even in many highly developed countries, youth transitions have faltered or been delayed, and young people are increasingly experiencing a "failure to launch" into adulthood (Bell and others, 2007). Unfortunately, in the face of life's overwhelming difficulties, some youth choose socially inappropriate options such as violence, drug use or other forms of delinquency with negative consequences for their future.

The core areas identified by this report as requiring attention—education, employment, poverty reduction, health, and promoting the rights of young women—apply to all world regions to varying degrees. National policy action inevitably requires adjustment to reflect specific regional and domestic circumstances. However, key interventions in all of these areas have been identified by the World Programme of Action for Youth (see box 8.1), and they constitute the minimum set of actions upon which to build more specific recommendations. The recommendations presented in the succeeding sections must be considered in the light of the Millennium Development Goals, which provide the overall framework for the global development agenda in the next decade.

When the areas highlighted above are not addressed in a comprehensive manner with attention to all youth, regardless of their background, young people's ability to participate meaningfully in development is compromised. Although second chances to make up for missed opportunities are important, it is even more critical to take advantage of first chances. Losing out on these opportunities the first time around can be costly.

Many of the recommendations presented in this chapter reflect those emanating from the development dialogue and recognized analytical works. The recommendations do not address each region specifically; the fact that countries are at different stages with respect to the progress young people have achieved and the challenges they face must be taken into account in policy development and implementation, as there are no "one-size-fits-all" solutions.

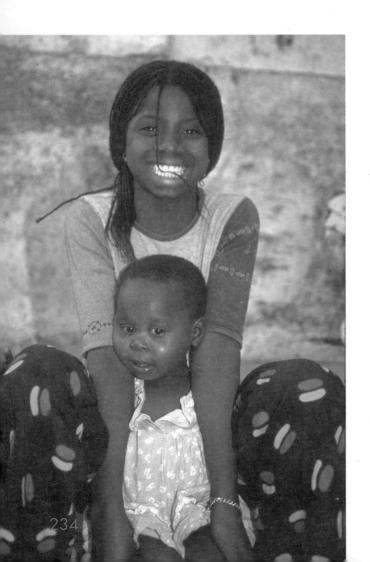

Box 8.1

Education

1. Improve technical, secondary and higher education, maximizing the use of new technologies.
2. Preserve cultural heritage and diversity and encourage participatory dialogue.
3. Increase vocational, professional and life-skills training.
4. Promote human rights education, including among migrant and indigenous youth.
5. Facilitate the transition from school to work.
6. Train skilled guidance and vocational counsellors, as well as youth workers.

Employment

1. Increase microfinance and entrepreneurship programmes to benefit young people.
2. Target the unemployment of vulnerable and marginalized youth.
3. Encourage youth-led and youth-run voluntary service projects.
4. Promote youth employment and skill development in the context of globalization.

Poverty

1. Empower young people as key contributors in poverty reduction strategies.
2. Promote decent work with social protection schemes, even in the informal economy.
3. Increase vocational training and employment opportunities.
4. Foster rural development to include youth in strengthening food security and sustainable agriculture.

Health

1. Ensure the provision of youth-friendly basic health services, including sexual and reproductive health care.
2. Further the development of health education, including sexual and reproductive health education.
3. Scale up the prevention and treatment of HIV infection and AIDS among youth.
4. Promote good hygiene and sanitary practices.
5. Reduce preventable diseases and illnesses.
6. Eliminate the trafficking and sexual abuse of young people.
7. Reduce obesity, hunger and malnutrition.

Rights of girls and young women

1. Eliminate discrimination and ensure equal participation at all levels of society.
2. Increase levels of education and literacy, including non-formal education.
3. Develop gender-sensitive health programmes, including sexual and reproductive health programmes.
4. Increase employment opportunities and ensure equal representation at decision-making levels.
5. Eliminate all forms of violence against girls and young women and strengthen the family.

Source: Drawn from the World Programme of Action for Youth (A/RES/50/81).

EDUCATION

Access to basic education has improved, but youth need a higher-quality education, including greater access to tertiary education, to succeed in the global economy. In developing education policies, particular attention must be given to providing opportunities for disadvantaged groups in society. Young women in many regions continue to have limited access to quality education in relevant specializations.

Worldwide, perhaps the greatest progress with respect to youth development has been made in the area of education. More young people are completing basic education, making this the best-educated generation of youth ever. Although public sector funding for education has not kept up with demand, in many regions, private and transnational ventures have played a vital complementary role, and distance learning opportunities have expanded as well.

Many of the deficiencies in educational performance and attainment among youth reflect past and present inadequacies in education systems. Wide, entrenched gender gaps in access, the relatively poor quality of instruction in many settings, and the lack of relevant, up-to-date curricula prevent many students from acquiring the knowledge and skills they need to function effectively in society. Even the developed market economies, which offer many and varied opportunities for education, have not been universally successful in addressing the wide intracountry and intercountry disparities in access to schooling. Youth from disadvantaged backgrounds are particularly vulnerable to exclusion.

High educational qualifications do not necessarily guarantee decent employment. Increasingly, it is not just those with little education and training who are left behind, but also educated youth, whose knowledge, skills and attitudes may not be compatible with the needs of the global economy.

Recommendations

- Interventions in education must be geared towards providing students with the basic knowledge they need to function in society, but also towards furnishing the skills required to enter the world of work. In particular, there is a need to ensure that educational provision is aligned with and tailored to the needs of the global economy.

- Countries that have concentrated on providing basic education must now focus on improving quality and performance levels. Policies and programmes need to be geared not only towards ensuring universal primary education and strengthening literacy, but also towards improving instructional quality, educational facilities, and student proficiency levels. In the context of rapid globalization, it is especially important to ensure that secondary education becomes the new minimum level of attainment.

- To encourage the development of education and training systems that are better aligned with the current and future needs of young people and their societies, a wide range of learning options—including formal and non-formal education, literacy instruction, job-skills training, and lifelong education—should be made available.

- In developing countries in particular, education policies have too long focused on providing basic education as a sort of panacea for young people's development problems. Opportunities for young people to pursue university or other advanced studies, engage in research, or receive training for self-employment should be expanded in the developing world.

- Disparities in access to education prevent many young people, especially those from minority groups and migrant backgrounds, from participating fully in society. The educational needs of vulnerable and disadvantaged groups must be specifically addressed in national policies.

- Secondary and tertiary qualifications are becoming increasingly necessary for meaningful participation in an evolving global economy. Although undue emphasis on academic degrees must be avoided, it should be recognized that there is a basic level of academic competence youth must achieve if they are to succeed in today's globalizing world.

- Governments and intergovernmental and non-governmental organizations in both developed and developing countries should work to create a supportive, enabling environment in which young people can obtain an education and pursue various forms of training at all levels. Arrangements should also be made to facilitate mutual academic exchanges among developing countries.

- There is a need for greater "youth sensitivity" and a "youth perspective" in a number of policy areas. Particular attention must be given to easing the school-to-work transition for young people. The needs of the job market should guide educational provision, since obtaining productive, decent employment is necessary for socio-economic stability and success.

- Public education is necessary and must be adequately supported and monitored. Governments must also introduce or strengthen quality assurance mechanisms for private education.

- A review and revision of educational curricula may be necessary to ensure that young people are provided with the academic, professional, entrepreneurial and job-search skills they need for the workplace. There should be close monitoring of labour market needs and trends, and educational curricula should be adjusted periodically to ensure continued relevance. Schools and other educational institutions should also provide youth with social, personal and other life skills that will benefit them and the wider community. Education must support active citizenship, intercultural learning, and social solidarity, ensuring equitable development, social justice, peace and social cohesion.

EMPLOYMENT

Many youth seek work but remain unemployed; many are well-educated but cannot find work in an increasingly competitive and rapidly changing global labour market.

Productive employment represents one of the most fundamental and rewarding ways in which young people can become engaged in their communities while also making a positive contribution to development. Earning an income through paid employment strengthens self-esteem and independence and is an essential component of the transition to responsible adulthood.

Unemployment and underemployment among youth constitute a global problem. All over the world, young people are finding it increasingly difficult to break into the labour market. Youth make up 25 per cent of the global working-age population but account for 43.7 per cent of the unemployed, which means that almost every other jobless person in the world is between the ages of 15 and 24. A global deficit of decent work opportunities has resulted in a situation in which one out of every three youth in the world is either seeking but unable to find work, has given up the job search entirely, or is working but still living on less than US$ 2 a day. To circumvent the difficulties associated with unemployment, growing numbers of young people are staying in full-time education for longer periods.

The disturbing reality is that economic growth is not always accompanied by growth in employment, especially decent employment. When jobs are scarce, large numbers of young people are deprived of the opportunity to secure independent housing or the accommodations necessary to establish and support a family and participate fully in society. Advances in technology and communications, coupled with improved productivity, have created new challenges but have also provided new (if somewhat limited) employment opportunities. If effective solutions to the perils of jobless growth are not found, the cost to society is likely to be extremely high in the long run. Unemployment contributes to a wide range of social ills, and young people are particularly susceptible to its damaging effects; lacking marketable skills, young people may experience low self-esteem, marginalization and impoverishment. Ultimately, to society, such a situation represents an enormous waste of valuable human resources and lost productivity.

Keeping up with an ever-changing job market is a challenge for even the most advanced educational systems. Schools and universities must not only provide academic, professional, and technical qualifications; they must also equip potential labour force entrants with the social, moral and attitudinal skills needed for meaningful employment.

Evidence indicates that educational gains among females around the world have not necessarily improved their position in the labour market. Young women face higher rates of unemployment and underemployment and are typically paid lower wages than their male peers.

Many young people throughout the world have limited options in the formal economy and may be compelled to work in the informal economy for low pay. Apart from inadequate remuneration, informal employment typically offers little social protection or job security, and working conditions may be dangerous. Youth often have trouble finding ways to build upon their education so that they can be better prepared to participate in a rapidly changing job market. Young women and young men are active participants in the labour force, yet opportunities for decent work are limited. Many young workers, aware that they are at a disadvantage in the labour market, accept lower wages than older workers and are more willing to accept short-term contracts.

Recommendations

- Governments, with the support of the international community and other stakeholders, should design and implement programmes aimed at reducing the proportion of youth in vulnerable employment. The term "vulnerable employment" refers to inadequate working conditions and to the work of own-account workers, unpaid family labour and others without social protection. It is important to ensure that policies established to address this issue do not simply move youth from vulnerable employment to unemployment but rather create viable decent employment options for them. Only through decent employment do young people have the opportunity to work themselves out of poverty.

- The persistence of unemployment among youth vividly demonstrates that economic growth alone is not a panacea for youth employment problems. Policies must focus on improving the overall context of development as well as providing opportunities in the labour market for those who are most vulnerable to unemployment. It is important for Governments to offer incentives to private sector enterprises that are labour-intensive and could contribute to the alleviation of youth unemployment.

- Volunteer work should be promoted and encouraged. Efforts are required to ensure that these experiences are mutually beneficial for the volunteer and the entity benefiting from the assistance. Recognizing that volunteer opportunities help to hone the skills of youth while also enabling them to contribute to development, Governments should devise incentives for businesses that provide such opportunities for young people. The provision of inducements also allows better monitoring of how youth fare in these work situations and may protect those who are vulnerable to exploitation.

- Governments should involve youth, represented by youth-led organizations, in identifying those subgroups of young people in need of special attention. Youth should also be involved in developing innovative approaches to, and assist with the implementation of strategies for, creating opportunities for decent and productive work for young people.

- Policies designed to support youth employment must be tailored to individual circumstances, as the contexts in which youth live and the solutions required to address employment challenges differ. Youth living in slums require different employment policies than youth living in rural areas. Similarly, specific policies are needed to address the employment needs of young women, the youngest members of the youth cohort, migrant youth, young people with disabilities, youth from ethnic minorities, and youth living in areas affected by armed conflict.

- Governments should contribute to easing the school-to-work transition by creating a supportive learning environment and facilitating the provision of ongoing skills training that translates into poverty-reducing employment.

- Partnerships between educational institutions and the public and private sectors should be established to facilitate the exchange of information on labour market needs and trends. Educational institutions can then focus on providing skills in high demand in order to facilitate the flow of labour to expanding industries where youth will be most productive.

- Every effort should be made to ensure that young people have access to information, knowledge and financial services that will enable them to establish their own business enterprises if they so choose.

- The private sector must be encouraged to make apprenticeship opportunities available for youth. Adequate remuneration must be provided to ensure equal access.

- Active labour market policies for youth need to be carefully and objectively evaluated to determine which are particularly effective in promoting youth employment.

- In many countries, facilities for vocational training are insufficient and need to be scaled up. Technical and vocational training is an important bridge between education and the world of work. Vocational education can provide targeted training for those young people who lack marketable skills, improving their chances of securing productive employment.

POVERTY

Youth in many regions experience poverty; many decide to migrate, regardless of the costs, to find greener pastures.

The World Programme of Action for Youth identifies poverty and hunger as one core priority area, noting that more than 1 billion people in the world today live in unacceptable conditions of poverty, mostly in developing countries. Poverty has multiple manifestations, including hunger and malnutrition, ill health, a lack of (or limited) access to education and other basic services, increased morbidity and mortality from illness, homelessness or inadequate housing, unsafe living conditions, and social discrimination and exclusion; it is also characterized by the absence of opportunities to participate in decision-making and in civil and sociocultural affairs. Hunger and malnutrition remain among the most serious and intractable threats faced by humanity, often preventing children and youth from taking part in society. Hunger is the result of many factors, including incompatibilities between traditional and modern production systems, excessive population growth, the mismanagement of food production and distribution, poor accessibility, the maldistribution of financial resources, the inefficient or excessive exploitation of natural resources, unsustainable patterns of consumption, environmental pollution, natural and man-made disasters, and armed conflict.

Poverty is inseparably linked to a lack of access to, or the loss of control over, resources, including land, skills, knowledge, capital and social connections. Without those resources, individuals and their families have limited access to institutions, markets, employment and public services. Young people are particularly affected by this situation.

In the context of poverty and lack of opportunities, migration has become one of the coping mechanisms used by young people across the world to improve their livelihoods. Though much of this migration may initially be for educational purposes, many youth remain in their host countries in search of better-paying jobs than they would find back home. The exploitation of young migrants by traffickers, unscrupulous employers, and agents needs to be addressed as a stand-alone policy issue. Unfortunately, both internal and international migration among youth tends to be neglected by policy makers and researchers, even though members of this age group are known to be among the most mobile.

Recommendations

- Poverty among youth is closely tied to their unemployment and underemployment. Policies to address youth poverty must therefore focus, as a matter of priority, on eliminating barriers to youth employment.

- It is imperative that the multidimensional aspects of poverty be addressed to ensure that a deepening of poverty does not occur during the transition from youth to adulthood. A broad approach should reflect the understanding that monetary poverty among youth can interact with and intensify other aspects of poverty in significant ways.

- Governments, with the help of the international community, should intensify efforts to provide all households with access to clean water, sanitation, electricity, adequate health care, and other basic services in order to relieve the burden on youth—especially young women, who often suffer most from the lack of access to these facilities. Special attention must be given to improving access for youth living in rural areas and young people with disabilities.

- Youth perspectives should be considered in evaluating the progress achieved in addressing poverty issues, and especially in the preparation of Poverty Reduction Strategy Papers (PRSPs). Youth poverty should be specifically addressed in these policy papers.

HEALTH

All regions have made progress, but young people remain vulnerable to many modern health risks. Health policies must evolve in response to changing global challenges; in all regions, policy makers must respond to the growing HIV/AIDS-related threat among youth.

The period between the ages of 15 and 24 is typically one of the healthiest in the life course of an individual. However, young people in both developed and developing countries are currently facing a number of serious health risks that can derail their transition to healthy, productive adulthood. In developing countries, and in many of the economies in transition, HIV/AIDS represents perhaps the greatest risk. Around the world, the reproductive health needs of adolescents have been largely ignored. In many countries, regardless of the level of development or well-being, there is a lack of information and services to protect youth from unwanted pregnancy and sexually transmitted diseases, including HIV/AIDS.

Young people around the world are also exposed to other health threats that can seriously affect their welfare. Many are associated with contemporary lifestyles; for example, poor nutritional practices are contributing to the growing incidence of obesity and related diseases among youth. The prevalence of tobacco, alcohol and drug use and the high rates of morbidity and mortality associated with accidents and violence among youth are also a source of grave concern.

The recommendations regarding health in the World Youth Report 2005 (United Nations, 2005) remain valid today. In order to reduce the vulnerability of young people to infection, steps must be taken to ensure the provision of high-quality primary health care (including sexual and reproductive health care) that is accessible, available and affordable. Community-based interventions should be used more effectively to ensure that an appropriate environment exists for reducing young people's vulnerability to HIV/AIDS and for implementing targeted interventions. The findings of the present report suggest additional areas of attention that should be addressed by Governments, the private sector, individuals, and other stakeholders.

Recommendations

- Countries should work on developing and implementing policies aimed at improving youth access to information on nutrition and healthy lifestyles. The promotion of poor dietary practices and unfavourable lifestyles and behaviours—especially tobacco and alcohol advertising—should be the focus of regular attention among national authorities and in many cases should be regulated, with appropriate taxation of the tobacco and alcohol industries.

- Demand reduction is a critical component of any drug control strategy. National efforts should involve collaboration with young people and their communities in identifying the factors that encourage young people's drug habits, with a view to arriving at a comprehensive and realistic intervention strategy.

- In regions where the HIV/AIDS epidemic is severe, the prevention and treatment of HIV/AIDS and other sexually transmitted diseases must be the mainstay of health services targeted at young people, especially young women. Health education and ensuring access to condoms are essential elements of any prevention strategy.

- Strategies and programmes designed for specific purposes, such as preventing mother-to-child transmission of HIV or reducing HIV transmission among injecting drug users, are appropriate in all contexts. It is important to establish an environment in which youth can receive confidential HIV testing without prejudice so that those who are infected can be treated early and reduce the risk of spreading the virus.

- Sexually transmitted disease prevention and treatment efforts must be youth-sensitive. Experience has shown that peers are often the most effective deliverers of HIV prevention messages and services if the social environment is conducive to prevention strategies and efforts.

- Continued international cooperation and collective global efforts are necessary for the containment of HIV/AIDS among youth. A full range of prevention options should be presented to youth, with messages focusing broadly on developing a healthy lifestyle and more specifically on abstinence, delayed sexual debut, reducing the number of sexual partners, and correct and consistent condom use.

RIGHTS OF GIRLS AND YOUNG WOMEN

Progress has been achieved in many areas, but young women still face greater employment and wage discrimination than young men.

Young women continue to face barriers in many areas of development. Although progress has been made in providing schooling opportunities for girls and young women, secondary and tertiary education remain elusive for many. Young women face special challenges with respect to education. In developing regions, levels of educational attainment still tend to be higher among young men than among young women. In many developing countries, young females are more likely than young males to drop out of school at times of acute financial need or during family crises. Early marriage and childbearing remain impediments to school completion for young women. In some areas, substantial numbers of young women drop out of school to help with domestic and other chores.

In most regions, unemployment is higher and wages are lower among young women than among young men. The educational choices made by (or for) girls and young women often limit their access to certain types of employment and cause wage differentials to become entrenched. These choices are sometimes encouraged by the stereotypical casting of women in textbooks and other teaching materials in primarily domestic roles. Even in regions where levels of educational attainment in primary and secondary education are higher for females than for males (such as in Latin America), labour force participation rates are much lower and unemployment rates much higher for female youth than for male youth.

Recommendations

- Gender analysis must be incorporated into all youth development strategies. Special attention should be focused on marginalized young women, especially those living in rural areas.

- Governments should devise effective policies to enhance the involvement of girls and young women in the global economy and ensure that educational and employment policies and practices do not discriminate against young people on the basis of gender.

- Governments and other development partners should strive to adopt and implement innovative policies that create an enabling environment for young women to break out of poverty. These policies should be sensitive to the social and cultural contexts in which young women live while also enabling them to take action regarding their own welfare.

- Effective strategies should be developed for the provision of training at the national, regional and international levels to enable young women to acquire business-related, financial management and technical skills and to participate in economic policy-making in their communities. Approaches must be designed to enhance the capacity of young women who wish to return to work after childbearing to take full advantage of opportunities in the labour market, and policies and programmes that support maternity leave should be implemented or strengthened.

- Governments and civil society should contribute to efforts to achieve gender equality, in part by promoting women's studies and by keeping abreast of the results of gender research and studies in all areas, including economic, scientific and technological fields.

YOUTH PARTICIPATION: A KEY TO FUNDAMENTAL CHANGE IN YOUTH DEVELOPMENT

Youth participation is more than just political engagement. It includes the empowerment of young people through capacity-building and increased access to human development opportunities. It represents a situation in which young people are no longer seen as passive recipients of resources or as the cause of society's problems, but rather as important contributors to their countries' development—contributors whose efforts are recognized and whose involvement is nurtured.

Young people's ability to contribute to development and reap the "demographic dividend" is hindered where investments in youth are limited or where the doors to their development are closing as a result of changing global markets or restrictive national development policies. Because young people constitute a relatively large share of the population, especially in developing countries, the failure to ensure that young people—and the families in which they are raised—have access to resources and opportunities for health, education, employment, leisure, poverty reduction, and the development of girls and young women will derail future national and global development.

The effective engagement of youth as equal partners requires recognition of the rights of all young people to participate at all levels of decision-making and to make productive use of their knowledge, perspectives and experience. It is a process from which both youth and non-youth stakeholders benefit. It also represents a situation in which young people are no longer seen as passive recipients of national resources or the root cause of society's problems; instead, they are regarded as vital participants in society who can make an important contribution to their countries' development and whose involvement must therefore be appropriately nurtured and cultivated.

Youth participation must be regarded as the active and meaningful involvement of young people in all aspects of their own development and that of their communities, including their empowerment to contribute to decisions about their personal, family, social, economic and political development. Although civic participation, political decision-making, and opportunities to vote for elected officials are important channels for youth to become involved in development, full participation requires their empowerment through capacity-building to ensure that they have the skills needed to participate in society in their capacity as individuals, as members of families, communities and organizations, and as citizens. Youth participation is incomplete without adequate empowerment through access to human development opportunities such as education and health, and to adequate resources through opportunities for productive employment and poverty alleviation.

One of the most striking and positive aspects of the recent behaviour of young people in all regions is their increasing involvement in volunteerism. Youth today are ardent volunteers in many sectors, contributing to societal development while also gaining valuable skills and experience that can facilitate their transition to the world of work. Whether pursued as a way to gain practical skills, as a form of leisure, or as an avenue to influence the community, volunteerism has become a key part of youth life cycles. Young people in both developed and developing countries are increasingly volunteering for various causes, and many participate, with little or no remuneration, in activities that shape their societies.

In developed market economies, young people often treat volunteer work as an intermediate activity in the transition from school to further studies or regular paid employment. Even in sub-Saharan Africa, where youth poverty is high, many young people engage in volunteerism and, in the process, contribute to development. Although volunteers may earn little or no income, they gain important workplace skills and experience that can improve their chances for securing decent employment. The emotional dividend, including the deep sense of satisfaction that accompanies giving, also constitutes an important part of the transition to responsible adulthood.

Volunteerism is a clear manifestation of youth participation in society—one that is often altruistic and devoid of immediate selfish interests. Given its enormously important role in building interpersonal and social skills and in strengthening individual human potential, it is essential for society to promote volunteerism and to expand other opportunities for youth participation in development. Ensuring adequate and appropriate volunteer and other participatory opportunities for youth is highly beneficial to society and can form part of a strategy to combat social ills such as drug abuse, juvenile delinquency and other deviant behaviour. Where possible, Governments, the private sector, civil society, and other stakeholders should provide support for youth who cannot undertake volunteer activities because of the private costs associated with such endeavours. Communities should also develop low-cost volunteer programmes that enable youth to provide services in businesses and locations close to where they live so that the costs of transportation can be eliminated or reduced for participants.

It should be emphasized that there is no single effective practice or structure for youth participation. Participation is, in essence, a way of thinking that incorporates young people as partners all the time and in as many ways as possible. The focus should be not on one specific approach to or level of involvement, but rather on creating channels for the expression of young people's opinions and their dynamic participation in daily interactions, in service delivery or project implementation, and in more formal structures at all levels. Giving young people a chance to take part in decision-making contributes to their own development; this, in turn, enables them to contribute to the development of their societies, eventually creating a better environment for youth participation—a virtuous circle. One-time interventions or isolated structures that support youth participation are not sustainable; there must be broader, synergistic feedback mechanisms that include input from and dialogue between young people, their families, local councils and other community institutions, national Governments, and the international community.

Given the varied nature and intensity of some of the problems faced by youth around the world, it is clear that interventions should be tailored to individual circumstances within a particular country or region. Policies should be designed, however, with full acknowledgement of the fact that young people do not constitute a passive group, waiting for resources and opportunities to be handed to them; in all regions, there is clear evidence of young people's determination to make a better life for themselves, their communities and their countries. What young people need in this process is an enabling environment that provides opportunities for them to be seen and be heard. Giving youth greater visibility and a role in the development process strengthens their resolve to contribute to the advancement of a world in which they are equal stakeholders—a world for which they will be responsible for many decades to come.

References

Bell, Lisa, and others (2007). Failure to launch: cross-national trends in the transition to economic independence. Luxembourg Income Study Working Paper Series, No. 456.

United Nations (1995). World Programme of Action for Youth to the Year 2000 and Beyond. General Assembly resolution 50/81 of 14 December 1995 (A/RES/50/81).

_____ (2005). World Youth Report 2005: Young People Today, and in 2015. Sales No. E.05.IV.6.

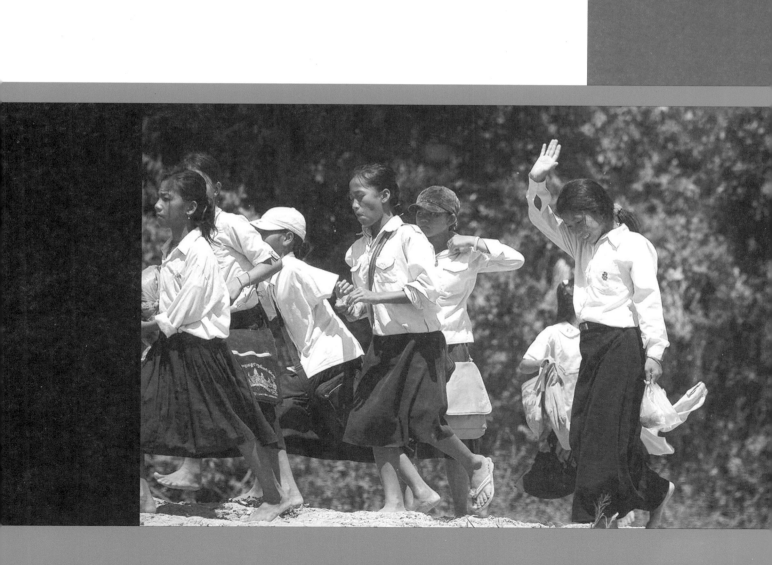

Statistical Annex

INTRODUCTION

*S*ince the adoption of the World Programme of Action for Youth in 1995, Governments, the international community, civil society and other actors have increasingly recognized the importance of investing in youth, and many have joined with youth-led organisations to address key constraints to youth development. While the World Programme of Action for Youth has been instrumental in guiding the formulation and implementation of national youth policies, assessing the impact of interventions and investments made in youth development remains difficult because youth-related age-disaggregated data are not always available. Where these data do exist, they are often part of a larger compilation on other population groups and youth-specific issues and trends remain hidden or are glossed over.

The purpose of this Annex is to collate existing data related to core areas of youth development in an effort to present a synopsis of the situation of youth and the challenges they face across countries and regions. The data also complement the analysis presented in this Report by providing a compilation of indicators related to youth for as many countries and regions as possible to facilitate planning and evaluation of youth programmes and policies. The data reflect several basic demographic indicators as well as youth specific statistics that can guide the tracking of progress in various priority areas of the World Programme of Action for Youth. While the Annex brings together existing data that are available from various sources, in certain cases new calculations are made to highlight specific aspects of youth development.

It is important to note that the data presented here are by no means exhaustive. Many gaps remain that need to be filled through new data collection. Further, even existing data are often not fully reliable. However, the data do provide a picture of the global, regional and national context in which youth live and make a transition into adulthood. Existing gaps in the data should stimulate interest and investment in data collection to help elucidate and clarify some of the issues that are addressed in the present Report.

The Annex tables that follow cover nine broad areas and issues:

Basic Demographics: The indicators in Annex table 1 give a sense of the numbers of youth and the change in these numbers over time, by country and world region. These data define the magnitude of the youth development challenge in terms of the size and share of the population that youth represent. Although at the global level youth constitute 18 per cent of the population, in many developing countries this share is above 20 per cent. This is in sharp contrast to the situation in many European countries where the share of youth is around 12 per cent.

249

Marriage: The percentage of youth aged 15-19; 20-24 and 15-24 years who have ever been married or are in some form of consensual union gives insight into youth marriage trends, including whether youth are delaying marriage. Youth around the world are delaying marriage, but there are still major differences across countries and regions in the proportions of youth who do marry. This may reflect choices that youth make, but it may also be an indication of difficulties in the transition into marriage.

Literacy: According to UNESCO's 1958 definition, literacy is measured by the ability of an individual to read and write, with understanding, a simple short statement related to his/her everyday life. Though youth around the world are the best educated generation ever, differences in literacy across countries persist. As seen in Annex table 3, literacy rates generally exceed 70 per cent for many countries; but rates lower than 50 per cent are still evident in some countries. Females also continue to be disadvantaged in many contexts.

Education: Various indicators are used in Annex tables 4, 5 and 6 to capture the coverage of education in a country. The Gross Enrolment Ratio (GER) refers to the total enrolment in a level of education, regardless of age, expressed as a percentage of the theoretical school-age population in a given school-year. The GER can exceed 100 per cent due to early or late entry and/or grade repetition. This indicator, which is shown for primary, secondary and tertiary education, by sex, is widely used to show the general level of participation in secondary education. It can be a complementary indicator to the NER by indicating the extent of over-aged and under-aged enrolment.

Similarly, the Net Enrolment Rate (NER) refers to the number of pupils in the theoretical age-group for the particular level of education (primary or secondary, in this case) expressed as a percentage of the total population in that age-group. The rates shown in Annex table 5 show the extent of participation in primary and secondary education of youth belonging to the official age-group for the particular level of schooling. A high NER denotes a high degree of participation of the official school-age population. The NER for tertiary education is not pertinent because of the difficulties in determining an appropriate age-group due to the wide variations in the ages of students at this level of education.

A sharp discrepancy between the GER and NER indicates that enrolled children do not progress regularly through the grades and that the system's internal efficiency could be improved. Female/male ratios that are shown in Annex tables 4 and 5 also show how females fare relative to males with respect to the gross and net enrolment ratios at each level. A ratio which is lower than 1 indicates that there is a female disadvantage in school enrolment. It is interesting to note the disparity in the female to male ratio across countries and across education levels. In many countries, females appear to outnumber males at the tertiary level, but in many other contexts, females face a major disadvantage at tertiary as well as lower levels of education.

Annex table 6 shows primary to secondary school transition rates, by sex and country. This rate is calculated by dividing the number of new entrants in the first grade of secondary education by the number of pupils who were enrolled in the final grade of primary education in the previous school year, multiplied by 100. A transition rate thus measures the degree of progression to a given level of education from the previous level of education. It can reflect difficulties with accessibility or problems related to student performance in the lower level of schooling. From the perspective of the level of education from which a student is leaving, it is considered as an output indicator, and from the perspective of the level of education to which a student is entering, it is an indicator of access. It can also help in assessing the relative selectivity of an education system, which can be due to pedagogical or financial requirements.

Labour force participation and employment: There is no doubt from the analysis presented in the chapters in this book that labour force participation and employment issues are among the most pressing in practically all countries of the world. Table 7 thus presents some indicators of the situation in individual countries. The percent of youth in the labour force is a measure of the proportion of a country's youth population that engages actively in the labour market, either by working or looking for work; it provides an indication of the relative size of the youth labour force available to engage in the production of goods and services. Labour force activity among the young may reflect the availability of educational facilities as well as the degree to which young workers are discouraged from joining the labour force. Female/male labour force participation rates show sex differentials in labour force participation by sex. Ratios less than one suggest that females are less likely than males to participate in the labour force.

Annex tables 7 and 8 suggest a complex global picture with respect to labour force participation and employment. For some countries, virtually all youth—including the younger subgroup aged 15 to 19 years—are in the labour force. In other countries, most youth do not enter the labour force until later. Gender differentials in participation also vary, with some countries showing little difference and other showing much lower female participation in the labour force. The age transition in labour force participation rates show how labour force participation of youth changes as youth progress from the younger to the older age group. The data suggest, as would be expected, that in all countries labour force participation is higher for older youth. The degree of increase is, however, variable across countries and by sex. In the Czech Republic, for example, labour force participation rates increase eleven fold between ages 15 to 19 and 20 to 24 years. Similar increases are also recorded for Macao China SAR, and Kuwait.

In Annex table 8 which presents various indicators of youth unemployment, the youth labour force is the number of youth who are either actively looking for work or who are unemployed; and unemployed youth are those who do not have a job but are actively looking for work. Youth are considered to be employed if they performed some work—for at least one hour during the specified reference period—for wage or salary (paid employment) or for profit or family gain (self-employment). It should be noted that while a high unemployment rate indicates that a large share of the labour force is actively looking for work but cannot locate one, it does not say anything about those who have given up on the job search (discouraged people) or people who are outside the labour force for other reasons. Nor does it indicate underemployment.

Annex table 8 also shows the ratios of the youth to adult unemployment rate. This ratio is the youth unemployment rate as a percentage of the adult (aged 25 and over) unemployment rate. The indicator provides an indication of how youth fare in labour markets relative to adults. For example, in a country where the youth unemployment rate is high and the ratio of the youth unemployment rate to the adult unemployment rate is close to one, it may be concluded that the problem of unemployment is not specific to youth, but is country-wide. In all countries, it is normal for the youth unemployment rate to be higher than the adult unemployment rate to some extent. Young people often have less work experience than adults, they may lack job search expertise, and they might be "shopping around" for the right job.

The youth employment-to-population ratio, which is shown in the last column of Annex table 8, is calculated by dividing the number of employed youth by the total youth population. Although it may be assumed that a high employment rate among youth could be positive, this is not always the case. If low employment-to-population rates are due to large numbers of youth remaining in education to build their human capital, they are preferable to high rates, which might be an indication of limited education options and the need for young people to take up any work available. Employment-to-population ratios are of particular interest when broken down by sex, as the ratios for males and females can provide information on gender differences in labour market activity in a given country.

Hunger and poverty: The most widely known poverty indicators are the number or proportion of people living below the poverty lines of one and two dollars a day. Table 9 presents extrapolated estimates of youth poverty for countries. The table applies estimates of the proportion of national populations living in poverty to the size of the youth population of individual countries in order to estimate the numbers of youth living under various conditions of monetary poverty. While the estimates shown in the last two columns of Annex table 9 are approximations, they are likely to be fairly close to the actual degree of poverty among youth. This is because of the tendency for poverty to be transmitted across generations; this means that youth are likely to reflect the particular poverty situation within their households.

Nutrition and shelter and sanitation and water: Annex tables 10 and 11 present additional estimates of youth welfare. There is debate over whether poverty should be measured by income only. A broader approach to measurement is often called for to characterize the severe deprivation of basic human needs, including food, safe drinking water, sanitation facilities, health, shelter, education and information. The indicators shown in Annex table 10 and 11 present these estimates, showing poverty in access to nutrition, shelter and sanitation and water. These data, derived by the Townsend Centre for International Poverty Research, University of Bristol, based on household surveys, including Demographic and Health Surveys (DHS) and Multiple Indicator Cluster Surveys (MICS), show large proportions of youth in many countries to be deprived of access to basic needs.[1]

The criteria for the calculations are the following:

- Food Deprivation: Body Mass Index of 18.5 or below (underweight).

- Severe Food Deprivation: Body Mass Index of 16 or below (severe underweight).

- Shelter Deprivation: living in dwellings with three or more people per room (overcrowding), or in a house with no flooring (e.g. a mud floor), or inadequate roofing (e.g. natural roofing materials).

- Deprivation of Sanitation Facilities: access only to unimproved sanitation facilities e.g.: pour flush latrines; covered pit latrines; open pit latrines; and buckets or no access to a toilet of any kind.

- Water Deprivation: access only to unimproved source such as open wells, open springs or surface water, or having to walk for more than 15 minutes to their water source (30 minutes round-trip).

Leading causes of death for youth: Annex table 12 provides insight into the primary cause of mortality for young people in various countries. Variations in these causes across countries indicate a need for differences in policy responses. Although these data are undoubtedly incomplete because of the difficulty in obtaining reliable cause of death data for many countries, land transport accidents and intentional self-harm are important causes of death for youth. The tendency for youth to take more risks and also be less experienced with motorized vehicles may account for the importance of motor vehicle accidents among causes of death. Suicide is also of increasing concern as youth struggle to find their place and acceptance in an increasingly complex world.

Reproductive health and HIV/AIDS: Annex tables 13 and 14 present a sense of youth sexual behaviour and practices and their vulnerability to HIV/AIDS and reproductive health challenges. These data have been drawn from a number of surveys from MEASURE DHS (Demographic and Health Surveys—accessed at http://www.measuredhs.org). The picture of youth sexual behaviour varies across countries. Table 13 suggests for the countries for which data are available that high risk sex continues to be a problem in a number of countries, and large proportions of youth continue to engage in unprotected high risk sexual intercourse. Also, as suggested by table 14, the use of condoms at first sexual encounter is not yet universal among youth.

---

[1] The proposed indicators described above build on the work undertaken on behalf of UNICEF and the United Kingdom's Department for International Development to operationalize measures of deprivation and severe deprivation for children and adults.

Annex table 1: Youth population indicators, 2007

Country, region or major area*	Notes	Total youth population (thousands) by age and sex						Total youth population aged 15 - 24 years	Youth as percentage of total population	Percentage change (1995-2015)
		Males			Females					
		Age (years)		15-24 years	Age (years)		15-24 years			
		15 - 19	20 - 24		15 - 19	20 - 24				
WORLD		315 052	297 036	612 088	298 080	282 892	580 972	1 193 060	17.6	14.6
More developed regions	a	40 786	43 134	83 919	38 893	41 516	80 409	164 328	12.9	-13.0
Less developed regions	b	274 267	253 903	528 170	259 187	241 376	500 563	1 028 733	18.7	18.4
Least developed countries (LDCs)	c	44 045	38 242	82 287	43 089	37 592	80 682	162 969	20.2	39.1
Less developed regions, excluding LDCs		230 221	215 661	445 882	216 098	203 783	419 881	865 763	18.5	13.8
Less developed regions, excluding China		214 444	197 097	411 541	205 031	189 661	394 692	806 233	19.5	25.2
AFRICA		52 897	46 441	99 338	52 212	46 242	98 455	197 793	20.4	37.7
Sub-Saharan Africa		44 513	38 278	82 790	44 101	38 206	82 307	165 098	20.4	41.2
Eastern Africa	1	17 178	14 753	31 931	17 126	14 778	31 904	63 835	20.7	42.3
Burundi		494	431	925	495	436	931	1 856	21.7	45.6
Comoros	2	45	42	86	44	41	85	171	20.3	37.9
Djibouti		48	42	90	48	41	89	179	21.4	37.3
Eritrea		262	239	501	264	245	509	1 010	20.8	36.0
Ethiopia		4 603	3 801	8 404	4 583	3 809	8 392	16 796	20.1	45.3
Kenya		2 123	1 956	4 079	2 108	1 953	4 061	8 140	21.6	35.5
Madagascar		1 054	879	1 933	1 054	881	1 935	3 868	19.6	45.6
Malawi		758	634	1 392	754	633	1 387	2 779	19.9	46.3
Mauritius	3	51	49	100	50	48	98	198	15.5	-0.5
Mozambique		1 144	979	2 123	1 149	979	2 128	4 251	19.8	39.1
Réunion		34	33	67	34	32	66	133	16.3	14.0
Rwanda		618	561	1 179	630	576	1 206	2 385	24.4	58.6
Somalia		436	375	810	437	377	814	1 624	18.6	37.7
Uganda		1 754	1 418	3 172	1 736	1 412	3 149	6 321	20.4	50.4
Tanzania, United Republic of		2 205	1 917	4 122	2 194	1 916	4 109	8 231	20.3	39.4
Zambia		685	587	1 272	681	584	1 265	2 537	21.2	38.5
Zimbabwe		862	808	1 670	862	811	1 673	3 343	24.9	25.7
Middle Africa		6 454	5 455	11 908	6 444	5 473	11 917	23 825	19.9	43.0
Angola		940	774	1 713	949	786	1 735	3 448	20.2	44.8
Cameroon		1 049	920	1 969	1 038	914	1 952	3 921	21.0	38.3
Central African Republic		242	204	446	247	210	456	902	20.7	39.1
Chad		575	480	1 055	571	480	1 051	2 106	19.5	49.6
Congo		202	177	379	202	178	380	759	20.1	37.2
Congo, Democratic Republic of the		3 336	2 803	6 139	3 329	2 810	6 139	12 278	19.5	43.6
Equatorial Guinea		26	22	49	26	22	49	97	19.1	42.7
Gabon		75	66	141	74	65	139	280	20.9	33.5
São Tomé and Príncipe		9	9	17	9	8	17	35	21.8	30.1
Northern Africa		10 489	10 000	20 489	10 150	9 825	19 974	40 464	20.5	20.3
Algeria		1 892	1 899	3 791	1 814	1 829	3 643	7 433	21.8	7.7
Egypt		4 006	3 782	7 788	3 874	3 713	7 588	15 376	20.2	22.8
Libyan Arab Jamahiriya		284	340	624	272	327	599	1 223	19.7	1.9
Morocco		1 638	1 576	3 214	1 617	1 626	3 243	6 457	20.5	9.0
Sudan		2 105	1 837	3 941	2 039	1 789	3 827	7 768	20.1	38.1
Tunisia		541	542	1 083	512	517	1 029	2 112	20.3	0.1
Western Sahara		24	25	49	23	23	46	94	19.6	53.6
Southern Africa		2 900	2 791	5 691	2 881	2 768	5 650	11 340	20.3	17.4
Botswana		111	109	219	110	107	217	437	23.1	23.3
Lesotho		124	110	234	125	116	242	476	23.5	28.2
Namibia		131	108	239	131	107	239	478	22.9	38.3
South Africa		2 458	2 398	4 855	2 439	2 370	4 809	9 665	19.8	15.1
Swaziland		76	67	142	76	67	143	286	24.9	33.3
Western Africa	4	15 877	13 443	29 319	15 611	13 398	29 010	58 329	20.3	43.6
Benin		499	437	936	482	421	904	1 840	20.3	48.4
Burkina Faso		820	695	1 516	797	677	1 474	2 989	20.1	44.0
Cape Verde		32	29	60	32	28	60	120	22.5	37.5
Côte d'Ivoire		1 119	985	2 104	1 119	983	2 101	4 205	21.8	41.4
Gambia		86	74	160	85	73	157	317	18.5	48.3
Ghana		1 330	1 181	2 511	1 277	1 143	2 421	4 932	20.9	35.2
Guinea		507	431	939	490	417	907	1 845	19.6	39.0
Guinea-Bissau		88	71	159	88	72	161	320	18.8	46.2
Liberia		202	173	375	200	171	371	746	19.9	57.0
Mali		685	565	1 250	688	574	1 262	2 512	20.2	45.5
Mauritania		168	149	317	159	141	300	616	19.6	39.3
Niger		705	495	1 200	716	592	1 308	2 507	17.5	51.7
Nigeria		8 286	6 998	15 284	8 133	6 945	15 078	30 363	20.4	43.8
Senegal		689	592	1 281	682	591	1 273	2 554	20.5	42.1
Sierra Leone		301	255	556	302	257	560	1 116	19.0	43.0
Togo		360	311	670	362	313	675	1 345	20.4	46.1

Annex table 1: Youth population indicators, 2007

Country, region or major area*	Notes	Total youth population (thousands) by age and sex						Total youth population aged 15 - 24 years	Youth as percentage of total population	Percentage change (1995-2015)
		Males			Females					
		Age (years)		15-24 years	Age (years)		15-24 years			
		15 - 19	20 - 24		15 - 19	20 - 24				
ASIA		197 208	185 072	382 280	183 038	172 479	355 517	737 797	18.1	12.1
Eastern Asia		65 874	63 388	129 262	59 885	57 957	117 842	247 104	15.8	-13.8
China	5	59 583	56 548	116 131	53 928	51 460	105 388	221 519	16.5	-11.5
Hong Kong, China SAR	6	218	238	456	208	233	441	897	12.1	-7.3
Korea, Democratic People's Republic of		987	959	1 945	945	918	1 863	3 809	15.9	9.2
Korea, Republic of		1 693	1 826	3 519	1 565	1 687	3 252	6 771	13.8	-28.8
Japan		3 215	3 651	6 866	3 066	3 494	6 560	13 426	10.0	-51.8
Macao, China SAR	7	21	20	41	20	21	41	82	16.8	15.6
Mongolia		157	146	303	153	144	297	600	22.7	0.2
South-central Asia		92 278	84 257	176 534	85 374	78 194	163 568	340 102	19.9	26.8
Afghanistan		1 532	1 261	2 792	1 417	1 158	2 575	5 367	19.7	52.0
Bangladesh		8 587	7 923	16 511	8 162	7 498	15 660	32 170	20.2	27.1
Bhutan		39	41	80	39	34	72	152	22.9	37.0
India		61 507	56 328	117 835	56 188	51 678	107 866	225 701	19.2	25.2
Iran, Islamic Republic of		4 441	4 548	8 989	4 219	4 350	8 569	17 559	24.5	10.4
Kazakhstan		783	747	1 530	753	725	1 478	3 008	19.3	-14.5
Kyrgyzstan		302	272	574	293	268	561	1 135	21.2	20.7
Maldives		20	18	38	19	18	37	75	24.5	32.3
Nepal		1 593	1 353	2 946	1 501	1 298	2 800	5 746	20.3	39.1
Pakistan		10 249	8 813	19 062	9 658	8 258	17 915	36 977	22.4	41.5
Sri Lanka		865	916	1 781	832	906	1 738	3 518	18.0	-18.9
Tajikistan		430	349	779	422	350	772	1 551	22.9	34.6
Turkmenistan		293	258	551	287	254	541	1 092	21.8	22.4
Uzbekistan		1 636	1 430	3 066	1 585	1 400	2 984	6 050	21.9	25.8
South-eastern Asia		27 958	26 868	54 826	27 045	26 312	53 357	108 182	18.7	9.9
Brunei Darussalam		17	18	36	16	18	34	69	17.7	28.9
Cambodia		900	841	1 742	875	824	1 699	3 441	23.7	47.6
Timor-Leste		62	55	117	59	52	112	229	19.8	46.3
Indonesia		10 770	10 795	21 565	10 451	10 618	21 069	42 635	18.3	2.9
Lao People's Democratic Republic		368	293	661	359	291	649	1 310	22.3	37.3
Malaysia		1 315	1 247	2 562	1 267	1 223	2 491	5 053	18.9	28.2
Myanmar		2 375	2 356	4 732	2 322	2 312	4 634	9 366	19.0	-1.3
Philippines		4 689	4 197	8 886	4 512	4 066	8 579	17 464	19.8	27.6
Singapore		165	142	307	154	132	286	593	13.1	26.8
Thailand		2 503	2 554	5 057	2 388	2 499	4 887	9 944	15.3	-23.1
Viet Nam		4 793	4 368	9 161	4 641	4 277	8 918	18 078	20.5	13.5
Western Asia		11 098	10 561	21 659	10 734	10 016	20 750	42 409	19.2	27.1
Armenia		155	146	301	151	152	303	604	19.7	-6.9
Azerbaijan		479	431	910	457	421	878	1 788	20.9	11.4
Bahrain		31	33	64	29	28	57	121	16.0	30.6
Cyprus		34	34	68	32	33	64	132	15.0	14.2
Georgia		191	180	372	183	179	362	733	16.3	-30.2
Iraq		1 635	1 365	3 000	1 575	1 315	2 890	5 890	20.2	39.3
Israel		284	276	560	271	264	535	1 095	15.4	20.7
Jordan		314	297	611	301	286	587	1 198	20.1	27.1
Kuwait		103	139	241	94	107	201	442	15.5	39.2
Lebanon		189	181	370	182	178	361	731	17.6	13.2
Occupied Palestinian Territory		222	180	402	212	171	383	785	19.4	51.7
Oman		144	140	284	137	131	268	553	21.2	37.9
Qatar		26	43	69	24	22	46	115	13.6	42.9
Saudi Arabia		1 195	1 142	2 336	1 219	1 037	2 256	4 593	18.5	40.5
Syrian Arab Republic		1 142	1 134	2 276	1 100	1 098	2 198	4 474	22.3	28.7
Turkey		3 441	3 444	6 885	3 337	3 367	6 704	13 589	18.0	7.3
United Arab Emirates		148	265	412	119	150	269	681	15.5	47.8
Yemen		1 368	1 130	2 498	1 311	1 078	2 389	4 887	21.8	51.3
EUROPE		24 161	26 343	50 504	23 075	25 445	48 520	99 024	13.0	-26.7
Eastern Europe		10 976	12 538	23 514	10 528	12 164	22 692	46 206	15.3	-46.9
Belarus		377	417	794	358	404	763	1 557	15.7	-36.9
Bulgaria		241	272	513	230	258	488	1 001	12.7	-70.1
Czech Republic		328	342	670	312	327	639	1 309	12.4	-60.5
Hungary		320	323	643	306	310	616	1 259	12.1	-45.5
Poland		1 394	1 618	3 012	1 329	1 563	2 891	5 904	15.1	-37.2
Republic of Moldova		193	195	388	182	184	366	754	19.5	-30.3
Romania		780	830	1 609	748	797	1 545	3 154	14.3	-68.4
Russian Federation		5 444	6 396	11 840	5 247	6 259	11 507	23 347	16.0	-45.4
Slovakia		199	219	417	190	210	401	818	14.8	-39.7
Ukraine		1 701	1 926	3 627	1 624	1 852	3 476	7 103	14.9	-49.1

Annex table 1: Youth population indicators, 2007

Country, region or major area*	Notes	Total youth population (thousands) by age and sex						Total youth population aged 15 - 24 years	Youth as percentage of total population	Percentage change (1995-2015)
		Males			Females					
		Age (years)		15-24 years	Age (years)		15-24 years			
		15 - 19	20 - 24		15 - 19	20 - 24				
Northern Europe	8	3 305	3 259	6 563	3 138	3 133	6 271	12 834	12.6	1.4
Channel Islands	9	5	4	9	4	4	9	17	11.3	-4.8
Denmark		170	149	318	160	143	303	622	11.0	1.8
Estonia		50	54	104	48	52	100	205	14.8	-44.0
Finland	10	166	168	335	159	160	320	654	11.9	1.2
Iceland		11	11	22	11	11	21	44	14.1	6.1
Ireland		148	169	317	143	166	308	625	14.2	-8.4
Latvia		87	94	181	84	90	174	355	15.1	-48.3
Lithuania		135	135	270	129	129	258	528	15.1	-26.5
Norway	11	159	145	303	151	139	290	593	12.1	8.9
Sweden		317	284	601	301	271	573	1 173	12.2	3.8
United Kingdom		2 052	2 042	4 094	1 943	1 963	3 906	8 000	12.6	4.9
Southern Europe	12	4 177	4 668	8 845	3 972	4 458	8 430	17 274	10.9	-39.1
Albania		162	142	303	156	143	299	602	18.6	1.3
Bosnia and Herzegovina		134	138	273	130	136	265	538	13.5	-12.6
Croatia		140	156	296	135	150	284	580	12.3	-25.9
Greece		298	363	661	280	333	613	1 274	11.0	-45.8
Italy		1 456	1 539	2 995	1 387	1 476	2 863	5 858	9.4	-40.5
Malta		14	15	30	14	15	28	58	13.9	-8.7
Montenegro		24	24	48	22	24	47	94	15.4	-31.5
Portugal		297	349	646	284	336	621	1 266	11.5	-39.8
Serbia		353	375	728	335	360	695	1 423	14.1	-24.0
Slovenia		60	70	130	57	67	124	253	12.2	-50.4
Spain		1 154	1 410	2 563	1 093	1 336	2 428	4 991	10.8	-50.9
The former Yugoslav Republic of Macedonia	13	81	84	165	77	79	156	321	15.4	-14.8
Western Europe	14	5 703	5 878	11 581	5 438	5 690	11 128	22 709	11.6	-4.5
Austria		251	265	516	239	257	496	1 012	11.6	-5.6
Belgium		321	321	642	308	313	620	1 262	11.5	-3.4
France		1 955	1 983	3 938	1 872	1 943	3 815	7 753	12.0	-5.0
Germany		2 410	2 568	4 978	2 287	2 458	4 744	9 722	11.2	-6.3
Luxembourg		14	14	29	14	14	27	56	11.6	24.4
Netherlands		512	493	1 005	491	479	970	1 975	11.6	-1.5
Switzerland		237	232	469	225	226	451	920	11.8	7.2
LATIN AMERICA AND THE CARIBBEAN		26 881	25 603	52 484	26 533	25 731	52 264	104 748	18.1	11.6
Caribbean	15	1 899	1 774	3 674	1 844	1 750	3 595	7 268	17.3	9.3
Aruba		4	3	7	4	3	7	13	12.7	23.0
Bahamas		14	14	29	14	15	29	58	17.2	12.6
Barbados		11	11	22	10	11	21	43	14.2	-24.9
Cuba		421	400	822	399	376	774	1 596	13.8	-23.9
Dominican Republic		471	426	897	465	426	891	1 788	18.1	17.7
Grenada		7	5	12	6	5	11	23	21.5	18.5
Guadeloupe		16	14	30	16	13	29	59	13.0	-10.8
Haiti		541	500	1 041	527	507	1 034	2 076	21.5	32.0
Jamaica		140	122	262	136	121	257	519	18.8	10.5
Martinique		15	14	29	15	13	28	57	13.9	-8.4
Netherlands Antilles		7	5	12	7	5	12	24	12.1	-35.7
Puerto Rico		155	154	310	150	151	300	610	14.8	-6.1
Saint Lucia		8	8	17	8	8	17	33	19.7	2.9
Saint Vincent and the Grenadines		6	6	13	6	6	13	25	20.7	-17.5
Trinidad and Tobago		64	74	139	62	73	135	274	20.3	-21.0
U.S. Virgin Islands		5	4	9	5	4	9	19	16.3	10.1
Central America		7 103	6 231	13 334	7 342	6 732	14 075	27 408	18.4	11.5
Belize		16	14	30	15	14	29	59	20.2	33.5
Costa Rica		229	221	450	216	210	426	876	19.4	26.4
El Salvador		338	302	640	332	301	633	1 273	18.4	10.8
Guatemala		725	599	1 324	732	634	1 366	2 690	20.0	40.2
Honduras		408	350	757	403	354	757	1 516	21.2	35.6
Mexico		4 909	4 314	9 224	5 176	4 792	9 967	19 191	17.8	3.1
Nicaragua		322	284	606	320	286	606	1 212	21.4	24.6
Panama		155	146	301	149	141	290	591	17.5	16.9
South America	16	17 879	17 598	35 477	17 346	17 249	34 595	70 071	18.0	11.9
Argentina		1 736	1 650	3 385	1 683	1 613	3 296	6 682	16.5	11.0
Bolivia		513	435	948	496	426	922	1 870	19.5	32.5
Brazil		8 583	9 018	17 601	8 345	8 841	17 186	34 787	17.9	6.5
Chile		759	703	1 463	735	684	1 419	2 881	17.0	14.4
Colombia		2 250	2 084	4 334	2 177	2 056	4 233	8 567	18.4	16.7
Ecuador		674	608	1 282	653	595	1 249	2 531	18.7	13.5
French Guiana		10	8	18	9	8	17	35	17.3	50.6
Guyana		30	29	58	31	29	60	118	15.9	-22.2
Paraguay		334	308	641	324	300	624	1 265	20.5	33.6
Peru		1 446	1 311	2 757	1 403	1 288	2 691	5 448	19.3	14.6

Annex table 1: Youth population indicators, 2007

Country, region or major area*	Notes	Total youth population (thousands) by age and sex						Total youth population aged 15 - 24 years	Youth as percentage of total population	Percentage change (1995-2015)
		Males			Females					
		Age (years)		15-24 years	Age (years)		15-24 years			
		15 - 19	20 - 24		15 - 19	20 - 24				
Suriname		22	22	44	20	22	43	86	18.7	2.0
Uruguay		133	121	255	128	118	247	501	14.5	-2.3
Venezuela		1 390	1 301	2 691	1 340	1 268	2 608	5 299	19.0	22.6
NORTHERN AMERICA	17	12 516	12 253	24 769	11 904	11 731	23 636	48 405	13.8	17.3
Canada		1 129	1 131	2 260	1 074	1 090	2 164	4 424	13.0	8.8
United States of America		11 383	11 118	22 500	10 825	10 637	21 462	43 962	13.9	18.1
OCEANIA		1 390	1 324	2 713	1 317	1 264	2 581	5 295	15.0	17.5
Australia/New Zealand		893	887	1 780	847	847	1 694	3 474	13.4	7.8
Australia	18	732	738	1 470	694	703	1 398	2 867	13.3	7.4
New Zealand		162	149	311	153	143	296	607	14.1	9.7
Melanesia		433	382	815	411	362	773	1 588	19.5	34.6
Fiji		43	41	84	40	39	79	163	19.3	11.0
New Caledonia		11	10	21	11	10	20	41	16.9	19.8
Papua New Guinea		339	294	633	322	281	603	1 236	19.5	37.3
Solomon Islands		28	25	53	25	23	48	101	20.2	35.1
Vanuatu		13	11	24	12	11	23	47	20.7	42.6
Micronesia	19	27	24	51	26	27	53	104	18.7	26.0
Guam		8	7	14	7	6	14	28	16.0	26.5
Micronesia, Federated States of		7	6	13	6	6	12	26	22.8	15.3
Polynesia	20	36	31	67	33	28	61	128	19.3	19.2
French Polynesia		13	13	26	13	12	25	51	19.2	17.4
Samoa		11	8	19	10	7	16	35	18.7	18.4
Tonga		6	6	12	5	5	10	22	21.6	15.9

Source: United Nations, Department of Economic and Social Affairs, Population Division, *World Population Prospects: The 2006 Revision*. CD-ROM edition: Extended Dataset (New York, 2007).

Notes:

Two dots (..) indicate that data are not available or are not separately reported.

* Countries or areas listed individually are those with 100,000 inhabitants or more in 2005; other countries and areas are included in the regional groups but are not listed separately.

(a) More developed regions comprise Europe, Northern America, Australia/New Zealand, and Japan.

(b) Less developed regions comprise all regions of Africa, Asia (except Japan), Latin America and the Caribbean, plus Melanesia, Micronesia and Polynesia.

(c) The least developed countries, as defined by the United Nations General Assembly in 2003, include 50 States: 34 are in Africa, 10 in Asia, 1 in Latin America and the Caribbean, and 5 in Oceania.

(1) Including Seychelles.

(2) Including the island of Mayotte.

(3) Including Agalega, Rodrigues, and Saint Brandon.

(4) Including Saint Helena, Ascension, and Tristan da Cunha.

(5) For statistical purposes, the data for China do not include Hong Kong and Macao, Special Administrative Regions of China.

(6) On 1 July 1997, Hong Kong became a Special Administrative Region of China.

(7) On 20 December 1999, Macao became a Special Administrative Region of China.

(8) Including the Faeroe Islands and the Isle of Man.

(9) Refers to Guernsey and Jersey.

(10) Including Åland Islands.

(11) Including Svalbard and Jan Mayen Islands.

(12) Including Andorra, Gibraltar, the Holy See, and San Marino.

(13) The former Yugoslav Republic of Macedonia.

(14) Including Liechtenstein and Monaco.

(15) Including Anguilla, Antigua and Barbuda, British Virgin Islands, Cayman Islands, Dominica, Montserrat, Saint Kitts and Nevis, and Turks and Caicos Islands.

(16) Including the Falkland Islands (Malvinas).

(17) Including Bermuda, Greenland, and Saint Pierre et Miquelon.

(18) Including Christmas Island, the Cocos (Keeling) Islands, and Norfolk Island.

(19) Including Kiribati, the Marshall Islands, Nauru, the Northern Mariana Islands, and Palau.

(20) Including American Samoa, the Cook Islands, Niue, Pitcairn, Tokelau, Tuvalu, and the Wallis and Futuna Islands.

Annex table 2. Youth that have ever been married as a proportion of the total population (most recent data available)

Region and subregion	Country	Percentage of youth that have ever married by age (years) and sex				
		Year	15-19 Female	15-19 Male	20-24 Female	20-24 Male
AFRICA						
Eastern Africa						
	Burundi	1990	6.9	0.7	60.2	26.6
	Comoros	1996	11.5	3.0	48.4	15.0
	Djibouti	..	..	..	..	..
	Eritrea	2002	31.1	..	72.7	..
	Ethiopia	2000	29.9	3.3	73.0	23.8
	Kenya	1998	16.6	0.7	65.1	22.6
	Madagascar	1997	33.7	..	74.3	..
	Malawi	2000	36.7	4.0	87.7	41.7
	Mauritius	2000	9.7	0.6	49.7	11.4
	Mozambique	1997	47.1	3.8	88.8	57.6
	Réunion	1990	2.0	0.1	19.5	6.8
	Rwanda	2000	7.2	1.6	58.5	28.7
	Seychelles	1994	6.9	1.2	33.0	17.9
	Somalia	..	..	..	..	..
	Uganda	2001	32.2	6.5	84.7	45.4
	Tanzania, United Republic of	1996	25.3	2.8	75.5	29.2
	Zambia	2001	26.9	1.8	75.3	31.3
	Zimbabwe	1999	22.6	0.6	71.7	23.3
Middle Africa						
	Angola	1970	35.7	7.6	82.8	41.7
	Cameroon	1998	35.8	4.2	73.6	28.0
	Central African Republic	1995	42.4	8.1	81.2	45.6
	Chad	1996	48.6	5.9	92.2	43.7
	Congo	1984	18.1	1.4	53.5	12.9
	Congo, Democratic Republic of the	1984	32.3	4.7	74.1	33.9
	Equatorial Guinea	1983	26.4	2.1	62.8	21.9
	Gabon	2000	22.4	4.0	61.3	29.2
	Sao Tome and Principe	1991	19.9	1.9	61.6	27.9
Northern Africa						
	Algeria	1992	96.4	..	71.6	..
	Egypt	2000	12.0	..	54.4	..
	Libyan Arab Jamahiriya	1995	0.9	0.1	12.3	1.3
	Morocco	1995	10.5	..	39.8	..
	Sudan	1993	20.4	1.8	55.0	14.1
	Tunisia	1994	3.0	—	27.7	3.7
	Western Sahara	1970	60.3	1.3	80.3	23.5
Southern Africa						
	Botswana	1991	5.4	2.4	27.2	9.0
	Lesotho	1986	18.1	1.6	70.4	25.9
	Namibia	1992	7.7	..	30.9	..
	South Africa	1996	3.4	0.8	22.3	8.6
	Swaziland	1991	9.0	1.0	39.7	14.6
Western Africa						
	Benin	1996	29.1	—	79.5	27.3
	Burkina Faso	1999	34.9	1.4	90.3	22.1
	Cape Verde	1990	6.6	1.1	32.3	14.6
	Côte d'Ivoire	..	..	..	..	..
	Gambia	1993	38.9	1.7	74.9	12.4
	Ghana	1998	16.4	3.0	71.1	25.6
	Guinea	1999	46.0	2.3	84.7	19.7
	Guinea-Bissau	..	..	..	..	..
	Liberia	1986	36.0	..	75.3	..
	Mali	1996	49.7	4.8	87.5	28.9
	Mauritania	2001	27.7	0.5	60.5	8.1
	Niger	1998	61.9	4.1	88.9	41.8
	Nigeria	1999	27.5	3.1	63.5	17.2
	St. Helena	..	..	..	..	..
	Senegal	1997	29.0	..	62.8	8.1
	Sierra Leone	1992	45.5	4.7	72.4	19.6
	Togo	1998	19.9	2.4	63.4	18.3
ASIA						
Eastern Asia						
	China	..	..	..	..	..
	Hong Kong, China SAR	..	..	..	..	..
	Japan	2000	0.9	0.4	12.0	7.0
	Korea, Democratic People's Republic of	..	..	..	..	..
	Korea, Republic of	1995	0.8	0.2	16.7	3.6
	Macao, China SAR	..	..	..	..	..
	Mongolia	2000	5.5	1.3	48.3	29.2

Annex table 2. Youth that have ever been married as a proportion of the total population (most recent data available)

Region and subregion	Country	Percentage of youth that have ever married by age (years) and sex				
		Year	15-19 Female	15-19 Male	20-24 Female	20-24 Male
South-central Asia						
	Afghanistan	1979	53.6	9.2	90.7	36.5
	Bangladesh	2000	48.1	..	81.5	..
	Bhutan	1990	25.5	7.7	69.2	45.3
	India	1998	29.9	4.1	78.1	32.8
	Iran, Islamic Republic of	1996	17.8	2.6	60.5	27.3
	Kazakhstan	1999	7.5	1.4	52.7	25.9
	Kyrgyzstan	1999	11.5	1.0	65.8	28.3
	Maldives	2000	12.0	1.3	64.1	25.0
	Nepal	2001	40.2	11.3	82.9	56.5
	Pakistan	1998	20.6	6.2	61.4	30.1
	Sri Lanka	1993	7.1	..	38.8	..
	Tajikistan	1989	11.6	1.2	76.8	44.1
	Turkmenistan	1989	6.4	1.4	53.3	36.6
	Uzbekistan	1996	13.0	..	77.2	..
South-eastern Asia						
	Brunei Darussalam	1991	8.0	1.2	38.2	18.6
	Cambodia	2000	12.9	..	55.5	..
	Democratic Republic of Timor-Leste		..	..	..	..
	Indonesia	1997	8.4	1.1	45.5	17.7
	Lao People's Democratic Republic		..	..	..	..
	Malaysia	2000	4.9	1.0	31.5	11.8
	Myanmar	1991	10.7	3.3	43.9	30.1
	Philippines	1998	8.5	..	43.7	..
	Singapore	2000	1.0	0.1	16.1	4.7
	Thailand	1995	17.8	3.9	61.0	33.3
	Viet Nam	1997	7.7	..	53.1	..
Western Asia						
	Armenia	2000	8.6	1.2	52.5	26.0
	Azerbaijan	1999	12.8	2.4	49.1	16.9
	Bahrain	1992	5.2	0.4	34.7	11.1
	Cyprus	1992	7.5	0.6	50.8	18.1
	Georgia		..	..	..	..
	Iraq	1987	20.8	5.8	56.6	27.6
	Israel	2002	3.8	0.4	32.6	12.0
	Jordan	1997	8.2	..	38.8	..
	Kuwait	1996	13.2	1.2	47.8	21.9
	Lebanon	1970	13.2	1.0	49.1	11.9
	Occupied Palestinian Territory	1997	24.2	2.0	63.9	27.9
	Oman	1995	15.5	1.3	61.3	22.4
	Qatar	1998	4.2	0.2	32.2	9.6
	Saudi Arabia	1996	7.4	0.4	40.2	9.9
	Syrian Arab Republic	1981	24.9	3.8	64.5	25.4
	Turkey	2000	12.8	2.1	53.0	20.8
	United Arab Emirates	1987	18.5	2.5	52.2	26.6
	Yemen	1997	26.9	..	72.8	..
EUROPE						
Eastern Europe						
	Belarus	1999	6.2	0.9	54.9	29.9
	Bulgaria		..	..	..	..
	Czech Republic		..	..	..	..
	Hungary	2002	1.0	0.2	11.7	5.3
	Poland		..	..	..	..
	Republic of Moldova	1997	12.0	..	72.4	..
	Romania	2003	4.3	0.2	34.0	10.2
	Russian Federation	2002	7.6	1.6	12.9	2.8
	Slovakia		..	..	..	..
	Ukraine	1989	15.4	2.7	70.7	41.3
Northern Europe						
	Channel Islands		..	..	..	..
	Denmark	2002	0.5	0.1	8.8	3.4
	Estonia	2000	4.7	1.0	40.5	21.7
	Faeroe Islands	1992	1.0	—	19.0	6.4
	Finland	2003	0.5	0.1	9.7	4.5
	Iceland	2002	13.6	2.7	64.3	46.9
	Ireland	2002	0.3	0.1	3.9	1.7
	Isle of Man	1991	1.5	0.3	22.2	10.5
	Latvia	2002	1.1	0.2	18.9	9.4
	Lithuania	2001	..	..	34.9	17.3
	Norway	2002	0.5	0.1	8.8	3.3
	Sweden	2002	0.4	0.1	6.7	2.2
	United Kingdom		..	..	..	..

Annex table 2. Youth that have ever been married as a proportion of the total population (most recent data available)

Region and subregion	Country	Percentage of youth that have ever married by age (years) and sex				
		Year	15-19 Female	15-19 Male	20-24 Female	20-24 Male
Southern Europe						
	Albania	1955	23.2	4.7	75.6	27.3
	Andorra	2001	2.3	0.3	25.8	7.7
	Bosnia and Herzegovina	..	..	..	..	..
	Croatia	..	..	..	..	..
	Gibraltar	1991	8.4	2.3	50.7	25.4
	Greece	1999	..	..	23.2	6.9
	Holy See	..	..	..	..	..
	Italy	2000	0.9	0.1	12.8	2.9
	Malta	1985	3.0	0.4	33.1	13.1
	Portugal	..	..	..	..	..
	San Marino	1997	0.4	—	18.1	2.9
	Serbia and Montenegro (former)	1991	11.3	1.8	50.9	20.6
	Slovenia	2002	5.7	1.0	50.1	28.6
	Spain	1995	..	..	24.3	9.3
	The former Yugoslav Republic of Macedonia	1994	9.1	1.5	51.3	21.6
Western Europe						
	Austria	1996	..	..	41.1	23.3
	Belgium	2001	0.1	..	5.7	..
	France	2002	0.3	0.2	0.4	1.1
	Germany	2001	0.3	—	8.7	2.6
	Liechtenstein	..	..	..	..	..
	Luxembourg	..	..	..	..	..
	Monaco	1982	1.0	0.1	26.2	8.8
	Netherlands	2003	0.7	0.1	11.0	3.5
	Switzerland	2001	0.7	0.1	12.6	5.2
LATIN AMERICA AND THE CARIBBEAN						
Caribbean						
	Anguilla	2001	1.4	—	15.0	5.1
	Antigua and Barbuda	1991	0.5	0.1	8.0	3.2
	Aruba	1991	3.2	0.4	29.1	15.0
	Bahamas	1990	3.7	0.8	25.2	13.7
	Barbados	1990	0.6	0.2	6.6	2.2
	British Virgin Islands	1991	1.3	0.2	14.3	7.1
	Cayman Islands	1989	5.8	1.8	36.2	19.8
	Cuba	1981	28.9	6.7	73.5	40.5
	Dominica	2001	0.2	0.2	4.7	1.0
	Dominican Republic	1996	28.9	4.4	66.1	32.3
	Grenada	1991	0.6	0.1	6.3	1.1
	Guadeloupe	1999	0.7	0.2	7.0	1.5
	Haiti	2000	19.4	2.6	57.3	29.8
	Jamaica	1997	6.9	..	27.8	..
	Martinique	1999	0.4	0.1	3.9	0.9
	Montserrat	1980	0.3	0.5	8.8	2.2
	Netherlands Antilles	2001	0.8	0.2	12.3	4.5
	Puerto Rico	1995	19.5	..	55.0	..
	Saint Kitts and Nevis	1980	0.5	0.1	7.7	2.4
	Saint Lucia	2001	5.5	1.0	26.9	12.3
	Saint Vincent and the Grenadines	2002	16.4	4.5	47.9	25.6
	Trinidad and Tobago	1990	9.0	1.1	27.4	10.6
	Turks and Caicos Islands	1980	3.0	0.4	40.0	13.7
	U.S. Virgin Islands	1995	3.2	4.1	15.5	5.5
Central America						
	Belize	1991	7.8	1.4	30.9	18.0
	Costa Rica	2003	11.5	3.1	44.4	23.3
	El Salvador	2000	15.9	4.4	49.9	34.4
	Guatemala	1998	26.0	..	69.5	..
	Honduras	1996	30.5	..	68.3	..
	Mexico	2000	17.2	5.9	52.3	37.9
	Nicaragua	1998	34.3	..	75.1	..
	Panama	2000	22.0	4.8	57.6	32.9
South America						
	Argentina	1991	12.5	2.7	45.3	25.6
	Bolivia	1998	12.2	5.2	53.4	33.5
	Brazil	1996	16.7	4.3	52.6	29.1
	Chile	1992	11.6	5.3	43.9	25.4
	Colombia	2000	17.5	3.4	50.0	26.8
	Ecuador	2001	22.0	7.1	57.0	38.0
	Falkland Islands (Malvinas)	1986	..	..	..	..
	French Guiana	1999	0.8	—	6.5	1.5
	Guyana	1991	6.9	0.8	26.7	12.0
	Paraguay	1998	16.9	..	56.7	..
	Peru	2000	11.3	..	47.1	..
	Suriname	1964	19.7	2.8	61.3	35.9
	Uruguay	1996	12.7	3.4	44.7	26.8
	Venezuela	1990	14.0	4.2	43.5	26.2

Annex table 2. Youth that have ever been married as a proportion of the total population (most recent data available)

Region and subregion	Country	Percentage of youth that have ever married by age (years) and sex				
		Year	15-19 Female	15-19 Male	20-24 Female	20-24 Male
NORTHERN AMERICA						
	Bermuda	2000	0.4	0.2	13.9	5.4
	Canada	2003	3.0	1.0	25.0	13.0
	Greenland	1999	0.5	0.1	12.0	3.6
	Saint-Pierre et Miquelon	1982	2.1	—	45.2	16.0
	United States of America	2000	..	..	27.2	16.3
OCEANIA						
Australia/New Zealand						
	Australia	2001	0.5	0.1	13.1	5.7
	New Zealand	1996	6.2	2.7	33.5	21.4
Melanesia						
	Fiji	1996	10.3	1.7	54.1	22.5
	New Caledonia	1996	1.2	0.1	13.1	4.1
	Papua New Guinea	1980	17.6	4.2	73.3	36.0
	Solomon Islands	1986	19.1	3.1	65.0	31.2
	Vanuatu	1989	12.0	2.3	56.9	29.1
Micronesia						
	Guam	1990	5.9	2.1	45.2	29.3
	Kiribati	1990	19.2	6.1	65.5	38.6
	Marshall Islands	1999	14.3	7.7	57.7	40.2
	Micronesia (Federated States of)	1994	10.2	4.1	43.4	28.9
	Nauru	..	..	..	..	..
	Northern Mariana Islands	..	..	..	..	..
	Palau	..	..	..	..	..
Polynesia						
	American Samoa	1990	4.7	1.6	35.1	16.0
	Cook Islands	1996	2.1	1.3	17.4	12.1
	French Polynesia	1962	—	—	0.7	0.1
	Niue	..	..	..	..	..
	Samoa	1999	8.3	1.1	50.7	19.0
	Tokelau	1976	1.4	2.6	24.1	30.4
	Tonga	1996	4.9	1.8	33.4	17.7
	Tuvalu	1979	3.2	0.2	33.4	14.5
	Wallis and Futuna Islands	1990	2.8	0.1	25.8	8.8

Source: United Nations, Population Division, *World Marriage Patterns 2005* (POP/DB/Marr/Rev.2005).

Notes:
Two dots (..) indicate that data are not available or are not separately reported.
An dash (—) indicates that the amount is nil or negligible.

Annex table 3. Youth literacy rates (most recent data available)

Region and subregion	Country	Year	Percentage of youth population that is literate, by age and sex									Source/year
			15-19 years			20-24 years			15-24 years			
			Female	Male	Total	Female	Male	Total	Female	Male	Total	
AFRICA	*Regional average*	2005	..	..	..	..	..	..	70.2	80.3	75.2	
Eastern Africa	*Regional average*	2005	..	..	..	..	..	..	67.4	75.6	71.5	
	Burundi	2000	..	..	..	..	..	..	70.4	76.8	73.3	MICS 2000
	Comoros	..	..	..	..	..	..	..	..	..	..	..
	Djibouti	..	..	..	..	..	..	..	..	..	..	..
	Eritrea	..	..	..	..	..	..	..	..	..	..	..
	Ethiopia	..	..	..	..	..	..	..	..	..	..	..
	Kenya	2000	..	..	..	..	..	..	80.7	79.8	80.3	MICS 2000
	Madagascar	2000	..	..	..	..	..	..	68.2	72.7	70.2	MICS 2000
	Malawi	1998	76.6	83.3	79.9	64.6	80.6	71.7	70.7	82.1	76.0	c 1998
	Mauritius	2000	96.4	94.4	95.4	94.5	93.0	93.8	95.4	93.7	94.5	c 2000
	Mozambique	..	..	..	..	..	..	..	..	..	..	..
	Réunion	..	..	..	..	..	..	..	..	..	..	..
	Rwanda	2000	..	..	..	..	..	..	76.9	78.5	77.6	MICS 2000
	Seychelles	2002	99.4	98.9	99.1	99.4	98.7	99.0	99.4	98.8	99.1	c 2002
	Somalia	..	..	..	..	..	..	..	..	..	..	..
	Tanzania, United Republic of	2002	75.9	79.9	77.8	76.5	82.3	79.0	76.2	80.9	78.4	c 2002
	Uganda	2002	..	..	..	..	..	..	71.2	82.7	76.6	c 2002
	Zambia	1999	..	..	..	..	..	..	66.2	72.6	69.5	MICS 1999
	Zimbabwe	..	..	..	..	..	..	..	..	..	..	..
Middle Africa	*Regional average*	2005	..	..	..	..	..	..	60.5	77.6	68.6	
	Angola	2001	..	..	..	..	..	..	63.2	83.7	72.2	MICS 2001
	Cameroon	..	..	..	..	..	..	..	..	..	..	..
	Central African Republic	2000	..	..	..	..	..	..	46.9	70.3	58.5	MICS 2000
	Chad	2000	..	..	..	..	..	..	23.2	55.7	37.6	MICS 2001
	Congo	..	..	..	..	..	..	..	..	..	..	..
	Congo, Democratic Republic of the	2001	..	..	..	..	..	..	63.1	78.0	70.4	MICS 2001
	Equatorial Guinea	2000	..	..	..	..	..	..	94.9	94.8	94.9	MICS 2000
	Gabon	..	..	..	..	..	..	..	..	..	..	..
	Sao Tome and Principe	..	..	..	..	..	..	..	..	..	..	..
Northern Africa	*Regional average*	2005	..	..	..	..	..	..	77.2	89.0	83.1	
	Algeria	2002	88.8	93.9	91.3	83.1	94.3	88.8	86.1	94.1	90.1	s 2002
	Egypt	2005	84.6	90.5	87.7	72.3	89.7	81.9	78.9	90.1	84.9	s 2005
	Libyan Arab Jamahiriya	..	..	..	..	..	..	..	..	..	..	..
	Morocco	2004	67.3	84.3	75.7	53.4	77.0	64.8	60.5	80.8	70.5	c 2004
	Sudan*	2000	..	..	..	..	..	..	71.4	84.6	77.2	MICS 2000
	Tunisia	2004	94.3	96.9	95.7	90.1	95.8	93.0	92.2	96.4	94.3	c 2004
	Western Sahara	..	..	..	..	..	..	..	..	..	..	..
Southern Africa	*Regional average*	2005	..	..	..	..	..	..	94.0	92.4	93.2	
	Botswana	2003	94.9	92.5	93.7	96.4	91.6	94.2	95.6	92.1	94.0	s 2003
	Lesotho	..	..	..	..	..	..	..	..	..	..	..
	Namibia	2001	94.0	91.1	92.6	92.8	91.2	92.0	93.5	91.2	92.3	c 2001
	South Africa	1996	95.3	94.0	94.7	93.3	92.9	93.1	94.3	93.5	93.9	c 1996
	Swaziland	2000	..	..	..	..	..	..	89.8	87.0	88.4	MICS 2000
Western Africa	*Regional average*	2005	..	..	..	..	..	..	67.1	77.5	72.1	
	Benin	2002	38.0	61.5	49.6	28.4	56.2	40.3	33.2	59.2	45.3	c 2002
	Burkina Faso	2003	27.5	38.1	32.7	21.6	38.8	29.3	24.8	38.4	31.2	s 2003
	Cape Verde	..	..	..	..	..	..	..	..	..	..	..
	Côte d'Ivoire	2000	..	..	..	..	..	..	52.1	70.8	60.7	MICS 2000
	Gambia	..	..	..	..	..	..	..	..	..	..	..
	Ghana	2000	70.8	77.4	74.2	59.6	74.2	66.6	65.5	75.9	70.7	c 2000
	Guinea	2003	..	..	..	..	..	..	33.7	58.7	46.6	MICS 2003
	Guinea-Bissau	..	..	..	..	..	..	..	..	..	..	..

Annex table 3. Youth literacy rates (most recent data available)

Region and subregion	Country	Year	15-19 years			20-24 years			15-24 years			Source/year
			Female	Male	Total	Female	Male	Total	Female	Male	Total	
Western Africa (cont'd)	Liberia	..	..	..	..	..	..	..	..	..	..	..
	Mali	1998	18.2	33.7	25.7	15.1	30.3	22.3	16.9	32.3	24.2	c 1998
	Mauritania	2000	58.0	68.3	63.0	52.3	66.9	59.2	55.5	67.7	61.3	c 2000
	Niger	2005	26.3	53.9	39.4	19.8	50.5	33.1	23.2	52.4	36.5	s 2005
	Nigeria	..	..	..	..	..	..	..	..	..	..	..
	St. Helena	..	..	..	..	..	..	..	..	..	..	..
	Senegal	2002	41.3	57.8	49.0	40.5	59.3	49.3	41.0	58.5	49.1	s 2002
	Sierra Leone	2004	43.4	63.1	52.9	29.6	53.6	40.5	37.2	59.1	47.6	c 2004
	Togo	2000	..	..	..	..	..	..	63.6	83.7	74.4	MICS 2000
ASIA	Regional average	2005							82.4	90.4	86.5	
Eastern Asia	Regional average	2005	..	..	..	..	..	..	98.5	99.2	98.9	
	China	2000	98.8	99.3	99.1	98.2	99.1	98.6	98.5	99.2	98.9	c 2000
	Hong Kong, China SAR	..	..	..	..	..	..	..	..	..	..	..
	Japan	..	..	..	..	..	..	..	..	..	..	..
	Macao, China SAR	2001	99.8	99.7	99.7	99.8	99.1	99.5	99.8	99.4	99.6	c 2001
	Korea, Democratic People's Republic of	..	..	..	..	..	..	..	..	..	..	..
	Korea, Republic of	..	..	..	..	..	..	..	..	..	..	..
	Mongolia	2000	97.9	95.8	96.8	99.1	98.4	98.7	98.4	97.0	97.7	c 2000
South-central Asia	Regional average	2005	..	..	..	..	..	..	64.8	81.0	73.2	
	Afghanistan	2000	..	..	..	..	..	..	18.4	50.8	34.3	MICS 2000
	Bangladesh	..	..	..	..	..	..	..	..	..	..	..
	Bhutan	..	..	..	..	..	..	..	..	..	..	..
	India	2001	72.7	85.0	79.3	62.5	83.3	73.2	67.7	84.2	76.4	c 2001
	Iran, Islamic Republic of	..	..	..	..	..	..	..	..	..	..	..
	Kazakhstan	2005	99.9	99.8	99.8	99.9	99.8	99.9	99.9	99.8	99.8	c 1999
	Kyrgyzstan	2005	99.7	99.6	99.7	99.8	99.7	99.7	99.7	99.7	99.7	c 1999
	Maldives	2000	98.3	97.9	98.1	98.3	98.2	98.3	98.3	98.0	98.2	c 2000
	Nepal	2001	66.2	82.5	74.3	53.4	78.2	65.0	60.1	80.6	70.1	c 2001
	Pakistan	2005	58.1	76.7	67.8	50.5	74.6	62.6	54.7	75.8	65.5	s 2005
	Sri Lanka	2001	96.7	95.6	96.1	95.5	94.5	95.0	96.1	95.1	95.6	c 2001
	Tajikistan	2005	99.9	99.8	99.9	99.8	99.8	99.8	99.8	99.8	99.8	c 2000
	Turkmenistan	2005	99.8	99.8	99.8	99.8	99.8	99.8	99.8	99.8	99.8	c 1995
	Uzbekistan	..	..	..	..	..	..	..	..	..	..	..
South-eastern Asia	Regional average	2005	..	..	..	..	..	..	95.9	96.5	96.2	
	Brunei Darussalam	2001	99.4	99.4	99.4	98.5	98.4	98.5	98.9	98.9	98.9	c 2001
	Cambodia	2004	82.9	89.6	86.3	74.5	85.9	80.0	78.9	87.9	83.4	s 2004
	Timor-Leste	..	..	..	..	..	..	..	..	..	..	..
	Indonesia	2004	98.8	98.9	98.8	98.3	98.8	98.6	98.5	98.9	98.7	s 2004
	Lao People's Democratic Republic	2001	77.1	83.6	80.3	71.1	80.9	75.6	74.7	82.6	78.5	s 2001
	Malaysia	2000	97.8	97.8	97.8	96.6	96.6	96.6	97.3	97.2	97.2	c 2000
	Myanmar	2000	..	..	..	..	..	..	93.4	95.7	94.5	MICS 2000
	Philippines	2000	95.5	94.1	94.8	96.0	94.9	95.4	95.7	94.5	95.1	c 2000
	Singapore	2000	..	..	..	..	..	..	99.6	99.4	99.5	c 2000
	Thailand	2000	..	..	..	..	..	..	97.8	98.1	98.0	c 2000
	Viet Nam	1999	94.5	94.9	94.7	93.1	93.7	93.4	93.6	94.2	93.9	c 1999
Western Asia	Regional average	2005	..	..	..	..	..	..	88.5	95.2	91.9	
	Armenia	2005	99.8	99.7	99.8	99.9	99.8	99.8	99.9	99.8	99.8	c 2001
	Azerbaijan	2005	99.9	99.9	99.9	99.9	99.8	99.8	99.9	99.9	99.9	c 1999
	Bahrain	2001	99.4	99.4	99.4	95.2	94.8	95.0	97.3	96.8	97.0	c 2001
	Cyprus	2001	99.9	99.8	99.8	99.8	99.7	99.7	99.8	99.7	99.8	c 2001
	Georgia	..	..	..	..	..	..	..	..	..	..	..
	Iraq	2000	..	..	..	..	..	..	80.5	88.9	84.8	MICS 2000
	Israel	2004	100.0	100.0	100.0	99.1	100.0	99.6	99.6	100.0	99.8	s 2004
	Jordan	2003	99.2	99.5	99.4	98.6	99.1	98.9	98.9	99.3	99.1	s 2003
	Kuwait	2005	99.9	99.9	99.9	99.7	99.5	99.6	99.8	99.7	99.7	c 2005
	Lebanon	2005	..	..	..	..	..	..	..	..	..	..
	Occupied Palestinian Territory	2005	99.2	99.1	99.2	98.3	99.2	98.8	98.8	99.1	99.0	s 2004
	Oman	2003	97.5	98.7	98.1	95.7	97.0	96.4	96.7	97.9	97.3	c 2003
	Qatar	2004	97.7	98.5	98.1	97.3	92.9	94.3	97.5	94.9	95.9	c 2004
	Saudi Arabia	2000	95.5	98.4	97.0	91.6	97.7	94.7	93.7	98.1	95.9	s 2000

Annex table 3. Youth literacy rates (most recent data available)

| Region and subregion | Country | Year | Percentage of youth population that is literate, by age and sex | | | | | | | | | Source/year |
| | | | 15-19 years | | | 20-24 years | | | 15-24 years | | | |
			Female	Male	Total	Female	Male	Total	Female	Male	Total	
Western Asia (cont'd)	Syrian Arab Republic	2004	91.8	95.0	93.4	88.4	93.5	90.9	90.2	94.3	92.2	s 2002
	Turkey	2004	93.7	98.2	96.0	93.0	97.9	95.2	93.3	98.0	95.6	s 2004
	United Arab Emirates	..	..	..	..	..	..	..	..	..	..	..
	Yemen	..	..	..	..	..	..	..	..	..	..	..
EUROPE	*Regional average*	2005							99.7	99.6	99.6	
Eastern Europe	*Regional average*	2005							99.6	99.5	99.5	
	Belarus	1999	99.8	99.8	99.8	99.8	99.8	99.8	99.8	99.8	99.8	c 1999
	Bulgaria	2001	97.8	98.0	97.9	98.4	98.6	98.5	98.1	98.3	98.2	c 2001
	Czech Republic	..	..	..	..	..	..	..	..	..	..	..
	Hungary	..	..	..	..	..	..	..	..	..	..	..
	Poland	..	..	..	..	..	..	..	..	..	..	..
	Republic of Moldova	2004	99.7	99.5	99.6	99.4	99.5	99.4	99.5	99.5	99.5	s 2004
	Romania	2002	97.8	97.6	97.7	97.8	97.8	97.8	97.8	97.7	97.8	c 2002
	Russian Federation	2002	99.8	99.7	99.7	99.8	99.7	99.7	99.8	99.7	99.7	c 2002
	Slovakia	..	..	..	..	..	..	..	..	..	..	..
Northern Europe	*Regional average*	2005	..	..	..	..	..	..	99.7	99.7	99.7	
	Channel Islands	..	..	..	..	..	..	..	..	..	..	..
	Denmark	..	..	..	..	..	..	..	..	..	..	..
	Estonia	2000	99.8	99.7	99.8	99.8	99.7	99.7	99.8	99.7	99.8	c 2000
	Faeroe Islands	..	..	..	..	..	..	..	..	..	..	..
	Finland	..	..	..	..	..	..	..	..	..	..	..
	Iceland	..	..	..	..	..	..	..	..	..	..	..
	Ireland	..	..	..	..	..	..	..	..	..	..	..
	Isle of Man	..	..	..	..	..	..	..	..	..	..	..
	Latvia	2000	99.8	99.7	99.7	99.8	99.7	99.8	99.8	99.7	99.8	c 2000
	Lithuania	2001	99.8	99.7	99.7	99.7	99.6	99.6	99.7	99.7	99.7	c 2001
	Norway	..	..	..	..	..	..	..	..	..	..	..
	Sweden	..	..	..	..	..	..	..	..	..	..	..
	United Kingdom	..	..	..	..	..	..	..	..	..	..	..
Southern Europe	*Regional average*	2005	..	..	..	..	..	..	99.6	99.6	99.6	
	Albania	2001	99.5	99.4	99.4	99.5	99.4	99.4	99.5	99.4	99.4	c 2001
	Andorra	..	..	..	..	..	..	..	..	..	..	..
	Bosnia and Herzegovina	2000	..	..	..	..	..	..	99.8	99.7	99.8	MICS 2000
	Croatia	2001	99.7	99.6	99.6	99.7	99.6	99.7	99.7	99.6	99.6	
	Gibraltar	..	..	..	..	..	..	..	..	..	..	..
	Greece	2005	99.1	99.2	99.2	98.9	98.6	98.7	99.5	99.5	99.5	c 2001
	Holy See	..	..	..	..	..	..	..	..	..	..	..
	Italy	2001	99.9	99.8	99.9	99.8	99.8	99.8	99.8	99.8	99.8	c 2001
	Malta	1995	98.1	94.6	96.3	97.5	94.1	95.7	97.8	94.4	96.0	c 1995
	Portugal	..	..	..	..	..	..	..	..	..	..	..
	San Marino	..	..	..	..	..	..	..	..	..	..	..
	Serbia and Montenegro** (former)	2003	99.3	99.4	99.3	99.3	99.4	99.4	99.3	99.4	99.4	c 2003
	Slovenia	..	..	..	..	..	..	..	..	..	..	..
	Spain	..	..	..	..	..	..	..	..	..	..	..
	The former Yugoslav Republic of Macedonia	2002	98.5	99.0	98.7	98.5	99.0	98.7	98.5	99.0	98.7	c 2002

Annex table 3. Youth literacy rates (most recent data available)

Region and subregion	Country	Year	15-19 years Female	Male	Total	20-24 years Female	Male	Total	15-24 years Female	Male	Total	Source/year
Western Europe	Regional average	2005	..	..	..	..	..	..	99.9	99.7	99.8	
	Austria	..	..	..	..	..	..	..	..	..	..	..
	Belgium	..	..	..	..	..	..	..	..	..	..	..
	France	..	..	..	..	..	..	..	..	..	..	..
	Germany	..	..	..	..	..	..	..	..	..	..	..
	Liechtenstein	..	..	..	..	..	..	..	..	..	..	..
	Luxembourg	..	..	..	..	..	..	..	..	..	..	..
	Monaco	..	..	..	..	..	..	..	..	..	..	..
	Netherlands	..	..	..	..	..	..	..	..	..	..	..
	Switzerland	..	..	..	..	..	..	..	..	..	..	..
LATIN AMERICA AND THE CARIBBEAN	Regional average	2005	..	..	..	..	..	..	96.4	95.6	96.0	
Caribbean	Regional average	2005	..	..	..	..	..	..	88.7	86.9	87.8	
	Anguilla	..	..	..	..	..	..	..	..	..	..	..
	Antigua and Barbuda	..	..	..	..	..	..	..	..	..	..	..
	Aruba	2000	99.2	99.1	99.1	99.1	98.6	98.9	99.2	98.9	99.0	c 2000
	Bahamas	..	..	..	..	..	..	..	..	..	..	..
	Barbados	..	..	..	..	..	..	..	..	..	..	..
	British Virgin Islands	..	..	..	..	..	..	..	..	..	..	..
	Cayman Islands	..	..	..	..	..	..	..	..	..	..	..
	Cuba	2002	100.0	100.0	100.0	99.9	99.9	99.9	100.0	100.0	100.0	c 2002
	Dominica	..	..	..	..	..	..	..	..	..	..	..
	Dominican Republic	2002	96.6	94.4	95.5	94.2	91.5	92.8	95.4	93.0	94.2	c 2002
	Grenada	..	..	..	..	..	..	..	..	..	..	..
	Guadeloupe	..	..	..	..	..	..	..	..	..	..	..
	Haiti	..	..	..	..	..	..	..	..	..	..	..
	Jamaica***	1999	..	..	..	..	..	..	85.9	74.1	79.9	s 1999
	Martinique	..	..	..	..	..	..	..	..	..	..	..
	Montserrat	..	..	..	..	..	..	..	..	..	..	..
	Netherlands Antilles	..	..	..	..	..	..	..	..	..	..	..
	Puerto Rico	..	..	..	..	..	..	..	..	..	..	..
	Saint Kitts and Nevis	..	..	..	..	..	..	..	..	..	..	..
	Saint Lucia	..	..	..	..	..	..	..	..	..	..	..
	Saint Vincent and the Grenadines	..	..	..	..	..	..	..	..	..	..	..
	Trinidad and Tobago	..	..	..	..	..	..	..	..	..	..	..
	Turks and Caicos Islands	..	..	..	..	..	..	..	..	..	..	..
	U.S. Virgin Islands	..	..	..	..	..	..	..	..	..	..	..
Central America	Regional average	2005	..	..	..	..	..	..	94.8	95.1	95.0	
	Belize	..	..	..	..	..	..	..	..	..	..	..
	Costa Rica	2000	98.3	97.4	97.9	97.7	96.9	97.3	98.0	97.2	97.6	c 2000
	El Salvador	..	..	..	..	..	..	..	..	..	..	..
	Guatemala	2002	81.2	87.4	84.2	75.3	85.2	79.9	78.4	86.4	82.2	c 2002
	Honduras	2001	92.0	87.3	89.7	89.6	86.3	88.1	90.9	86.9	88.9	c 2001
	Mexico	2004	97.9	98.1	98.0	97.3	96.8	97.1	97.6	97.5	97.6	s 2004
	Nicaragua	2001	90.7	84.7	87.7	86.4	82.1	84.3	88.8	83.6	86.2	s 2001
	Panama	2000	95.9	96.6	96.3	95.3	96.5	95.9	95.6	96.5	96.1	c 2000
South America	Regional average	2005	..	..	..	..	..	..	97.9	96.7	97.3	
	Argentina	2001	99.2	98.9	99.0	99.0	98.6	98.8	99.1	98.7	98.9	c 2001
	Bolivia	2001	97.1	98.8	98.0	95.0	98.3	96.6	96.1	98.5	97.3	c 2001
	Brazil	2004	98.5	96.7	97.6	97.3	94.8	96.1	97.9	95.8	96.8	s 2004
	Chile	2002	99.2	98.9	99.0	99.2	98.7	98.9	99.2	98.8	99.0	c 2002
	Colombia	2004	98.8	97.5	98.1	98.0	97.6	97.8	98.4	97.6	98.0	s 2004
	Ecuador	2001	96.6	96.3	96.4	96.4	96.5	96.4	96.5	96.4	96.4	c 2001
	Falkland Islands (Malvinas)	..	..	..	..	..	..	..	..	..	..	..

Annex table 3. Youth literacy rates (most recent data available)

Region and subregion	Country	Year	Percentage of youth population that is literate, by age and sex									Source/year
			15-19 years			20-24 years			15-24 years			
			Female	Male	Total	Female	Male	Total	Female	Male	Total	
South America (cont'd)	French Guiana	..	..	..	..	..	..	..	..	..	..	..
	Guyana	..	..	..	..	..	..	..	..	..	..	..
	Paraguay	..	..	..	..	..	..	..	..	..	..	..
	Peru	2004	96.1	98.0	97.1	95.1	97.5	96.3	95.7	97.8	96,8	s 2004
	Suriname	2004	94.8	95.5	95.2	93.5	95.7	94.6	94.1	95.6	94.9	c 2004
	Uruguay	..	..	..	..	..	..	..	..	..	..	..
	Venezuela	2001	98.3	96.5	97.4	97.8	96.1	97.0	98.1	96.3	97.2	c 2001
NORTHERN AMERICA	*Regional average*	2005	..	..	..	..	..	..	99.2	99.3	99.3	
	Bermuda	..	..	..	..	..	..	..	..	..	..	..
	Canada	..	..	..	..	..	..	..	..	..	..	..
	Greenland	..	..	..	..	..	..	..	..	..	..	..
	Saint-Pierre et Miquelon	..	..	..	..	..	..	..	..	..	..	..
	United States of America	..	..	..	..	..	..	..	..	..	..	..
OCEANIA	*Regional average*	2005	..	..	..	..	..	..	91.4	92.5	92.0	
Australia/New Zealand	*Regional average*	2005							99.8	99.8	99.8	
	Australia	..	..	..	..	..	..	..	..	..	..	..
	New Zealand	..	..	..	..	..	..	..	..	..	..	..
Melanesia	*Regional average*	2005	..	..	..	..	..	..	70.1	74.4	72.3	
	Fiji	..	..	..	..	..	..	..	..	..	..	..
	New Caledonia	..	..	..	..	..	..	..	..	..	..	..
	Papua New Guinea	2000	67.0	66.0	64.8	71.8	67.5	63.2	69.1	66.7	64.1	c 2000
	Solomon Islands	..	..	..	..	..	..	..	..	..	..	..
	Vanuatu	..	..	..	..	..	..	..	..	..	..	..
Micronesia	*Regional average*	2005	..	..	..	..	..	..	87.8	91.2	89.4	
	Guam	..	..	..	..	..	..	..	..	..	..	..
	Kiribati	..	..	..	..	..	..	..	..	..	..	..
	Marshall Islands	..	..	..	..	..	..	..	..	..	..	..
	Micronesia, Federated States of	..	..	..	..	..	..	..	..	..	..	..
	Nauru	..	..	..	..	..	..	..	..	..	..	..
	Northern Mariana Islands	..	..	..	..	..	..	..	..	..	..	..
	Palau	..	..	..	..	..	..	..	..	..	..	..
Polynesia	*Regional average*	2005	..	..	..	..	..	..	99.5	99.4	99.5	
	American Samoa	..	..	..	..	..	..	..	..	..	..	..
	Cook Islands	..	..	..	..	..	..	..	..	..	..	..
	French Polynesia	..	..	..	..	..	..	..	..	..	..	..
	Niue	..	..	..	..	..	..	..	..	..	..	..
	Pitcairn	..	..	..	..	..	..	..	..	..	..	..
	Samoa	..	..	..	..	..	..	..	..	..	..	..
	Tokelau	..	..	..	..	..	..	..	..	..	..	..
	Tonga	1996	99.4	99.5	99.6	99.1	99.1	99.1	99.3	99.3	99.4	c 1996
	Tuvalu	..	..	..	..	..	..	..	..	..	..	..
	Wallis and Futuna Islands	..	..	..	..	..	..	..	..	..	..	..

Source: UNESCO Institute for Statistics, 2006 data release.
Calculations based on population data drawn from:
United Nations Population Division estimate (2004 revision). The population estimate used corresponds to the year of the census/survey.
Symbols used:
c: census
MICS: Multiple Indicator Cluster Survey (UNICEF: http://www.unicef.org/statistics).
s: survey
Notes:
Two dots (..) indicate that data are not available or are not separately reported.
* Sudan: data are for northern Sudan only.
** Serbia and Montenegro: data exclude Kosovo and Metohia.
*** Jamaica: data are based on a literacy assessment.
Explanatory note:
Data for the UNESCO Institute of Statistics literacy table are for the reference period 2000-2004. For this time interval, the latest available data point is presented in each case. Most of these data are obtained from national surveys and censuses that were undertaken during the reference period 2000-2004 unless otherwise indicated in the last column of the table. The use of one literacy rate to represent a five-year period has been adopted because literacy rates do not fluctuate significantly over the short term, and, therefore, year-to-year estimates of short-term change can be unreliable in the absence of observed data. Please refer to the list of literacy definitions (http://www.uis.unesco.org/glossary/) and other metadata when interpreting the data.

Annex table 4. Gross primary, secondary and tertiary enrolment ratios, 2004

Gross enrolment ratios

Region and subregion	Country	Primary — Total	Primary — Male	Primary — Female	Primary — Female/male ratio*	Primary — Note	Secondary — Total	Secondary — Male	Secondary — Female	Secondary — Female/male ratio*	Secondary — Note	Tertiary — Total	Tertiary — Male	Tertiary — Female	Tertiary — Female/male ratio*	Tertiary — Note
AFRICA																
Eastern Africa	Burundi	79.9	87.2	72.6	0.83		12.1	13.9	10.4	0.75		2.3	3.4	1.3	0.37	
	Comoros	85.5	90.8	80.0	0.88		35.1	39.9	30.2	0.76		2.3	2.6	2.0	0.77	**
	Djibouti	39.1	43.7	34.5	0.79		21.5	25.5	17.5	0.69	+1	1.6	1.7	1.4	0.82	
	Eritrea	64.1	71.0	57.2	0.81	+1	31.4	39.6	23.4	0.59	+1	1.1	2.0	0.3	0.15	
	Ethiopia	93.4	100.5	86.1	0.86	+1	30.9	37.5	24.3	0.65	+1	2.5	3.7	1.3	0.34	
	Kenya	111.3	114.5	108.1	0.94		48.0	49.6	46.4	0.93	**	2.9	3.6	2.2	0.60	
	Madagascar	133.5	136.2	130.8	0.96		..	..	..	..		2.5	2.7	2.4	0.90	
	Malawi	124.9	123.4	126.5	1.02		28.9	32.0	25.7	0.81	**,+1	0.4	0.5	0.3	0.54	
	Mauritius	102.2	102.1	102.3	1.00	+1	88.4	88.9	88.0	0.99		17.2	14.5	20.1	1.39	
	Mozambique	94.9	103.5	86.2	0.83		10.8	12.7	8.9	0.70		1.2	1.6	0.7	0.46	
	Reunion	..	..	..	..		..	..	..	..		..	..	..	..	
	Rwanda	119.2	118.2	120.2	1.02		14.3	15.2	13.5	0.89		2.7	3.4	2.1	0.62	***
	Seychelles	109.7	109.4	109.9	1.00	***	102.2	98.4	106.1	1.08	***	..	..	..	..	
	Somalia	..	..	..	..		..	..	..	..		..	..	..	..	
	Tanzania, United Republic of	106.0	108.0	104.1	0.96	+1	..	..	..	..		1.2	1.7	0.7	0.41	**,-1
	Uganda	117.5	117.7	117.3	1.00	+1	16.0	17.9	14.1	0.79	**,+1	3.4	4.2	2.6	0.62	
	Zambia	98.8	101.1	96.6	0.96		25.8	28.7	22.8	0.79		..	..	..	..	
	Zimbabwe	96.0	96.9	95.2	0.98	-1	36.4	38.2	34.6	0.91	-1	3.7	4.5	2.8	0.63	
Middle Africa	Angola	..	..	..	..		..	..	..	..		0.8	1.0	0.7	0.66	
	Cameroon	116.8	126.0	107.5	0.85		43.8	51.5	36.0	0.70	***	5.3	6.5	4.1	0.64	
	Central African Republic	55.6	67.0	44.3	0.66		11.6	23.4	7.7	0.33		1.2	2.1	0.3	0.14	
	Chad	80.2	97.2	63.3	0.65		15.5	..	..	..		..	..	..	..	
	Congo	88.7	91.9	85.5	0.93		38.6	42.1	35.2	0.84	**	3.6	6.2	1.1	0.19	**,-1
	Congo, Democratic Republic of the	61.7	69.2	54.1	0.78	**,-1	22.1	28.0	16.2	0.58	**,-1	..	..	..	..	
	Equatorial Guinea	127.2	133.4	121.1	0.91	-2	29.7	37.9	21.6	0.57	**,-2	..	..	..	..	
	Gabon	129.5	129.9	129.2	0.99	**	50.1	..	..	..		..	..	..	..	
	Sao Tome and Principe	132.9	134.2	131.7	0.98		40.2	39.3	41.2	1.05		..	..	..	..	
Northern Africa	Algeria	111.7	115.9	107.4	0.93		80.7	77.9	83.5	1.07		19.6	18.8	20.4	1.08	
	Egypt	100.7	102.8	98.5	0.96	**	87.1	89.8	84.2	0.94	**	32.6	..	..	..	**
	Libyan Arab Jamahiriya	112.5	112.6	112.4	1.00	**,-1	103.9	100.8	107.1	1.06	**,-1	56.2	53.7	58.8	1.09	**,-1
	Morocco	105.9	111.5	100.2	0.90		47.6	51.6	43.4	0.84		10.6	11.4	9.9	0.87	
	Sudan	60.1	64.3	55.7	0.87		32.8	34.0	31.6	0.93		..	..	..	..	
	Tunisia	109.9	111.7	108.0	0.97		81.3	74.0	80.1	1.08	-1	28.6	24.3	33.1	1.36	
	Western Sahara	..	..	..	..		..	..	..	..		..	..	..	..	
Southern Africa	Botswana	104.5	105.3	103.8	0.99		75.1	73.2	77.1	1.05	**	6.2	6.7	5.7	0.85	
	Lesotho	131.1	131.0	131.1	1.00		36.4	32.1	40.7	1.27		2.8	2.2	3.3	1.51	
	Namibia	100.9	100.2	101.6	1.01	-1	58.2	54.4	62.0	1.14	-1	6.1	5.7	6.5	1.15	
	South Africa	105.0	106.7	103.3	0.97	-1	90.5	87.3	93.6	1.07	-1	15.3	14.1	16.5	1.17	
	Swaziland	100.6	103.3	97.8	0.95	-1	41.9	41.7	42.0	1.01	-1	5.0	4.8	5.2	1.08	
Western Africa	Benin	98.9	111.2	86.1	0.77		26.4	35.6	17.0	0.48		1.7	2.6	0.8	0.29	**
	Burkina Faso	53.0	59.3	46.5	0.78		12.1	14.4	9.8	0.68		..	..	..	..	
	Cape Verde	110.6	113.5	107.8	0.95		65.7	62.7	68.7	1.10	**	5.5	5.3	5.8	1.10	
	Côte d'Ivoire	71.8	80.1	63.4	0.79	***,-1	24.9	32.0	17.7	0.55	**,-2	..	..	..	..	
	Gambia	81.4	79.2	83.7	1.06		46.9	51.2	42.6	0.83	**	1.2	1.9	0.5	0.23	
	Ghana	88.4	90.0	86.6	0.96	+1	43.6	47.0	40.0	0.85	**,+1	3.1	4.2	2.0	0.48	
	Guinea	79.1	86.9	70.7	0.81		25.9	34.5	16.7	0.48		2.2	3.6	0.7	0.20	
	Guinea-Bissau	..	..	..	..		..	..	..	..		..	..	..	..	
	Liberia	..	..	..	..		..	..	..	..		..	..	..	..	
	Mali	63.8	71.2	56.1	0.79		22.3	27.7	16.8	0.61		2.1	2.8	1.3	0.47	
	Mauritania	94.1	95.0	93.3	0.98		20.2	22.0	18.3	0.83		3.5	5.3	1.6	0.31	
	Niger	44.7	51.8	37.1	0.72		7.9	9.4	6.3	0.67		0.8	1.1	0.4	0.40	
	Nigeria	99.2	107.1	91.0	0.85		34.6	38.1	30.9	0.81	-1	10.2	13.1	7.2	0.55	

Annex table 4. Gross primary, secondary and tertiary enrolment ratios, 2004

Region and subregion	Country	Primary					Secondary					Tertiary				
		Total	Male	Female	Female/male ratio*	Note	Total	Male	Female	Female/male ratio*	Note	Total	Male	Female	Female/male ratio*	Note
Western Africa (cont'd)	Saint Helena	..	..	..	..		..	..	..	..		..	..	..	..	
	Senegal	76.0	77.9	74.1	0.95		19.4	22.4	16.2	0.72		4.9	..	..	..	
	Sierra Leone	145.1	168.6	121.9	0.72		13.8	13.7	14.0	1.03		2.1	3.1	1.2	0.40	**,-2
	Togo	101.1	110.2	92.1	0.84		38.9	52.1	25.8	0.50		..	..	..	..	
ASIA																
Eastern Asia	China	117.6	117.8	117.4	1.00		72.5	72.5	72.5	1.00		19.1	20.6	17.4	0.85	**
	Hong Kong, China SAR	108.1	111.3	104.9	0.94		84.9	86.4	83.4	0.97		32.1	32.6	31.6	0.97	
	Japan	100.4	100.3	100.5	1.00		101.6	101.5	101.7	1.00		54.0	57.1	50.7	0.89	
	Korea, Democratic People's Republic of	..	..	..	..		..	..	..	..		..	..	..	..	
	Korea, Republic of	104.8	105.1	104.5	0.99	+1	92.9	92.8	93.1	1.00	+1	89.6	109.9	68.6	0.62	+1
	Macao, China SAR	105.6	109.8	101.1	0.92		95.9	94.1	97.7	1.04		68.8	83.8	54.4	0.65	
	Mongolia	104.4	103.7	105.3	1.02		89.5	83.9	95.2	1.14		38.9	29.5	48.5	1.64	
South-central Asia	Afghanistan	92.9	127.4	55.9	0.44		15.6	25.2	5.3	0.21		1.1	1.7	0.5	0.28	
	Bangladesh	108.9	107.3	110.7	1.03		51.3	48.7	54.0	1.11	-1	6.5	8.6	4.3	0.50	-1
	Bhutan	..	..	..	..		..	..	..	..		..	..	..	..	
	India	116.2	120.0	112.1	0.93	**	53.5	59.3	47.3	0.80		11.8	14.0	9.3	0.66	
	Iran, Islamic Republic of	103.0	98.3	108.0	1.10		81.9	84.5	79.1	0.94		22.5	21.4	23.6	1.11	
	Kazakhstan	109.2	109.8	108.5	0.99		98.1	99.2	97.0	0.98		48.0	40.5	55.7	1.38	
	Kyrgyzstan	98.0	98.2	97.9	1.00		88.0	87.5	88.5	1.01		39.7	36.3	43.2	1.19	
	Maldives	103.5	105.0	101.9	0.97		72.8	68.3	77.6	1.14	**	0.2	0.1	0.3	2.37	**
	Nepal	113.3	118.4	107.9	0.91	+1	45.7	49.0	42.1	0.86	**,+1	5.6	7.9	3.2	0.40	
	Pakistan	82.1	94.6	68.8	0.73		27.2	31.3	22.9	0.73		3.2	3.5	2.8	0.80	
	Sri Lanka	101.7	102.4	101.1	0.99	**,-1	82.5	82.4	82.6	1.00		..	24.5	8.1	0.33	
	Tajikistan	99.9	102.2	97.5	0.95		81.8	88.8	74.6	0.84	**	..	..	..	..	
	Turkmenistan	..	..	..	..		..	..	..	..		..	..	..	..	
	Uzbekistan	99.8	100.2	99.3	0.99	**	94.6	96.0	93.2	0.97	**	15.3	17.0	13.5	0.80	**
South-eastern Asia	Brunei Darussalam	109.2	109.4	109.0	1.00		93.6	91.5	96.0	1.05	**	14.8	9.8	20.0	2.03	+1
	Cambodia	136.6	142.5	130.5	0.92		29.4	34.7	23.9	0.69	**	2.9	4.0	1.8	0.46	**
	Indonesia	117.0	118.0	115.9	0.98		64.1	64.4	63.8	0.99		16.7	18.6	14.7	0.79	
	Lao People's Democratic Republic	116.4	123.7	108.8	0.88		45.9	52.2	39.4	0.76		5.9	7.2	4.5	0.63	
	Malaysia	93.5	93.6	93.3	1.00	-1	75.8	70.9	80.9	1.14	-1	32.4	27.0	38.0	1.41	-1
	Myanmar	99.6	98.7	100.6	1.02	+1	40.3	40.5	40.0	0.99	+1	11.3	..	..	..	+1
	Philippines	112.4	113.2	111.5	0.99		85.9	81.6	90.3	1.11		28.8	25.4	32.4	1.28	
	Singapore	..	..	..	..		..	..	..	..		..	..	..	..	
	Thailand	97.1	99.6	94.6	0.95	+1	73.2	72.2	74.2	1.03	+1	43.0	40.7	45.4	1.11	**
	Timor-Leste	146.5	..	..	..		34.2	..	..	..		10.2	8.4	12.4	1.48	***,-2
	Viet Nam	98.0	101.4	94.4	0.93		73.5	75.2	71.7	0.95		10.2	11.5	8.8	0.77	**
Western Asia	Armenia	100.9	99.3	102.7	1.03		91.4	90.2	92.7	1.03		26.2	23.7	28.6	1.21	
	Azerbaijan	96.8	97.7	95.9	0.98		83.1	84.4	81.8	0.97		14.8	15.8	13.7	0.87	
	Bahrain	104.0	103.9	104.0	1.00		98.8	96.1	101.6	1.06		34.4	24.5	45.1	1.84	**
	Cyprus	97.7	98.0	97.5	1.00	***	97.7	96.4	99.1	1.03	***	35.9	36.2	35.5	0.98	***
	Georgia	95.1	95.2	95.0	1.00		82.3	82.8	81.9	0.99		41.5	40.8	42.1	1.03	
	Iraq	98.5	107.7	88.9	0.83		44.8	53.7	35.5	0.66		15.4	19.3	11.4	0.59	
	Israel	110.2	109.9	110.5	1.01		92.7	92.8	92.6	1.00		56.5	48.6	64.7	1.33	
	Jordan	98.2	97.9	98.6	1.01		87.4	86.9	88.0	1.01		39.3	37.5	41.3	1.10	
	Kuwait	96.5	96.2	96.7	1.00		89.9	87.2	92.8	1.06		22.3	12.3	33.4	2.72	
	Lebanon	106.8	108.7	104.8	0.96		88.7	84.9	92.6	1.09		47.6	44.9	50.4	1.12	
	Oman	87.3	87.5	87.1	1.00		86.4	88.1	84.6	0.96		12.9	10.9	15.0	1.37	
	Palestinian Autonomous Territories	92.9	92.8	93.1	1.00	***	93.6	91.2	96.1	1.05	***	37.9	37.3	38.6	1.04	**
	Qatar	101.7	102.5	100.8	0.98		96.8	98.2	95.4	0.97		19.1	9.2	33.8	3.69	
	Saudi Arabia	67.3	68.7	65.8	0.96		67.8	71.8	63.6	0.88		27.7	22.2	33.4	1.50	
	Syrian Arab Republic	122.9	126.2	119.5	0.95		63.2	65.5	60.9	0.93		..	..	..	..	
	Turkey	93.3	96.1	90.4	0.94	**	79.2	90.5	67.6	0.75	**	29.0	33.5	24.3	0.73	**

Annex table 4. Gross primary, secondary and tertiary enrolment ratios, 2004

Region and subregion	Country	Primary Total	Primary Male	Primary Female	Primary Female/male ratio*	Primary Note	Secondary Total	Secondary Male	Secondary Female	Secondary Female/male ratio*	Secondary Note	Tertiary Total	Tertiary Male	Tertiary Female	Tertiary Female/male ratio*	Tertiary Note
Western Asia (cont'd)	United Arab Emirates	83.8	85.1	82.3	0.97		66.4	64.7	68.4	1.06		22.5	12.2	39.5	3.24	**,-1
	Yemen	87.5	102.1	72.2	0.71		47.8	64.2	30.5	0.48		9.4	13.5	5.1	0.38	
EUROPE																
Eastern Europe	Belarus	101.2	102.9	99.4	0.97		93.5	93.0	94.0	1.01		60.5	50.8	70.7	1.39	
	Bulgaria	104.8	105.7	103.8	0.98		102.1	104.3	99.8	0.96		41.1	38.1	44.3	1.16	
	Czech Republic	101.9	102.6	101.1	0.99		95.7	95.0	96.4	1.01		43.2	41.3	45.3	1.10	
	Hungary	97.9	98.6	97.2	0.99		96.5	96.8	96.2	0.99		59.6	49.9	69.8	1.40	
	Poland	98.9	99.1	98.6	0.99		96.7	96.2	97.3	1.01		61.0	50.8	71.6	1.41	
	Republic of Moldova	94.4	94.7	94.1	0.99	***	82.8	81.3	84.4	1.04	***	37.0	31.4	42.7	1.36	***
	Romania	106.5	107.4	105.6	0.98		85.1	84.6	85.6	1.01		40.2	35.6	45.0	1.26	
	Russian Federation	122.9	123.2	122.6	1.00		92.9	93.3	92.5	0.99		68.2	57.9	78.8	1.36	**
	Slovakia	99.1	99.7	98.3	0.99		94.2	93.6	94.9	1.01		36.1	32.5	39.8	1.23	
	Ukraine	94.8	94.9	94.6	1.00	***	92.9	93.8	91.9	0.98	***	65.5	59.8	71.4	1.19	***
Northern Europe	Denmark	101.0	100.9	101.0	1.00		124.2	121.5	127.1	1.05		73.9	61.3	86.8	1.42	
	Estonia	99.9	101.4	98.4	0.97		98.1	97.1	99.2	1.02		65.1	48.8	81.9	1.68	
	Faeroe Islands															
	Finland	100.5	100.9	100.1	0.99		109.4	106.9	112.1	1.05		89.5	81.6	97.8	1.20	
	Iceland	99.4	100.8	98.0	0.97		107.9	106.6	109.4	1.03		67.7	47.7	88.0	1.85	
	Ireland	106.5	107.1	105.8	0.99		111.6	107.5	115.9	1.08		58.5	51.4	66.0	1.28	
	Latvia	92.9	94.3	91.4	0.97		96.6	96.7	96.5	1.00		74.3	55.0	94.4	1.72	
	Lithuania	97.2	97.6	96.9	0.99		102.1	103.0	101.2	0.98		73.2	57.5	89.4	1.56	
	Norway	98.9	98.9	98.9	1.00		115.6	114.1	117.3	1.03		80.5	63.7	97.9	1.54	
	Sweden	99.1	99.2	99.0	1.00		102.6	100.7	104.6	1.04		83.7	66.1	102.3	1.55	
	United Kingdom	106.5	106.6	106.5	1.00		104.5	103.1	106.1	1.03		60.1	50.8	69.8	1.37	
Southern Europe	Albania	105.7	106.2	105.2	0.99		78.0	79.4	76.6	0.96		19.3	14.9	23.4	1.57	
	Andorra	101.4	102.4	100.4	0.98	**	81.3	79.9	82.7	1.03	**	9.4	9.4	9.4	1.00	**
	Bosnia and Herzegovina															
	Croatia	94.4	94.7	94.1	0.99	-1	88.2	87.5	88.9	1.02	-1	38.7	35.5	42.1	1.19	-1
	Gibraltar															
	Greece	101.6	102.1	101.0	0.99		96.3	96.0	96.6	1.01		79.4	73.3	86.0	1.17	
	Holy See					-1					-1					
	Italy	101.4	101.6	101.1	1.00		99.1	99.6	98.4	0.99		63.1	54.2	72.4	1.34	
	Malta	102.4	102.9	101.8	0.99		105.3	108.8	101.5	0.93		26.4	22.7	30.3	1.34	
	Portugal	116.2	118.8	113.5	0.96		96.7	92.0	101.6	1.11		56.6	48.9	64.6	1.32	
	San Marino															
	Serbia and Montenegro (former)															
	Slovenia	122.8	123.1	122.4	0.99		99.8	100.0	99.5	1.00		73.7	62.1	86.0	1.38	
	Spain	107.7	108.6	106.7	0.98		119.1	115.8	122.5	1.06		65.7	59.2	72.4	1.22	
	The former Yugoslav Republic of Macedonia	97.7	97.6	97.8	1.00		84.1	85.0	83.1	0.98		28.0	23.5	32.7	1.39	
Western Europe	Austria	105.9	105.9	105.9	1.00		100.9	103.6	98.1	0.95		49.8	45.6	54.1	1.19	
	Belgium	103.9	104.3	103.6	0.99		108.9	110.7	107.0	0.97		62.5	56.6	68.7	1.21	
	France	104.8	105.2	104.4	0.99		110.6	110.3	110.9	1.01		56.0	49.2	63.1	1.28	
	Germany	100.2	100.3	100.1	1.00		100.3	101.1	99.4	0.98						
	Liechtenstein	106.1	105.7	106.6	1.01	***	112.0	119.8	103.9	0.87	***	25.1	36.3	13.6	0.37	***
	Luxembourg	99.4	99.6	99.2	1.00		94.9	92.2	97.7	1.06		12.4	11.4	13.4	1.18	**
	Monaco															
	Netherlands	107.4	108.8	106.0	0.97		118.8	119.7	117.8	0.98		59.2	56.9	61.5	1.08	
	Switzerland	102.3	102.7	102.0	0.99		93.4	97.2	89.5	0.92		47.0	52.4	41.7	0.80	
LATIN AMERICA AND THE CARIBBEAN																
Caribbean	Anguilla	92.7	91.3	94.1	1.03	**	93.9	93.9	93.9	1.00	**					**
	Antigua and Barbuda															
	Aruba	114.5	117.4	111.5	0.95	***	98.4	97.3	99.5	1.02	***	28.6	22.8	34.4	1.51	***
	Bahamas	98.2	98.2	98.2	1.00	**	88.0	88.1	88.0	1.00	**					

Annex table 4. Gross primary, secondary and tertiary enrolment ratios, 2004

Region and subregion	Country	Primary					Secondary					Tertiary				
		Total	Male	Female	Female/male ratio*	Note	Total	Male	Female	Female/male ratio*	Note	Total	Male	Female	Female/male ratio*	Note
Caribbean (cont'd)	Barbados	107.0	107.8	106.3	0.99		110.1	109.4	110.7	1.01		:	:	:	:	:
	British Virgin Islands	107.7	110.1	105.2	0.96	***	95.7	92.9	98.5	1.06	***	:	:	:	:	***
	Cayman Islands	93.2	95.8	90.6	0.95	**	97.4	92.7	102.5	1.10	**	:	:	:	:	
	Cuba	100.4	103.0	97.7	0.95		92.5	92.2	92.9	1.01		53.6	53.7	53.4	1.00	
	Dominica	95.5	96.1	94.8	0.99	***	106.6	107.0	106.3	0.99	***	:	:	:	:	***
	Dominican Republic	112.0	114.7	109.1	0.95		68.4	61.5	75.6	1.23		32.9	25.0	41.0	1.64	**
	Grenada	91.7	93.8	89.6	0.96	***	100.7	96.4	105.1	1.09	***	:	:	:	:	***
	Guadeloupe	:	:	:	:		:	:	:	:		:	:	:	:	
	Haiti	:	:	:	:		:	:	:	:		:	:	:	:	
	Jamaica	95.3	95.2	95.5	1.00		88.1	87.3	89.0	1.02		19.0	11.5	26.3	2.29	**,-1
	Martinique	:	:	:	:		:	:	:	:		:	:	:	:	
	Montserrat	107.6	109.3	105.6	0.97	***	114.1	109.0	119.8	1.10	***	:	:	:	:	***
	Netherlands Antilles	125.8	127.1	124.4	0.98	**,-1	86.6	82.8	90.3	1.09	**,-1	23.6	19.0	28.2	1.49	-2
	Saint Kitts and Nevis	101.2	97.7	104.9	1.07	***	94.1	92.5	95.6	1.03	**	:	:	:	:	**
	Saint Lucia	105.6	107.9	103.2	0.96		81.3	76.6	86.1	1.12		1.2	0.6	1.8	2.85	-1
	Saint Vincent and the Grenadines	106.2	109.0	103.3	0.95		77.6	75.0	80.3	1.07	**	:	:	:	:	
	Trinidad and Tobago	102.3	103.8	100.6	0.97	***	83.8	81.2	86.5	1.07	***	11.9	10.5	13.3	1.26	***
	Turks and Caicos Islands	93.6	92.1	95.1	1.03	***	90.8	91.5	90.2	0.99	***	:	:	:	:	
	U. S. Virgin Islands	:	:	:	:		:	:	:	:		:	:	:	:	
Central America	Belize	124.1	125.5	122.6	0.98		85.3	83.6	87.1	1.04		2.6	1.5	3.7	2.43	
	Costa Rica	111.8	112.3	111.2	0.99		77.4	75.1	79.8	1.06		25.3	22.5	28.3	1.25	
	El Salvador	114.4	116.4	112.5	0.97		60.4	59.9	60.8	1.01	**	18.5	16.7	20.4	1.22	
	Guatemala	113.2	118.0	108.3	0.92		48.6	51.2	46.0	0.90		9.6	11.2	8.1	0.72	**,-1
	Honduras	113.0	113.1	112.8	1.00		65.5	58.5	72.7	1.24		16.4	13.4	19.6	1.46	**
	Mexico	109.2	110.2	108.1	0.98		79.7	77.1	82.4	1.07		23.4	23.6	23.2	0.98	
	Nicaragua	112.2	113.4	110.9	0.98		63.7	59.4	68.1	1.15		17.9	16.9	18.8	1.11	**,-1
	Panama	112.2	113.7	110.6	0.97		70.2	67.7	72.7	1.07		45.3	34.2	56.8	1.66	
South America	Argentina	112.2	112.6	111.8	0.99	-1	86.4	83.5	89.4	1.07	-1	63.9	51.0	77.0	1.51	-1
	Bolivia	113.5	113.8	113.2	0.99	**	88.5	89.8	87.1	0.97	**	40.6	:	:	:	
	Brazil	141.0	144.9	136.9	0.94	-1	102.0	97.0	107.3	1.11	-1	22.3	19.2	25.4	1.32	-1
	Chile	103.7	106.1	101.2	0.95		89.1	88.5	89.8	1.01		43.0	44.1	41.9	0.95	
	Colombia	111.3	111.9	110.6	0.99		74.5	70.7	78.5	1.11		26.9	25.8	28.0	1.09	
	Ecuador	116.9	117.0	116.7	1.00		61.1	61.0	61.1	1.00		:	:	:	:	
	Falkland Islands (Malvinas)	:	:	:	:		:	:	:	:		:	:	:	:	
	French Guiana	:	:	:	:		:	:	:	:		:	:	:	:	
	Guyana	129.5	133.9	124.9	0.93	**	89.9	91.6	94.8	1.03	**,-2	9.1	6.2	12.0	1.91	
	Paraguay	105.9	107.6	104.1	0.97	-1	62.9	62.4	63.3	1.01	-1	24.4	20.6	28.3	1.37	**,-1
	Peru	113.9	114.2	113.6	0.99		91.6	91.0	92.3	1.01		33.4	32.9	33.8	1.03	**
	Puerto Rico	:	:	:	:		:	:	:	:		:	:	:	:	
	Suriname	119.9	118.5	121.4	1.02	**,-1	73.2	62.8	84.1	1.34	**,-1	12.4	9.5	15.4	1.62	-2
	Uruguay	109.1	110.3	107.8	0.98	-1	108.0	100.4	115.8	1.15	-1	39.3	26.0	53.1	2.04	**,-1
	Venezuela	105.1	106.2	103.9	0.98		72.0	67.4	76.8	1.14		39.3	37.9	40.7	1.08	**,-1
NORTHERN AMERICA	Bermuda	102.8	99.8	105.9	1.06	***	89.0	84.4	93.5	1.11	***	61.2	56.0	66.2	1.18	**,-2
	Canada	100.2	100.4	100.0	1.00	**,-2	108.5	108.7	108.3	1.00	**,-2	60.2	51.2	69.7	1.36	-2
	Greenland	:	:	:	:		:	:	:	:		:	:	:	:	
	Saint-Pierre et Miquelon	:	:	:	:		:	:	:	:		:	:	:	:	
	United States of America	99.0	100.3	97.5	0.97		94.7	93.9	95.5	1.02		82.4	69.2	96.3	1.39	

Annex table 4. Gross primary, secondary and tertiary enrolment ratios, 2004

Region and subregion	Country	Primary					Secondary					Tertiary				
		Total	Male	Female	Female/male ratio*	Note	Total	Male	Female	Female/male ratio*	Note	Total	Male	Female	Female/male ratio*	Note
OCEANIA																
Melanesia	Australia	102.8	103.1	102.6	1.00		148.6	151.6	145.4	0.96		72.2	64.9	79.8	1.23	
	New Zealand	101.7	101.8	101.6	1.00		117.8	113.7	122.1	1.07		85.8	69.7	102.7	1.47	
	Fiji	106.0	107.2	104.7	0.98		87.7	84.9	90.6	1.07		15.3	13.9	16.7	1.20	
	New Caledonia	..	..	..	..		..	..	..	..		..	..	..	..	
	Papua New Guinea	75.4	80.1	70.4	0.88	**,-1	25.8	28.6	22.6	0.79	**,-1	..	..	..	..	
	Solomon Islands	95.1	97.9	92.2	0.94	**,-1	29.6	32.6	26.3	0.81	**,-1	..	..	..	..	
	Vanuatu	118.0	119.7	116.3	0.97		41.3	44.4	38.0	0.86		5.0	6.3	3.6	0.58	**
Micronesia	Guam	..	..	..	..		..	..	..	..		..	..	..	..	
	Kiribati	114.9	113.4	116.5	1.03	***	90.7	82.2	99.9	1.22	***	..	..	..	..	***
	Marshall Islands	112.7	115.9	109.4	0.94	**,-1	86.6	85.1	88.3	1.04	**,-1	17.0	14.8	19.1	1.30	**,-1
	Micronesia (Federated States of)	..	..	..	..		..	..	..	..		..	..	..	..	
	Nauru	83.7	83.9	83.4	0.99	**,-1	47.8	46.2	49.5	1.07	**,-1	..	..	..	..	***
	Palau	101.1	111.1	91.0	0.82	**	108.1	101.2	115.5	1.14	**	40.2	26.5	57.1	2.15	**,-2
Polynesia	American Samoa	..	..	..	..		..	..	..	..		..	..	..	..	
	Cook Islands	82.1	82.8	81.2	0.98	**,-1	63.9	63.3	64.6	1.02	**,-1	..	..	..	..	**
	French Polynesia	..	..	..	..		..	..	..	..		..	..	..	..	
	Niue	86.8	79.6	94.9	1.19	***	97.7	100.0	95.5	0.95	***	..	..	..	..	***
	Samoa	99.8	100.0	99.5	1.00		80.3	75.8	85.2	1.12		..	..	..	..	
	Tokelau	93.0	82.5	106.5	1.29	**,-1	100.5	107.5	93.8	0.87	**,-1	..	..	..	..	
	Tonga	114.7	117.5	111.7	0.95	***	97.8	94.1	101.8	1.08	**	6.1	4.6	7.7	1.67	**
	Tuvalu	98.5	95.1	102.2	1.07	***	..	..	..	..	***	..	..	..	..	***

Source: UNESCO Institute for Statistics.

Notes:
Two dots (..) indicate that data are not available or are not separately reported.

* A ratio of less than 1 means females are less likely to be enrolled.

** UNESCO Institute for Statistics estimation.

+/- n = Data refer to the school or financial year (or period) n years or periods in relation to the reference year or period.

*** National estimation.

Annex table 5. Net primary and secondary enrolment ratios, 2004

Region and subregion	Country	Note	Net enrolment ratios							
			Primary				Secondary			
			Total	Male	Female	Female/male ratio*	Total	Male	Female	Female/male ratio*
AFRICA										
Eastern Africa	Burundi		57.0	60.2	53.8	0.89	..	..	..	..
	Comoros									
	Djibouti	**,+1	32.2	35.9	28.5	0.79	18.7	22.1	15.4	0.70
	Eritrea	**,+1	46.0	49.6	42.4	0.86	25.6	30.9	20.4	0.66
	Ethiopia	**,+1	56.3	58.0	54.6	0.94	27.7	33.6	21.7	0.64
	Kenya		76.4	76.4	76.5	1.00	40.1	39.9	40.2	1.01
	Madagascar		88.8	88.8	88.7	1.00	..	..	..	..
	Malawi		95.3	93.1	97.6	1.05	24.7	26.6	22.9	0.86
	Mauritius	**,+1	94.5	93.6	95.4	1.02	82.5	82.3	82.7	1.01
	Mozambique		71.0	74.8	67.3	0.90	4.0	4.5	3.5	0.78
	Reunion									
	Rwanda		73.2	71.5	74.8	1.04	..	..	..	..
	Seychelles	***	96.4	96.0	96.9	1.01	93.1	90.0	96.4	1.07
	Somalia									
	Tanzania, United Republic of	+1	91.4	92.2	90.5	0.98	..	..	..	..
	Uganda		..	..	..	..	13.0	13.8	12.1	0.87
	Zambia		79.8	79.8	79.9	1.00	23.7	26.6	20.7	0.78
	Zimbabwe	-1	81.9	81.3	82.4	1.01	33.9	35.1	32.6	0.93
Middle Africa	Angola									
	Cameroon									
	Central African Republic									
	Chad	**,-1	56.9	67.8	45.9	0.68	10.8	16.2	5.3	0.33
	Congo									
	Congo, Democratic Republic of the									
	Equatorial Guinea	-2	85.3	92.2	78.4	0.85	..	..	..	..
	Gabon									
Northern Africa	Sao Tome and Principe		98.2	98.5	98.0	1.00	26.0	25.0	26.9	1.07
	Algeria	**	96.7	97.8	95.4	0.98	66.2	64.5	68.0	1.05
	Egypt		95.4	96.7	94.0	0.97	79.1	81.4	76.7	0.94
	Libyan Arab Jamahiriya									
	Morocco	-1	86.1	88.7	83.4	0.94	35.1	37.8	32.4	0.86
	Sudan									
	Tunisia		97.4	97.2	97.6	1.00	67.4	66.2	68.6	1.04
	Western Sahara									
Southern Africa	Botswana	**	82.1	80.9	83.3	1.03	60.9	57.9	64.0	1.10
	Lesotho		85.9	83.4	88.5	1.06	23.1	18.2	28.0	1.54
	Namibia	-1	73.7	70.9	76.5	1.08	37.5	31.9	43.1	1.35
	South Africa	-1	88.8	88.4	89.2	1.01	..	..	..	..
	Swaziland	-1	76.7	76.3	77.0	1.01	29.0	25.8	32.1	1.24

Education

Annex table 5. Net primary and secondary enrolment ratios, 2004

Region and subregion	Country	Note	Net enrolment ratios							
			Primary				Secondary			
			Total	Male	Female	Female/male ratio*	Total	Male	Female	Female/male ratio*
Western Africa	Benin		82.6	92.5	72.4	0.78	::	::	::	::
	Burkina Faso		40.5	45.6	35.3	0.77	9.5	11.3	7.7	0.68
	Cape Verde		91.8	92.2	91.4	0.99	55.0	51.9	58.0	1.12
	Côte d'Ivoire	***,-1	56.0	62.2	49.8	0.80	20.0	25.5	14.5	0.57
	Gambia	**	75.2	73.1	77.4	1.06	44.9	49.1	40.6	0.83
	Ghana	+1	65.0	65.3	64.7	0.99	37.0	39.0	35.0	0.90
	Guinea		63.8	69.0	58.2	0.84	21.2	27.8	14.1	0.51
	Guinea-Bissau		::	::	::	::	::	::	::	::
	Liberia		::	::	::	::	::	::	::	::
	Mali		46.5	50.1	42.7	0.85	::	::	::	::
	Mauritania		74.3	74.7	73.9	0.99	14.1	15.5	12.7	0.82
	Niger		39.2	45.7	32.4	0.71	6.8	8.1	5.4	0.68
	Nigeria	**	60.1	63.5	56.5	0.89	::	::	::	::
	Saint Helena		::	::	::	::	::	::	::	::
	Senegal		66.1	67.8	64.5	0.95	15.3	17.7	12.8	0.72
	Sierra Leone		::	::	::	::	::	::	::	::
	Togo		78.8	85.3	72.3	0.85	::	::	::	::
ASIA										
Eastern Asia	China		::	::	::	::	::	::	::	::
	Hong Kong, China SAR	***	93.0	95.6	90.4	0.95	77.7	78.7	76.7	0.97
	Japan		99.9	99.8	100.0	1.00	99.9	::	::	::
	Korea, Democratic People's Republic of		::	::	::	::	::	::	::	::
	Korea, Republic of	+1	99.4	99.6	99.1	1.00	90.4	90.3	90.6	1.00
	Macao, China SAR		89.2	90.5	87.8	0.97	76.8	73.8	80.0	1.08
	Mongolia		84.2	83.8	84.5	1.01	82.3	77.0	87.6	1.14
South-central Asia	Afghanistan		::	::	::	::	::	::	::	::
	Bangladesh	***	93.8	92.2	95.4	1.03	48.0	45.5	50.6	1.11
	Bhutan		::	::	::	::	::	::	::	::
	India	**	89.7	92.2	87.0	0.94	::	::	::	::
	Iran, Islamic Republic of		88.6	88.9	88.3	0.99	78.1	80.4	75.7	0.94
	Kazakhstan		92.6	93.3	92.0	0.99	92.1	92.6	91.6	0.99
	Kyrgyzstan		90.1	90.3	89.8	0.99	::	::	::	::
	Maldives	-2	89.7	89.3	90.0	1.01	51.3	47.8	55.0	1.15
	Nepal	***,-1	78.0	83.1	72.7	0.87	::	::	::	::
	Pakistan	***	66.2	76.3	55.5	0.73	21.8	25.1	18.3	0.73
	Sri Lanka	**	97.1	98.8	98.4	1.00	::	::	::	::
	Tajikistan		96.7	98.9	94.5	0.96	79.4	85.6	72.9	0.85
	Turkmenistan		::	::	::	::	::	::	::	::
	Uzbekistan		::	::	::	::	::	::	::	::
South-eastern Asia	Brunei Darussalam		::	::	::	::	::	::	::	::
	Cambodia		97.6	99.6	95.6	0.96	25.8	29.7	21.8	0.73
	Indonesia		94.3	95.3	93.3	0.98	56.9	57.1	56.7	0.99
	Lao People's Democratic Republic		84.4	86.9	81.7	0.94	37.1	40.2	34.0	0.85
	Malaysia	-1	93.2	93.3	93.1	1.00	75.5	70.5	80.7	1.14
	Myanmar	+1	90.2	89.4	91.0	1.02	37.2	37.5	37.0	0.98
	Philippines		94.0	93.0	95.0	1.02	61.1	55.7	66.7	1.20
	Singapore		::	::	::	::	::	::	::	::
	Thailand		::	::	::	::	::	::	::	::
	Timor-Leste		::	::	::	::	::	::	::	::
	Viet Nam	**,-2	92.9	::	::	::	64.8	::	::	::

Annex table 5. Net primary and secondary enrolment ratios, 2004

Region and subregion	Country	Note	Net enrolment ratios							
			Primary				Secondary			
			Total	Male	Female	Female/male ratio*	Total	Male	Female	Female/male ratio*
Western Asia	Armenia		93.7	92.1	95.5	1.04	88.7	87.5	90.0	1.03
	Azerbaijan		83.8	84.6	83.0	0.98	77.0	77.9	76.1	0.98
	Bahrain		96.8	96.3	97.3	1.01	89.9	87.1	92.9	1.07
	Cyprus	***	96.1	96.3	96.0	1.00	93.0	91.5	94.6	1.03
	Georgia		92.8	93.1	92.5	0.99	80.7	80.7	80.7	1.00
	Iraq		87.7	94.3	81.0	0.86	37.9	44.3	31.3	0.71
	Israel		97.6	97.3	97.9	1.01	89.1	88.9	89.2	1.00
	Jordan		91.1	90.4	92.0	1.02	81.1	80.5	81.8	1.02
	Kuwait	**	86.0	84.9	87.1	1.03	77.6	75.7	79.6	1.05
	Lebanon		93.2	93.6	92.7	0.99				
	Oman		77.9	77.2	78.5	1.02	74.7	74.4	75.0	1.01
	Palestinian Autonomous Territories		86.3	86.4	86.2	1.00	89.4	87.3	91.6	1.05
	Qatar		94.8	95.4	94.1	0.99	87.2	88.0	86.3	0.98
	Saudi Arabia	**	58.9	61.6	56.1	0.91	52.4	53.5	51.3	0.96
	Syrian Arab Republic	-2	94.5	97.0	91.9	0.95	58.1	60.1	56.1	0.93
	Turkey	**	89.3	91.8	86.8	0.95				
	United Arab Emirates		71.2	72.3	70.1	0.97	60.0	58.4	61.8	1.06
	Yemen	**	75.3	86.9	63.2	0.73				
EUROPE										
Eastern Europe	Belarus		89.9	91.5	88.3	0.97	87.3	86.8	87.8	1.01
	Bulgaria		95.1	95.5	94.8	0.99	88.5	89.5	87.4	0.98
	Czech Republic									
	Hungary		89.1	89.7	88.4	0.99	90.7	91.0	90.3	0.99
	Poland		97.3	97.2	97.5	1.00	90.0	88.6	91.5	1.03
	Republic of Moldova	***	86.2	86.4	85.9	0.99	77.2	75.6	78.8	1.04
	Romania		91.9	92.2	91.5	0.99	80.8	79.8	81.9	1.03
	Russian Federation	**	91.5	91.1	91.9	1.01				
	Slovakia									
	Ukraine		82.1	82.2	82.0	1.00	83.5	83.4	83.7	1.00
Northern Europe	Denmark		98.0	97.5	98.5	1.01	91.7	90.3	93.1	1.03
	Estonia		94.1	94.2	94.1	1.00	89.7	88.5	90.9	1.03
	Faeroe Islands									
	Finland		99.3	99.4	99.2	1.00	94.0	93.7	94.3	1.01
	Iceland		98.6	99.9	97.2	0.97	87.9	86.7	89.2	1.03
	Ireland		96.4	96.4	96.4	1.00	86.5	84.0	89.2	1.06
	Latvia									
	Lithuania		89.4	89.6	89.2	1.00	93.5	93.3	93.7	1.00
	Norway		98.9	98.9	98.9	1.00	96.3	95.8	96.9	1.01
	Sweden		98.6	98.8	98.5	1.00	98.4	96.9	100.0	1.03
	United Kingdom		98.7	98.7	98.7	1.00	94.9	93.4	96.6	1.03
Southern Europe	Albania	**	94.0	94.0	94.0	1.00	74.1	75.0	73.2	0.98
	Andorra		88.5	89.8	87.1	0.97	71.4	71.0	71.8	1.01
	Bosnia and Herzegovina									
	Croatia	-1	87.3	87.8	86.8	0.99	85.0	84.3	85.8	1.02
	Gibraltar									
	Greece		99.4	99.7	98.9	0.99	86.5	84.8	88.4	1.04
	Holy See									
	Italy		98.8	99.0	98.7	1.00	92.4	91.7	93.1	1.02
	Malta	**	94.0	94.2	93.8	1.00	87.6	85.0	90.3	1.06
	Portugal		98.5	98.7	98.2	0.99	82.3	78.2	86.5	1.11

Annex table 5. Net primary and secondary enrolment ratios, 2004

Region and subregion	Country	Note	Primary Total	Primary Male	Primary Female	Primary Female/male ratio*	Secondary Total	Secondary Male	Secondary Female	Secondary Female/male ratio*
Southern Europe (cont'd)	San Marino		..	..	..	..	..	..	..	..
	Serbia and Montenegro (former)		..	..	..	..	..	..	..	..
	Slovenia		97.8	97.9	97.6	1.00	94.7	94.5	94.9	1.00
	Spain		99.4	99.7	99.1	0.99	96.7	94.7	98.7	1.04
	The former Yugoslav Rep. of Macedonia		92.0	92.1	91.9	1.00	81.1	82.2	80.0	0.97
Western Europe	Austria		..	..	..	..	..	..	..	..
	Belgium		98.8	98.7	98.8	1.00	97.0	96.9	97.2	1.00
	France		98.9	98.8	99.1	1.00	96.2	95.3	97.0	1.02
	Germany		..	..	..	..	..	..	..	..
	Liechtenstein	***	88.2	87.0	89.4	1.03	65.2	62.0	68.6	1.11
	Luxembourg		90.9	90.7	91.0	1.00	79.2	76.5	82.1	1.07
	Monaco		..	..	..	..	..	..	..	..
	Netherlands		98.7	99.4	98.0	0.99	89.2	88.7	89.6	1.01
	Switzerland		93.9	94.1	93.7	1.00	83.1	86.2	79.9	0.93
LATIN AMERICA AND THE CARIBBEAN										
Caribbean	Anguilla	**	88.3	87.2	89.4	1.02	87.0	87.5	86.5	0.99
	Antigua and Barbuda		..	..	..	..	..	..	..	..
	Aruba	***	96.6	96.9	96.2	0.99	74.3	73.5	75.2	1.02
	Bahamas	**	88.7	87.6	89.9	1.03	81.2	80.2	82.1	1.02
	Barbados		97.2	97.6	96.8	0.99	95.1	92.7	97.6	1.05
	British Virgin Islands	**	94.7	94.7	94.6	1.00	79.5	75.4	83.5	1.11
	Cayman Islands	**	87.2	89.3	85.2	0.95	90.9	86.5	95.6	1.10
	Cuba		96.2	97.5	94.8	0.97	86.6	85.8	87.4	1.02
	Dominica	***	87.7	87.1	88.3	1.01	90.4	88.9	91.8	1.03
	Dominican Republic		86.0	85.3	86.8	1.02	49.3	44.6	54.1	1.21
	Grenada	***	83.9	84.2	83.6	0.99	78.2	74.7	81.8	1.10
	Guadeloupe		..	..	..	..	..	..	..	..
	Haiti		..	..	..	..	..	..	..	..
	Jamaica		90.6	90.2	91.1	1.01	79.2	77.9	80.6	1.03
	Martinique		..	..	..	..	..	..	..	..
	Montserrat	***	94.3	96.0	92.1	0.96	100.0	92.0	97.7	1.06
	Netherlands Antilles						76.9	73.3	80.6	1.10
	Saint Kitts and Nevis	***	94.3	90.8	97.9	1.08	86.8	85.6	88.0	1.03
	Saint Lucia		97.6	99.0	96.1	0.97	71.1	67.9	74.3	1.09
	Saint Vincent and the Grenadines	**	93.9	95.4	92.5	0.97	62.3	59.6	64.9	1.09
	Trinidad and Tobago	***	92.2	92.4	91.9	0.99	71.9	70.0	73.9	1.05
	Turks and Caicos Islands	***	81.5	78.2	84.7	1.08	77.7	77.7	77.6	1.00
	U. S. Virgin Islands		..	..	..	..	..	..	..	..
Central America	Belize		95.2	94.6	95.9	1.01	71.4	69.8	73.1	1.05
	Costa Rica		..	..	..	..	..	..	..	..
	El Salvador	**	92.3	92.1	92.5	1.00	48.1	47.4	48.7	1.03
	Guatemala		93.0	95.4	90.5	0.95	33.7	35.1	32.4	0.92
	Honduras		90.6	89.7	91.5	1.02				
	Mexico		97.8	97.8	97.8	1.00	63.8	62.7	64.8	1.03
	Nicaragua		87.9	88.5	87.4	0.99	40.7	38.3	43.3	1.13
	Panama		98.2	98.5	98.0	1.00	63.7	60.8	66.7	1.10

Annex table 5. Net primary and secondary enrolment ratios, 2004

| Region and subregion | Country | Note | Net enrolment ratios | | | | | | | | | | | |
| | | | Primary | | | | Secondary | | | | |
			Total	Male	Female	Female/male ratio*	Total	Male	Female	Female/male ratio*
South America	Argentina	-1	98.8	99.2	98.4	0.99	79.1	76.3	81.9	1.07
	Bolivia	**	95.2	94.8	95.7	1.01	73.6	74.1	73.1	0.99
	Brazil	-1	92.9	..	..	..	75.7	73.3	78.1	1.07
	Chile		..	..	..	..	..	..	..	..
	Colombia		83.2	82.7	83.7	1.01	54.9	52.1	57.9	1.11
	Ecuador	**	97.7	97.2	98.2	1.01	52.2	51.8	52.5	1.01
	Falkland Islands (Malvinas)		..	..	..	..	..	..	..	..
	French Guiana		..	..	..	..	..	..	..	..
	Guyana	**,-2	93.3	94.2	92.5	0.98	..	..	..	..
	Paraguay		..	..	..	..	..	..	..	..
	Peru		97.1	96.9	97.2	1.00	68.8	69.0	68.7	1.00
	Puerto Rico		..	..	..	..	..	..	..	..
	Suriname	**,-1	92.4	89.6	95.5	1.07	63.2	53.2	73.5	1.38
	Uruguay		..	..	..	..	..	..	..	..
	Venezuela		92.0	91.8	92.3	1.01	61.2	56.9	65.7	1.15
NORTHERN AMERICA	Bermuda		..	..	..	..	..	..	..	..
	Canada		..	..	..	..	..	..	..	..
	Greenland		..	..	..	..	..	..	..	..
	Saint-Pierre et Miquelon		..	..	..	..	..	..	..	..
	United States of America		92.4	94.3	90.5	0.96	89.3	88.1	90.6	1.03
OCEANIA	Australia		95.8	95.5	96.0	1.00	85.5	84.9	86.1	1.01
	New Zealand		99.3	99.3	99.2	1.00	91.1	89.5	92.7	1.04
Melanesia	Fiji		96.2	96.7	95.8	0.99	82.6	80.1	85.3	1.06
	New Caledonia		..	..	..	..	..	..	..	..
	Papua New Guinea		..	..	..	..	..	..	..	..
	Solomon Islands	**,-1	63.4	64.6	62.0	0.96	26.4	28.4	24.3	0.86
	Vanuatu		93.9	94.7	93.0	0.98	39.3	42.1	36.2	0.86
Micronesia	Guam		..	..	..	..	..	..	..	..
	Kiribati		..	..	..	..	70.4	64.9	76.5	1.18
	Marshall Islands	**,-1	89.6	89.9	89.3	0.99	74.4	72.3	76.5	1.06
	Micronesia, Federated States of		..	..	..	..	..	..	..	..
	Nauru		..	..	..	..	..	..	..	..
	Palau		..	..	..	..	..	..	..	..
Polynesia	American Samoa		..	..	..	..	..	..	..	..
	Cook Islands		..	..	..	..	..	..	..	..
	French Polynesia		..	..	..	..	..	..	..	..
	Niue		..	..	..	..	..	..	..	..
	Samoa	**	90.4	90.3	90.6	1.00	65.7	61.7	70.1	1.14
	Tokelau		..	..	..	..	..	..	..	..
	Tonga		..	..	..	..	67.7	61.2	75.0	1.23
	Tuvalu		..	..	..	..	..	..	..	..

Source: UNESCO Institute for Statistics.

Notes:

Two dots (..) indicate that data are not available or are not separately reported.

* A ratio of less than 1 means females are less likely to be enrolled than males.

** UNESCO Institute for Statistics estimation.

+/- n = Data refer to the school or financial year (or period) n years or periods in relation to the reference year or period.

*** National estimation.

Annex table 6. Primary to secondary school transition rates (most recent data available)

The number of pupils admitted to the first grade of secondary education in specified year, expressed as a percentage of the number of pupils enrolled in the final grade of primary education in the previous year, by region, country and sex							Female/male ratio*
Region and subregion	Country	Year	Note	Total	Male	Female	
AFRICA							
Eastern Africa	Burundi	2003		34.3	35.4	32.9	0.93
	Comoros	2003		66.7	71.6	60.7	0.85
	Djibouti	2003	**	59.2	60.4	57.5	0.95
	Eritrea	2004	**	80.6	80.5	80.7	1.00
	Ethiopia	2004		84.6	84.3	84.9	1.01
	Kenya	..		..	..	..	..
	Madagascar	2003		55.4	55.8	54.9	0.98
	Malawi	2001		76.0	78.5	73.2	0.93
	Mauritius	2004	**	66.5	61.0	72.4	1.19
	Mozambique	2001		44.5	43.3	46.4	1.07
	Reunion	..		..	..	..	..
	Rwanda	..		..	..	..	..
	Seychelles	2003		94.9	92.5	97.3	1.05
	Somalia	..		..	..	..	..
	Uganda	2003	**	36.2	36.1	36.4	1.01
	Tanzania, United Republic of	2004	**	33.2	33.6	32.8	0.98
	Zambia	2001	**	54.0	51.5	57.2	1.11
	Zimbabwe	2002	**	69.7	69.3	70.2	1.01
Middle Africa	Angola	..		..	..	..	..
	Cameroon	2003		48.0	46.9	49.4	1.05
	Central African Republic	..		..	..	..	..
	Chad	2003	**	55.5	59.7	46.4	0.78
	Congo	2003		78.2	78.5	77.9	0.99
	Democratic Republic of the Congo	..		..	..	..	..
	Equatorial Guinea	..		..	..	..	..
	Gabon	..		..	..	..	..
	Sao Tome and Principe	2003		55.2	57.2	53.2	0.93
Northern Africa	Algeria	2003		78.8	75.5	82.6	1.09
	Egypt	2003	**	86.1	83.2	89.4	1.08
	Libyan Arab Jamahiriya	..		..	..	..	..
	Morocco	2003		78.7	78.1	79.4	1.02
	Sudan	2003		89.8	88.0	91.8	1.04
	Tunisia	2003		88.0	85.7	90.4	1.05
	Western Sahara	..		..	..	..	..
Southern Africa	Botswana	2003	**	98.8	99.7	97.9	0.98
	Lesotho	2003		62.7	63.6	62.1	0.98
	Namibia	2002	**	87.9	87.4	88.5	1.01
	South Africa	2002		95.2	94.4	96.1	1.02
	Swaziland	2002		77.1	76.0	78.3	1.03
Western Africa	Benin	2002		51.1	51.1	51.0	1.00
	Burkina Faso	2003	**	39.8	41.6	37.5	0.90
	Cape Verde	2003		72.4	68.9	75.9	1.10
	Côte d'Ivoire	2001		39.7	41.9	36.3	0.87
	Gambia	1999	**	82.3	83.3	81.1	0.97
	Ghana	2004	**	97.3	95.1	100.0	1.05
	Guinea	2003		67.9	72.8	59.8	0.82
	Guinea-Bissau	2000	**	63.2	66.0	58.5	0.89
	Liberia	..		..	..	..	..
	Mali	2003		59.7	61.6	56.7	0.92
	Mauritania	2003		45.3	46.9	43.7	0.93
	Niger	2003		49.5	50.7	47.6	0.94
	Nigeria	..		..	..	..	..
	Saint Helena	..		..	..	..	..
	Senegal	2003		47.1	48.8	44.9	0.92
	Sierra Leone	..		..	..	..	..
	Togo	2003		64.4	67.0	60.7	0.91
ASIA							
Eastern Asia	China	..		..	..	..	..
	Hong Kong, China SAR	2003		99.8	99.8	99.7	1.00
	Japan			..	..	..	..
	Korea, Democratic People's Republic of	..		..	..	..	..
	Korea, Republic of	2004		98.7	99.1	98.2	0.99
	Macao, China SAR	2003		92.1	89.1	95.3	1.07
	Mongolia	2003		99.0	99.2	98.9	1.00
South-central Asia	Afghanistan	..		..	..	..	..
	Bangladesh	2002		95.4	91.8	98.9	1.08
	Bhutan	2000		82.5	82.3	82.6	1.00
	India	2003		85.1	87.5	82.2	0.94
	Iran, Islamic Republic of	2003		98.7	97.6	100.0	1.02
	Kazakhstan	2003		99.8	100.0	99.5	1.00
	Kyrgyzstan	2003		99.0	98.0	100.0	1.02
	Maldives	2002	**	60.2	54.5	66.0	1.21
	Nepal	2003	**	75.8	78.0	73.0	0.94

The number of pupils admitted to the first grade of secondary education in specified year, expressed as a percentage of the number of pupils enrolled in the final grade of primary education in the previous year, by region, country and sex							Female/male ratio*
Region and subregion	**Country**	**Year**	**Note**	**Total**	**Male**	**Female**	
South-central Asia (cont'd)	Pakistan	2004		69.0	67.0	72.0	1.07
	Sri Lanka	2002	**	97.0	96.4	97.7	1.01
	Tajikistan	2003	**	97.9	98.3	97.5	0.99
	Turkmenistan	..		..	..	..	..
	Uzbekistan	2002	**	99.6	100.0	99.2	0.99
South-eastern Asia	Brunei Darussalam	2003	**	89.4	86.7	92.7	1.07
	Cambodia	2003		83.0	85.3	80.3	0.94
	Indonesia	2003		83.5	83.5	83.5	1.00
	Lao People's Democratic Republic	2003		77.9	79.9	75.5	0.95
	Malaysia	2000		99.7	100.0	99.5	0.99
	Myanmar	2004	**	71.7	72.3	71.0	0.98
	Philippines	2003		96.6	97.1	96.1	0.99
	Singapore	..		..	..	..	..
	Thailand	..		..	..	..	..
	Timor-Leste	..		..	..	..	..
	Viet Nam	2002	**	99.7	99.4	100.0	1.01
Western Asia	Armenia	2003	**	98.8	97.7	100.0	1.02
	Azerbaijan	2003		99.0	98.8	99.2	1.00
	Bahrain	2003		97.3	95.5	99.2	1.04
	Cyprus	2003		99.8	99.6	100.0	1.00
	Georgia	2002		98.3	98.1	98.5	1.00
	Iraq	1999	**	72.6	78.9	64.2	0.81
	Israel	2003		74.1	74.1	74.1	1.00
	Jordan	2003		97.0	97.3	96.7	0.99
	Kuwait	2003	**	95.1	95.5	94.7	0.99
	Lebanon	2003		85.8	82.8	88.8	1.07
	Oman	2003		99.4	99.4	99.3	1.00
	Palestinian Autonomous Territories	2003		99.9	100.0	99.8	1.00
	Qatar	2000	**	95.5	91.4	100.0	1.09
	Saudi Arabia	2003		96.7	100.0	93.2	0.93
	Syrian Arab Republic	2003		93.8	92.8	94.8	1.02
	Turkey	2003	**	91.1	93.3	88.5	0.95
	United Arab Emirates	2003		96.3	96.4	96.3	1.00
	Yemen	..		..	..	..	..
EUROPE							
Eastern Europe	Belarus	2003		98.8	100.0	97.5	0.97
	Bulgaria	2003		95.7	95.6	95.7	1.00
	Czech Republic	2003		99.2	99.0	99.4	1.00
	Hungary	2003	**	98.6	98.1	99.0	1.01
	Poland	2003	**	98.5			
	Republic of Moldova	2003		98.1	97.2	99.1	1.02
	Romania	2003		98.2	98.0	98.3	1.00
	Russian Federation	..		..	..	..	..
	Slovakia	2003		98.2	98.0	98.5	1.01
	Ukraine	2001	**	99.4	98.9	100.0	1.01
Northern Europe	Denmark	2001		100.0	100.0	99.9	1.00
	Estonia	2003		96.3	94.3	98.6	1.05
	Faeroe Islands	..		..	..	..	..
	Finland	2003		99.9	99.8	100.0	1.00
	Iceland	2002		99.6	99.2	100.0	1.01
	Ireland	2002		100.0	..	..	..
	Latvia	2003		98.0	97.3	98.6	1.01
	Lithuania	2003		99.0	98.9	99.1	1.00
	Norway	2003		99.8	99.6	100.0	1.00
	Sweden	..		..	..	..	..
	United Kingdom	..		..	..	..	..
Southern Europe	Albania	2002	**	98.8	97.8	100.0	1.02
	Andorra	2003		95.5	95.2	95.9	1.01
	Bosnia and Herzegovina	..		..	..	..	..
	Croatia	2002		99.9	99.8	100.0	1.00
	Gibraltar	..		..	..	..	..
	Greece	..		..	..	..	..
	Holy See	..		..	..	..	..
	Italy	2003		99.7	100.0	99.3	0.99
	Malta	2003		97.0	94.3	100.0	1.06
	Portugal	..		..	..	..	..
	San Marino	..		..	..	..	..
	Serbia and Montenegro (former)	..		..	..	..	..
	Slovenia	2002	**	99.4	100.0	98.7	0.99
	Spain	..		..	..	..	..
	The former Yugoslav Republic of Macedonia	2003		98.3	98.8	97.8	0.99
Western Europe	Austria	..		..	..	..	..
	Belgium	..		..	..	..	..
	France	1999	**	98.7	99.1	98.3	0.99

Annex table 6. Primary to secondary school transition rates (most recent data available)

The number of pupils admitted to the first grade of secondary education in specified year, expressed as a percentage of the number of pupils enrolled in the final grade of primary education in the previous year, by region, country and sex							Female/male ratio*
Region and subregion	Country	Year	Note	Total	Male	Female	
Western Europe (cont'd)	Germany	2003		98.7	98.8	98.6	1.00
	Liechtenstein	2003		100.0	..	..	..
	Luxembourg	..		..	..	..	..
	Monaco	..		..	..	..	..
	Netherlands	2003	**	98.1	96.4	100.0	1.04
	Switzerland	2003		99.9	99.8	100.0	1.00
LATIN AMERICA AND THE CARIBBEAN							
Caribbean	Anguilla	2003		100.0	..	..	..
	Antigua and Barbuda	..		..	..	..	..
	Aruba	2003		99.2	98.4	100.0	1.02
	Bahamas	2003	**	95.0	96.5	93.6	0.97
	Barbados	2003		98.1	96.3	100.0	1.04
	British Virgin Islands	2001	**	69.0	62.2	76.2	1.22
	Cayman Islands	2001		90.8	89.0	92.9	1.04
	Cuba	2003		98.5	98.0	99.0	1.01
	Dominica	2002		93.6	93.6	93.6	1.00
	Dominican Republic	2003	**	87.4	87.5	87.4	1.00
	Grenada	2000	**	75.0	56.6	97.1	1.72
	Guadeloupe	..		..	..	..	..
	Haiti	..		..	..	..	..
	Jamaica	2000		94.4	96.5	92.4	0.96
	Martinique			..	..	..	..
	Montserrat	..		..	..	..	..
	Netherlands Antilles	1999	**	48.3	43.8	52.5	1.20
	Puerto Rico	..		..	..	..	..
	Saint Kitts and Nevis	2000		100.0	..	..	..
	Saint Lucia	2003	**	68.8	62.5	75.6	1.21
	Saint Vincent and the Grenadines	2003		73.7	68.4	78.5	1.15
	Trinidad and Tobago	2003	***	97.5	96.5	98.5	1.02
	Turks and Caicos Islands	2002		71.6	72.0	71.1	0.99
	U. S. Virgin Islands	..		..	..	..	..
Central America	Belize	2003		87.0	84.6	89.4	1.06
	Costa Rica	2002	**	91.6	91.7	91.4	1.00
	El Salvador	2003	**	94.1	94.2	94.1	1.00
	Guatemala	2003	**	96.1	97.1	95.0	0.98
	Honduras	..		..	..	..	..
	Mexico	2003		93.6	94.8	92.4	0.98
	Nicaragua	1999		99.2	100.0	98.3	0.98
	Panama	2003	**	64.1	63.3	65.0	1.03
South America	Argentina	2002		92.8	91.7	93.8	1.02
	Bolivia	2003	**	91.4	92.1	90.7	0.99
	Brazil	2000	**	84.0			
	Chile	2003		96.5	95.3	97.8	1.03
	Colombia	2003	**	99.8	99.5	100.0	1.00
	Ecuador	2003		73.6	76.0	71.2	0.94
	Falkland Islands (Malvinas)	..		..	..	..	..
	French Guiana	..		..	..	..	..
	Guyana	1999		67.6	64.7	70.7	1.09
	Paraguay	2002		90.8	90.9	90.6	1.00
	Peru	2003		94.9	95.8	94.0	0.98
	Suriname	2002	**	12.5	15.2	10.0	0.66
	Uruguay	2002		81.5	75.6	87.5	1.16
	Venezuela	2003		98.2	96.7	99.6	1.03
NORTHERN AMERICA							
	Bermuda	2001		100.0			
	Canada	..		..	..	..	..
	Greenland	..		..	..	..	..
	Saint-Pierre et Miquelon	..		..	..	..	..
	United States of America	..		..	..	..	..
OCEANIA							
	Australia	2002	**	99.9	99.9	99.8	1.00
	New Zealand	..		..	..	..	..
Melanesia	Fiji	2003		99.5	100.0	98.9	0.99
	New Caledonia	..		..	..	..	..
	Papua New Guinea	2002	**	76.8	77.0	76.5	0.99
	Solomon Islands	2002	**	69.8	71.4	67.9	0.95
	Vanuatu	2003	**	51.4	49.5	53.4	1.08
Micronesia	Guam	..		..	..	..	..
	Kiribati	..		..	..	..	..
	Marshall Islands	..		..	..	..	..
	Micronesia, Federated States of	..		..	..	..	..
	Nauru	2001		81.9	75.4	89.0	1.18
	Palau	..		..	..	..	..

Annex table 6. Primary to secondary school transition rates (most recent data available)

The number of pupils admitted to the first grade of secondary education in specified year, expressed as a percentage of the number of pupils enrolled in the final grade of primary education in the previous year, by region, country and sex							Female/male ratio*
Region and subregion	Country	Year	Note	Total	Male	Female	
Polynesia	American Samoa	..		..	..	..	..
	Cook Islands	..		..	..	..	..
	French Polynesia	..		..	..	..	..
	Niue	..		..	..	..	..
	Samoa	2003	**	96.3	95.3	97.4	1.02
	Tokelau	2002		87.5	91.7	82.1	0.90
	Tonga	2003	**	76.5	74.6	78.7	1.05
	Tuvalu	2001		69.3	84.6	53.4	0.63

Source: UNESCO Institute for Statistics.

Notes:

Two dots (..) indicate that data are not available or are not separately reported.

* A ratio of less than 1 means that girls are less likely to make the transition from primary to secondary school than boys.

** UIS estimation.

*** National estimation.

Annex table 7. Youth labour force participation rates, 2005

Region and subregion	Country	Percentage of youth in the labour force								Age transition in LFPR*		
		15-19 years				20-24 years						
		Total	Female	Male	Female/male LFPR**	Total	Female	Male	Female/male LFPR**	Total	Female	Male
AFRICA												
Eastern Africa	Burundi	81.7	83.9	79.5	1.1	94.3	94.1	94.6	1.0	1.2	1.1	1.2
	Comoros	47.9	44.6	51.2	0.9	73.2	56.8	89.4	0.6	1.5	1.3	1.7
	Djibouti	41.6	34.4	48.7	0.7	70.1	54.8	85.1	0.6	1.7	1.6	1.7
	Eritrea	59.3	50.4	68.2	0.7	79.6	66.0	93.5	0.7	1.3	1.3	1.4
	Ethiopia	70.9	68.0	73.7	0.9	84.2	77.1	91.4	0.8	1.2	1.1	1.2
	Kenya	62.0	56.8	67.1	0.8	80.1	66.3	93.9	0.7	1.3	1.2	1.4
	Madagascar	59.8	61.6	58.0	1.1	78.3	75.5	81.1	0.9	1.3	1.2	1.4
	Malawi	73.7	76.4	71.0	1.1	87.8	84.9	90.7	0.9	1.2	1.1	1.3
	Mauritius	25.7	18.6	32.6	0.6	66.6	49.9	82.9	0.6	2.6	2.7	2.5
	Mozambique	52.7	62.2	43.1	1.4	84.6	85.1	84.1	1.0	1.6	1.4	2.0
	Réunion	6.8	6.1	7.4	0.8	52.9	42.7	63.0	0.7	7.8	7.0	8.5
	Rwanda	60.9	61.5	60.3	1.0	83.8	80.1	87.7	0.9	1.4	1.3	1.5
	Somalia	70.0	60.6	79.4	0.8	85.1	72.3	97.9	0.7	1.2	1.2	1.2
	Tanzania, United Republic of	71.1	71.8	70.5	1.0	91.8	91.2	92.3	1.0	1.3	1.3	1.3
	Uganda	71.8	70.3	73.2	1.0	80.5	75.4	85.6	0.9	1.1	1.1	1.2
	Zambia	70.2	65.7	74.6	0.9	84.9	75.7	94.1	0.8	1.2	1.2	1.3
	Zimbabwe	45.5	35.4	55.7	0.6	75.8	62.0	89.7	0.7	1.7	1.8	1.6
Middle Africa	Angola	76.6	70.1	83.1	0.8	82.5	75.3	89.8	0.8	1.1	1.1	1.1
	Cameroon	37.5	34.2	40.8	0.8	69.3	53.8	84.7	0.6	1.8	1.6	2.1
	Central African Republic	64.1	60.8	67.4	0.9	77.4	65.9	89.3	0.7	1.2	1.1	1.3
	Chad	49.8	53.5	46.0	1.2	63.6	62.5	64.7	1.0	1.3	1.2	1.4
	Congo	52.1	46.7	57.6	0.8	66.0	49.0	83.1	0.6	1.3	1.0	1.4
	Congo, Democratic Republic of	64.0	55.6	72.4	0.8	81.0	69.0	93.0	0.7	1.3	1.2	1.3
	Equatorial Guinea	65.3	47.8	82.8	0.6	72.7	49.9	95.7	0.5	1.1	1.0	1.2
	Gabon	49.5	48.9	50.1	1.0	73.9	61.2	86.6	0.7	1.5	1.3	1.7
	Sao Tome and Principe	16.0	10.5	21.4	0.5	58.1	28.0	87.7	0.3	3.6	2.7	4.1
Northern Africa	Algeria	32.5	13.6	50.7	0.3	63.8	45.3	81.7	0.6	2.0	3.3	1.6
	Egypt	16.2	9.0	23.2	0.4	44.1	27.3	60.7	0.4	2.7	3.0	2.6
	Libyan Arab Jamahiriya	24.9	12.9	36.4	0.4	53.6	26.1	80.2	0.3	2.2	2.0	2.2
	Morocco	34.1	17.4	50.2	0.3	52.1	27.0	76.6	0.4	1.5	1.6	1.5
	Sudan	23.3	15.8	30.5	0.5	43.1	22.0	63.7	0.3	1.9	1.4	2.1
	Tunisia	28.5	21.6	35.0	0.6	52.9	41.0	64.3	0.6	1.9	1.9	1.8
	Western Sahara	44.8	34.0	55.3	0.6	77.3	56.7	97.5	0.6	1.7	1.7	1.8
Southern Africa	Botswana	16.1	15.8	16.4	1.0	58.5	51.3	65.6	0.8	3.6	3.2	4.0
	Lesotho	29.8	25.1	34.5	0.7	64.1	47.7	81.5	0.6	2.2	1.9	2.4
	Namibia	19.0	18.3	19.7	0.9	50.7	45.9	55.4	0.8	2.7	2.5	2.8
	South Africa	34.0	32.7	35.3	0.9	65.9	51.5	80.1	0.6	1.9	1.6	2.3
	Swaziland	24.6	19.5	29.7	0.7	62.1	37.6	87.3	0.4	2.5	1.9	2.9

Labour Force Participation and Employment

Annex table 7. Youth labour force participation rates, 2005

Region and subregion	Country	Percentage of youth in the labour force								Age transition in LFPR*		
		15-19 years				20-24 years						
		Total	Female	Male	Female/male LFPR**	Total	Female	Male	Female/male LFPR**	Total	Female	Male
Western Africa	Benin	53.8	43.3	63.9	0.7	67.9	51.8	83.4	0.6	1.3	1.2	1.3
	Burkina Faso	74.2	71.1	77.3	0.9	81.1	75.7	86.3	0.9	1.1	1.1	1.1
	Cape Verde	32.4	25.3	39.5	0.6	61.7	37.3	86.2	0.4	1.9	1.5	2.2
	Côte d'Ivoire	46.2	32.5	59.9	0.5	66.7	39.2	94.2	0.4	1.4	1.2	1.6
	Gambia	54.2	48.8	59.5	0.8	72.1	57.6	86.7	0.7	1.3	1.2	1.5
	Ghana	35.0	35.5	34.6	1.0	68.2	67.5	68.8	1.0	1.9	1.9	2.0
	Guinea	69.8	69.3	70.3	1.0	82.8	78.9	86.4	0.9	1.2	1.1	1.2
	Guinea-Bissau	70.1	61.8	78.5	0.8	79.5	66.8	92.4	0.7	1.1	1.1	1.2
	Liberia	48.2	47.4	49.0	1.0	70.0	56.1	83.6	0.7	1.5	1.2	1.7
	Mali	67.4	65.7	69.0	1.0	75.8	70.9	80.6	0.9	1.1	1.1	1.2
	Mauritania	45.0	37.5	52.4	0.7	71.5	57.2	85.9	0.7	1.6	1.5	1.6
	Niger	77.9	66.2	88.9	0.7	83.3	71.0	94.8	0.7	1.1	1.1	1.1
	Nigeria	47.6	32.3	62.3	0.5	60.5	38.3	82.0	0.5	1.3	1.2	1.3
	Senegal	48.7	46.5	50.8	0.9	71.2	54.6	87.8	0.6	1.5	1.2	1.7
	Sierra Leone	67.5	57.4	77.7	0.7	81.1	65.0	97.4	0.7	1.2	1.1	1.3
	Togo	56.4	44.6	68.3	0.7	72.4	50.5	94.4	0.5	1.3	1.1	1.4
ASIA												
Eastern Asia	China	52.7	56.4	49.3	1.1	87.9	85.9	89.8	1.0	1.7	1.5	1.8
	Hong Kong, China SAR	15.4	14.9	15.9	0.9	71.3	71.8	70.8	1.0	4.6	4.8	4.5
	Japan	17.1	16.9	17.2	1.0	69.4	69.3	69.5	1.0	4.1	4.1	4.0
	Korea, Democratic People's Republic	13.9	11.6	16.1	0.7	61.3	56.2	66.3	0.8	4.4	4.8	4.1
	Korea, Republic of	9.7	10.6	8.8	1.2	62.5	66.0	59.1	1.1	6.5	6.2	6.7
	Macau, China SAR	8.8	10.6	7.1	1.5	73.7	79.1	68.0	1.2	8.4	7.5	9.6
	Mongolia	35.2	32.9	37.4	0.9	75.1	64.9	85.2	0.8	2.1	2.0	2.3
South-central Asia	Afghanistan	49.4	34.4	63.4	0.5	66.8	42.4	89.4	0.5	1.4	1.2	1.4
	Bangladesh	53.3	43.9	62.3	0.7	69.2	57.5	80.2	0.7	1.3	1.3	1.3
	Bhutan	33.5	28.3	38.5	0.7	67.3	54.0	80.2	0.7	2.0	1.9	2.1
	India	33.2	22.4	43.3	0.5	57.5	30.7	82.5	0.4	1.7	1.4	1.9
	Iran, Islamic Republic of	27.1	21.4	32.6	0.7	60.7	48.8	72.1	0.7	2.2	2.3	2.2
	Kazakhstan	30.4	28.9	31.8	0.9	74.7	69.9	79.5	0.9	2.5	2.4	2.5
	Kyrgyzstan	33.1	28.6	37.5	0.8	65.9	54.6	77.1	0.7	2.0	1.9	2.1
	Maldives	22.1	20.0	24.2	0.8	71.5	62.8	80.0	0.8	3.2	3.1	3.3
	Nepal	46.8	47.6	46.1	1.0	67.1	53.6	80.1	0.7	1.4	1.1	1.7
	Pakistan	38.2	17.0	58.2	0.3	59.1	29.5	86.7	0.3	1.5	1.7	1.5
	Sri Lanka	24.9	16.7	32.8	0.5	65.1	45.7	83.9	0.5	2.6	2.7	2.6
	Tajikistan	14.7	14.9	14.6	1.0	60.3	52.5	68.2	0.8	4.1	3.5	4.7
	Turkmenistan	24.9	23.4	26.3	0.9	71.4	64.4	78.4	0.8	2.9	2.8	3.0
	Uzbekistan	26.5	24.3	28.6	0.8	67.8	58.9	76.5	0.8	2.6	2.4	2.7
South-eastern Asia	Brunei Darussalam	16.2	11.5	20.6	0.6	67.6	53.4	81.7	0.7	4.2	4.6	4.0
	Cambodia	50.0	59.2	41.0	1.4	83.3	81.1	85.4	0.9	1.7	1.4	2.1
	East Timor	52.1	48.9	55.1	0.9	71.8	60.3	82.3	0.7	1.4	1.2	1.5
	Indonesia	37.5	31.2	43.7	0.7	68.2	49.1	87.0	0.6	1.8	1.6	2.0
	Lao People's Democratic Republic	43.1	40.3	45.8	0.9	71.2	60.4	81.8	0.7	1.7	1.5	1.8

Labour Force Participation and Employment

Annex table 7. Youth labour force participation rates, 2005

| Region and subregion | Country | Percentage of youth in the labour force | | | | | | | | Age transition in LFPR* | | |
| | | 15-19 years | | | | 20-24 years | | | | | | |
		Total	Female	Male	Female/male LFPR**	Total	Female	Male	Female/male LFPR**	Total	Female	Male
South-eastern Asia (cont'd)	Malaysia	25.5	20.7	30.1	0.7	74.6	62.9	85.7	0.7	2.9	3.0	2.8
	Myanmar	53.5	52.6	54.4	1.0	73.8	59.9	87.6	0.7	1.4	1.1	1.6
	Philippines	37.6	28.0	46.9	0.6	69.2	57.2	80.8	0.7	1.8	2.0	1.7
	Singapore	15.1	15.4	14.8	1.0	75.3	77.9	72.8	1.1	5.0	5.1	4.9
	Thailand	26.7	19.8	33.5	0.6	71.0	64.4	77.5	0.8	2.7	3.3	2.3
	Viet Nam	52.8	59.3	46.4	1.3	87.8	84.4	91.2	0.9	1.7	1.4	2.0
Western Asia	Armenia	10.5	11.9	9.2	1.3	39.6	38.9	40.3	1.0	3.8	3.3	4.4
	Azerbaijan	28.2	26.5	29.8	0.9	72.1	64.6	79.5	0.8	2.6	2.4	2.7
	Bahrain	16.1	7.8	23.9	0.3	63.3	37.0	88.2	0.4	3.9	4.7	3.7
	Cyprus	19.6	13.0	25.8	0.5	72.0	70.0	73.9	0.9	3.7	5.4	2.9
	Georgia	25.2	19.6	30.5	0.6	42.1	29.0	55.3	0.5	1.7	1.5	1.8
	Iraq	25.8	10.4	40.6	0.3	55.1	28.1	81.2	0.3	2.1	2.7	2.0
	Israel	12.0	12.3	11.8	1.0	50.7	56.9	44.8	1.3	4.2	4.6	3.8
	Jordan	19.7	7.1	31.7	0.2	61.3	41.2	80.3	0.5	3.1	5.8	2.5
	Kuwait	6.3	3.9	8.6	0.5	64.3	52.8	73.9	0.7	10.1	13.5	8.6
	Lebanon	24.4	11.1	37.3	0.3	53.6	26.6	80.0	0.3	2.2	2.4	2.1
	Oman	15.5	7.6	23.0	0.3	54.7	24.6	83.0	0.3	3.5	3.2	3.6
	Qatar	5.8	0.7	10.5	0.1	55.0	11.0	75.2	0.1	9.5	15.7	7.2
	Saudi Arabia	12.0	1.9	21.7	0.1	46.2	14.6	75.2	0.2	3.9	7.7	3.5
	Syrian Arab Republic	48.3	35.3	60.9	0.6	68.5	43.9	92.3	0.5	1.4	1.2	1.5
	Turkey	38.4	26.4	50.0	0.5	59.2	33.6	84.3	0.4	1.5	1.3	1.7
	United Arab Emirates	16.2	5.3	24.7	0.2	74.3	44.1	89.2	0.5	4.6	8.3	3.6
	West Bank and Gaza Strip	13.8	1.2	25.8	0.0	40.2	11.8	67.0	0.2	2.9	9.8	2.6
	Yemen	28.5	12.4	43.8	0.3	55.1	32.2	76.9	0.4	1.9	2.6	1.8
EUROPE												
Eastern Europe	Belarus	16.3	13.0	19.5	0.7	72.0	66.3	77.4	0.9	4.4	5.1	4.0
	Bulgaria	7.0	7.8	6.2	1.3	45.2	38.1	51.9	0.7	6.5	4.9	8.4
	Czech Republic	5.6	5.5	5.7	1.0	64.7	61.3	68.0	0.9	11.6	11.1	11.9
	Hungary	5.8	4.6	7.0	0.7	51.6	45.9	57.0	0.8	8.9	10.0	8.1
	Poland	8.0	6.6	9.4	0.7	55.5	51.2	59.7	0.9	6.9	7.8	6.4
	Republic of Moldova	19.5	18.6	20.3	0.9	68.3	66.7	69.8	1.0	3.5	3.6	3.4
	Romania	10.5	9.9	11.0	0.9	49.7	44.3	54.9	0.8	4.8	4.5	5.0
	Russian Federation	13.9	11.3	16.5	0.7	62.7	57.7	67.7	0.9	4.5	5.1	4.1
	Slovakia	11.6	11.8	11.4	1.0	68.6	62.1	74.9	0.8	5.9	5.3	6.6
	Ukraine	12.2	11.4	12.9	0.9	65.3	58.2	72.4	0.8	5.4	5.1	5.6
Northern Europe	Channel Islands	26.0	16.5	35.3	0.5	68.7	62.7	74.7	0.8	2.6	3.8	2.1
	Denmark	56.1	58.3	54.1	1.1	78.8	72.3	85.2	0.8	1.4	1.2	1.6
	Estonia	9.2	6.7	11.5	0.6	61.7	51.8	71.3	0.7	6.7	7.7	6.2
	Finland	33.7	37.0	30.5	1.2	69.9	68.7	71.0	1.0	2.1	1.9	2.3
	Iceland	60.9	64.2	57.8	1.1	80.8	77.1	84.4	0.9	1.3	1.2	1.5
	Ireland	29.8	25.8	33.7	0.8	71.2	65.1	77.1	0.8	2.4	2.5	2.3
	Latvia	10.8	8.0	13.4	0.6	63.1	55.6	70.4	0.8	5.9	6.9	5.3
	Lithuania	5.5	4.8	6.2	0.8	54.0	47.2	60.5	0.8	9.8	9.8	9.8
	Norway	55.5	56.0	55.0	1.0	76.3	72.0	80.4	0.9	1.4	1.3	1.5
	Sweden	36.4	40.5	32.6	1.2	65.9	61.7	69.8	0.9	1.8	1.5	2.1
	United Kingdom	59.8	59.2	60.3	1.0	74.0	68.9	79.0	0.9	1.2	1.2	1.3

Annex table 7. Youth labour force participation rates, 2005

| Region and subregion | Country | Percentage of youth in the labour force | | | | | | | | Age transition in LFPR* | | |
| | | 15-19 years | | | | 20-24 years | | | | | | |
		Total	Female	Male	Female/male LFPR**	Total	Female	Male	Female/male LFPR**	Total	Female	Male
Southern Europe	Albania	42.6	41.5	43.7	0.9	60.7	50.1	71.8	0.7	1.4	1.2	1.6
	Bosnia and Herzegovina	22.9	21.9	23.9	0.9	76.2	73.3	79.0	0.9	3.3	3.3	3.3
	Croatia	16.7	15.8	17.6	0.9	63.3	60.1	66.4	0.9	3.8	3.8	3.8
	Greece	11.0	8.6	13.3	0.6	59.3	56.1	62.3	0.9	5.4	6.5	4.7
	Italy	14.0	11.7	16.1	0.7	53.1	45.8	60.2	0.8	3.8	3.9	3.7
	Malta	30.8	34.0	27.7	1.2	79.1	73.5	84.4	0.9	2.6	2.2	3.0
	Portugal	22.7	18.4	26.9	0.7	64.8	61.2	68.3	0.9	2.9	3.3	2.5
	Serbia and Montenegro (former)	23.8	21.7	25.8	0.8	70.7	61.4	79.4	0.8	3.0	2.8	3.1
	Slovenia	13.6	9.2	17.7	0.5	58.6	50.2	66.7	0.8	4.3	5.5	3.8
	Spain	24.2	18.2	30.0	0.6	60.5	54.7	66.1	0.8	2.5	3.0	2.2
	The former Yugoslav Republic of Macedonia	14.2	13.0	15.3	0.8	56.2	41.0	70.7	0.6	4.0	3.2	4.6
Western Europe	Austria	38.2	30.8	45.2	0.7	67.0	63.4	70.6	0.9	1.8	2.1	1.6
	Belgium	10.6	8.1	12.9	0.6	56.7	49.9	63.2	0.8	5.4	6.2	4.9
	France	9.0	6.0	11.9	0.5	50.4	45.6	54.9	0.8	5.6	7.6	4.6
	Germany	28.4	25.8	30.8	0.8	68.8	65.1	72.4	0.9	2.4	2.5	2.4
	Luxembourg	8.8	7.1	10.4	0.7	48.0	45.7	50.2	0.9	5.5	6.4	4.8
	Netherlands	66.6	66.6	66.6	1.0	84.7	80.3	89.0	0.9	1.3	1.2	1.3
	Switzerland	57.8	55.3	60.3	0.9	81.0	81.4	80.5	1.0	1.4	1.5	1.3
LATIN AMERICA AND THE CARIBBEAN												
Caribbean	Bahamas	33.0	28.6	37.5	0.8	74.5	78.5	70.4	1.1	2.3	2.7	1.9
	Barbados	32.2	25.9	38.4	0.7	88.5	86.9	90.1	1.0	2.7	3.4	2.3
	Cuba	16.6	8.7	24.1	0.4	62.9	47.5	77.6	0.6	3.8	5.5	3.2
	Dominican Republic	33.0	21.9	43.8	0.5	68.4	52.3	84.1	0.6	2.1	2.4	1.9
	Guadeloupe	23.6	22.4	24.8	0.9	80.3	81.0	79.6	1.0	3.4	3.6	3.2
	Haiti	45.4	39.4	51.3	0.8	72.4	62.6	82.1	0.8	1.6	1.6	1.6
	Jamaica	15.8	12.3	19.3	0.6	70.1	60.0	80.2	0.7	4.4	4.9	4.2
	Martinique	11.4	8.3	14.5	0.6	70.7	64.4	76.7	0.8	6.2	7.8	5.3
	Netherlands Antilles	24.1	21.1	27.1	0.8	75.3	70.4	80.2	0.9	3.1	3.3	3.0
	Saint Lucia	40.7	27.7	53.5	0.5	78.5	67.7	89.6	0.8	1.9	2.4	1.7
	Saint Vincent and the Grenadines	36.4	22.7	50.2	0.5	82.0	71.5	92.6	0.8	2.2	3.1	1.8
	Trinidad and Tobago	26.8	19.8	33.7	0.6	77.1	64.9	89.1	0.7	2.9	3.3	2.6
	U.S. Virgin Islands	25.0	20.2	30.0	0.7	72.8	63.0	83.0	0.8	2.9	3.1	2.8
Central America	Belize	33.4	21.4	45.1	0.5	70.2	51.8	88.3	0.6	2.1	2.4	2.0
	Costa Rica	34.1	21.6	46.0	0.5	69.7	55.2	83.4	0.7	2.0	2.6	1.8
	El Salvador	24.1	18.3	29.7	0.6	62.5	46.8	77.9	0.6	2.6	2.6	2.6
	Guatemala	44.3	31.2	57.6	0.5	60.8	35.2	88.0	0.4	1.4	1.1	1.5
	Honduras	53.6	35.9	70.7	0.5	74.6	56.6	92.1	0.6	1.4	1.6	1.3
	Mexico	31.9	24.9	38.8	0.6	59.1	41.4	77.4	0.5	1.9	1.7	2.0
	Nicaragua	41.6	21.5	61.2	0.4	59.4	32.3	86.0	0.4	1.4	1.5	1.4
	Panama	26.5	19.7	33.0	0.6	69.5	53.8	84.8	0.6	2.6	2.7	2.6

Labour Force Participation and Employment

Annex table 7. Youth labour force participation rates, 2005

Region and subregion	Country	Percentage of youth in the labour force								Age transition in LFPR*		
		15-19 years				20-24 years						
		Total	Female	Male	Female/male LFPR**	Total	Female	Male	Female/male LFPR**	Total	Female	Male
South America	Argentina	38.0	26.5	49.2	0.5	73.4	65.7	81.0	0.8	1.9	2.5	1.6
	Bolivia	45.3	42.6	48.0	0.9	66.9	53.4	80.2	0.7	1.5	1.3	1.7
	Brazil	46.3	39.5	52.9	0.7	76.0	65.4	86.4	0.8	1.6	1.7	1.6
	Chile	9.4	7.7	11.1	0.7	47.9	38.4	57.1	0.7	5.1	5.0	5.1
	Colombia	36.4	31.8	40.9	0.8	81.5	75.0	87.9	0.9	2.2	2.4	2.1
	Ecuador	41.2	35.0	47.3	0.7	72.8	63.4	82.0	0.8	1.8	1.8	1.7
	French Guiana	13.5	9.3	17.3	0.5	73.5	70.1	76.5	0.9	5.5	7.5	4.4
	Guyana	37.6	22.9	51.9	0.4	67.6	46.3	88.6	0.5	1.8	2.0	1.7
	Paraguay	52.6	50.2	55.0	0.9	84.4	78.1	90.6	0.9	1.6	1.6	1.6
	Peru	27.7	26.3	29.1	0.9	78.9	69.0	88.6	0.8	2.8	2.6	3.0
	Puerto Rico	17.8	14.2	21.2	0.7	58.1	44.5	71.3	0.6	3.3	3.1	3.4
	Suriname	12.4	4.7	19.8	0.2	42.4	23.7	61.3	0.4	3.4	5.0	3.1
	Uruguay	43.3	26.9	59.0	0.5	79.9	70.8	88.7	0.8	1.8	2.6	1.5
	Venezuela	31.3	10.0	51.9	0.2	84.6	82.7	86.5	1.0	2.7	8.3	1.7
NORTHERN AMERICA	Canada	53.9	54.3	53.5	1.0	78.1	75.1	81.0	0.9	1.4	1.4	1.5
	United States of America	46.4	46.8	46.1	1.0	76.6	72.9	80.1	0.9	1.6	1.6	1.7
OCEANIA	Australia	58.2	60.1	56.4	1.1	80.2	76.6	83.7	0.9	1.4	1.3	1.5
	New Zealand	55.0	55.2	54.9	1.0	72.2	67.2	77.0	0.9	1.3	1.2	1.4
Melanesia	Fiji	30.3	28.7	31.8	0.9	73.0	62.9	82.5	0.8	2.4	2.2	2.6
	New Caledonia	16.5	15.2	17.7	0.9	76.5	64.6	87.7	0.7	4.6	4.2	5.0
	Papua New Guinea	52.6	53.6	51.7	1.0	70.8	70.9	70.8	1.0	1.3	1.3	1.4
	Solomon Islands	44.7	43.2	46.0	0.9	72.9	61.2	83.8	0.7	1.6	1.4	1.8
	Vanuatu	71.1	70.2	72.0	1.0	85.5	80.1	90.8	0.9	1.2	1.1	1.3
Micronesia	Guam	24.4	18.6	30.2	0.6	69.8	60.3	79.1	0.8	2.9	3.2	2.6
Polynesia	French Polynesia	31.7	23.3	39.8	0.6	69.0	61.1	77.1	0.8	2.2	2.6	1.9
	Samoa	17.0	9.5	23.8	0.4	72.5	53.7	88.0	0.6	4.3	5.7	3.7
	Tonga	18.3	11.4	24.0	0.5	64.1	48.5	79.2	0.6	3.5	4.3	3.3

Source: International Labour Organization, Economically Active Population Estimates and Projections dataset for 2005.

Notes:

Two dots (..) indicate that data are not available or are not separately reported.

LFPR = labour force participation rate.

* Indicates the ratio of labour force participation among older youth aged 20-24 years to that of younger youth aged 15-19 years.
Transition ratios close to 1 suggest little change in youth labour force participation across age groups.

** A ratio of less than 1 means females are less likely to participate in the labour force than are males.

Labour Force Participation and Unemployment

Annex table 8. Youth unemployment indicators (most recent data available)

Region, country	Year	Numbers (in thousands) of: Youth population	Youth labour force	Unemployed youth	Youth unemployment rates by sex (percentages) Female	Male	Ratio of female to male youth unemployment	Total unemployment rates (percentage) Youth unemploy ment rate	Adult unemploy ment rate	Ratio of youth to adult unemployment rate	Share of unemployed youth in total unemployed (percentage)	Percentage of unemployed youth in youth population
AFRICA												
Algeria	2004	..	1 756.3	762.3	46.3	42.8	1.1	43.4	13.9	3.1	45.6	..
Botswana	2001	374.3	140.9	55.9	46.1	33.9	1.4	39.6	11.9	3.3	51.6	14.9
Burkina Faso	1985	1 351.5	1 112.3	23.7	..	4.1	..	2.1	0.8	2.6	55.6	1.8
Egypt	2003	..	..	1 476.9	..	..	..	..	..	..	65.9	..
Ethiopia	2005	11 712.8	9 237.9	713.5	11.2	4.1	2.7	7.7	4.2	1.8	47.0	6.1
Gabon	1993	..	..	27.3	..	..	..	..	..	..	41.2	..
Ghana	1999	3 170.0	2 160.0	343.4	19.4	12.7	1.5	15.9	8.0	2.0	41.4	10.8
Lesotho	1997	330.2	166.8	79.0	58.5	37.9	1.5	47.4	35.8	1.3	36.6	23.9
Madagascar	2003	3 058.1	2 066.6	144.3	7.3	6.7	1.1	7.0	4.3	1.6	38.1	4.7
Malawi	1987	1 441.6	808.5	6.7	0.3	1.6	0.2	0.8	0.5	1.6	32.1	0.5
Mauritius	2005	195.7	86.2	22.3	34.3	20.5	1.7	25.9	6.5	4.0	42.8	11.4
Morocco	2005	6 300.0	2 681.5	420.9	14.4	16.2	0.9	15.7	9.5	1.7	34.3	6.7
Namibia	2001	375.1	156.3	70.0	49.3	40.4	1.2	44.8	26.2	1.7	37.8	18.7
Réunion	2005	..	..	24.8	..	..	..	..	..	..	25.2	..
Rwanda	1996	1 161.6	917.5	6.8	0.5	1.0	0.5	0.7	0.5	1.4	45.3	0.6
South Africa	2003	9 601.0	2 856.0	1 717.0	64.7	55.8	1.2	60.1	25.3	2.4	32.7	17.9
Swaziland	1997	197.4	60.3	33.3	48.3	41.7	1.2	55.2	14.9	3.7	56.0	16.8
Tunisia	2005	2 043.1	671.1	205.9	29.3	31.4	0.9	30.7	10.2	3.0	42.3	10.1
Uganda	1992	..	..	55.9	..	..	..	..	..	..	82.8	..
Zambia	1990	2 186.0	868.0	181.0	21.0	20.7	1.0	20.9	7.3	2.9	63.4	8.3
Zimbabwe	2002	2 726.5	1 519.7	378.1	21.4	28.2	0.8	24.9	4.4	5.7	67.5	13.9
ASIA												
Bangladesh	2003	24 038.0	12 407.0	823.0	5.8	7.0	0.8	6.6	3.5	1.9	41.1	3.4
Cambodia	2001	..	..	62.1	..	..	..	..	..	..	59.6	..
China	1994	..	..	3 010.0	..	..	..	..	..	..	..	..
Hong Kong, China SAR	2005	903.6	393.5	42.7	8.0	13.8	0.6	10.9	4.9	2.2	21.3	4.7
India	2004	177 269.9	80 119.2	8 434.7	10.8	10.4	1.0	10.5	3.5	3.0	45.8	4.8
Indonesia	2005	42 316.5	22 995.4	6 597.1	33.8	25.2	1.3	28.7	5.1	5.6	60.8	15.6
Iran, Islamic Republic of	2005	16 028.0	5 633.0	1 303.0	32.1	20.3	1.6	23.1	7.5	3.1	51.4	8.1
Israel	2005	1 129.2	365.5	65.1	18.6	17.0	1.1	17.8	7.6	2.3	26.4	5.8
Japan	2005	14 210.0	6 340.0	550.0	7.4	9.9	0.7	8.7	4.0	2.2	18.8	3.9
Kazakhstan	2004	2 712.7	1 342.5	191.6	15.7	13.1	1.2	14.3	7.2	2.0	29.1	7.1
Korea, Republic of	2005	6 113.1	2 033.7	207.7	9.0	12.2	0.7	10.2	3.1	3.3	23.4	3.4
Kyrgyzstan	2004	1 048.6	476.3	72.6	17.8	13.5	1.3	15.2	6.7	2.3	39.1	6.9
Lao People's Democratic Republic	1995	819.8	607.8	30.5	3.9	6.4	0.6	5.0	0.9	5.6	56.8	3.7
Macau, China SAR	2005	84.7	29.3	2.4	5.8	10.8	0.5	8.2	3.5	2.3	23.5	2.8
Malaysia	2003	..	..	240.6	..	..	..	..	..	..	65.1	..
Maldives	2000	56.8	22.2	1.0	5.1	4.0	1.3	4.4	1.1	4.0	57.4	1.7
Mongolia	2003	456.8	199.3	39.9	20.7	19.5	1.1	20.0	12.7	1.6	28.0	8.7
Nepal	1999	3 456.0	2 818.0	84.0	2.2	4.0	0.6	3.0	1.4	2.1	47.2	2.4
Pakistan	2005	..	..	1 557.0	..	..	..	..	..	..	48.0	..
Papua New Guinea	2000	1 029.3	609.3	32.1	..	..	..	5.3	2.1	2.5	48.7	3.1
Philippines	2005	16 430.0	7 787.0	1 280.0	18.9	14.9	1.3	16.4	4.8	3.4	48.9	7.8
Qatar	2001	..	..	5.7	..	..	..	..	..	..	45.2	..
Saudi Arabia	2002	..	..	192.8	..	..	..	..	..	..	58.7	..
Singapore	2005	..	299.8	15.6	6.3	4.1	1.5	5.2	4.1	1.3	15.5	1.7
Sri Lanka	2005	3 641.2	1 521.0	398.3	37.1	20.1	1.8	26.2	3.3	7.9	64.3	10.9
Syrian Arab Republic	2002	3 640.0	1 895.0	498.8	38.9	21.4	1.8	26.3	3.9	6.7	78.2	13.7
Taiwan, Province of China	2000	..	..	94.0	..	..	..	..	..	..	32.1	..

Annex table 8. Youth unemployment indicators (most recent data available)

Region, country	Year	Numbers (in thousands) of:			Youth unemployment rates by sex (percentages)		Ratio of female to male youth unemployment	Total unemployment rates (percentage)		Ratio of youth to adult unemployment rate	Share of unemployed youth in total unemployed (percentage)	Percentage of unemployed youth in youth population
		Youth population	Youth labour force	Unemployed youth	Female	Male		Youth unemployment rate	Adult unemployment rate			
Thailand	2005	10 577.7	5 462.1	260.0	4.6	4.9	0.9	4.8	0.8	6.0	52.4	2.5
Turkey	2005	12 175.0	4 710.0	910.0	19.3	19.3	1.0	19.3	8.1	2.4	36.1	7.5
United Arab Emirates	2000	..	..	19.3	..	..	..	..	..	..	47.0	..
Viet Nam	2004	15 523.7	9 276.3	428.3	4.9	4.4	1.1	4.6	1.5	3.1	46.2	2.8
West Bank and Gaza Strip	2004	701.7	179.3	71.3	44.9	38.9	1.2	39.8	23.0	1.7	33.7	10.2
Yemen	1999	..	..	227.1	..	..	..	..	..	..	48.4	..
EUROPE												
Albania	2001	527.4	315.3	111.8	27.1	41.6	0.7	35.5	18.8	1.9	36.6	21.2
Austria	2005	983.3	581.7	60.1	9.9	10.7	0.9	10.3	4.3	2.4	28.9	6.1
Belgium	2005	1 263.6	419.0	83.3	19.1	20.6	0.9	19.9	6.9	2.9	22.5	6.6
Bulgaria	2005	1 048.5	292.0	65.2	21.1	23.3	0.9	22.3	8.9	2.5	19.5	6.2
Croatia	2005	..	205.7	66.9	35.5	30.4	1.2	32.5	10.2	3.2	29.2	..
Cyprus	2005	93.2	39.7	5.5	14.6	13.7	1.1	13.9	4.2	3.3	28.2	5.9
Czech Republic	2005	1 357.0	459.6	88.5	19.1	19.4	1.0	19.3	6.8	2.8	21.6	6.5
Denmark	2005	591.1	397.5	31.2	9.8	6.1	1.6	7.9	4.3	1.8	22.6	5.3
Estonia	2005	207.8	70.8	11.2	15.1	16.4	0.9	15.8	6.9	2.3	21.5	5.4
Finland	2005	653.0	321.0	64.0	19.3	20.6	0.9	19.9	6.8	2.9	29.0	9.8
France	2005	7 833.9	2 636.6	600.8	24.6	21.4	1.1	22.8	8.5	2.7	22.1	7.7
Georgia	2005	578.3	195.5	55.3	30.6	26.8	1.1	28.3	12.3	2.3	19.8	9.6
Germany	2005	9 783.0	4 911.0	746.0	14.0	16.1	0.9	15.2	10.6	1.4	16.3	7.6
Greece	2005	1 232.1	417.1	105.4	34.7	17.5	2.0	25.3	8.2	3.1	22.6	8.6
Hungary	2005	1 271.0	344.2	66.9	19.1	19.7	1.0	19.4	6.1	3.2	22.0	5.3
Iceland	2005	36.7	28.3	2.0	6.0	8.5	0.7	7.2	1.6	4.5	47.7	5.6
Ireland	2005	637.3	321.8	26.6	7.3	9.1	0.8	8.3	3.5	2.4	31.1	4.2
Italy	2005	6 103.0	2 044.0	490.0	27.4	21.5	1.3	24.0	6.2	3.9	25.9	8.0
Latvia	2005	359.6	134.6	17.5	14.2	11.9	1.2	13.0	8.2	1.6	17.7	4.9
Lithuania	2005	526.1	131.6	20.7	15.3	15.9	1.0	15.7	7.6	2.1	15.6	3.9
Luxembourg	2005	51.9	15.0	2.1	16.2	11.7	1.4	13.7	3.8	3.6	22.6	4.0
Malta	2004	61.0	33.8	5.6	17.4	15.8	1.1	16.6	4.5	3.7	48.6	9.2
Netherlands	2005	1 938.0	1 326.0	127.0	9.7	9.5	1.0	9.6	4.4	2.2	29.5	6.6
Norway	2005	508.4	306.0	36.8	11.5	12.5	0.9	12.0	3.5	3.4	33.3	7.2
Poland	2005	5 594.4	1 876.5	708.8	39.2	36.7	1.1	37.8	15.3	2.5	23.3	12.7
Portugal	2005	1 312.9	564.2	90.7	19.1	13.7	1.4	16.1	6.7	2.4	21.5	6.9
Republic of Moldova	2005	701.1	152.2	28.6	18.3	19.1	1.0	18.8	5.9	3.2	27.6	4.1
Romania	2005	3 354.3	1 068.7	210.3	18.4	20.5	0.9	19.7	5.6	3.5	29.9	6.3
Russian Federation	1999	22 162.4	9 284.0	2 296.0	25.9	23.9	1.1	24.7	11.6	2.1	24.6	10.4
Slovakia	2005	875.3	319.6	95.5	28.7	30.8	0.9	29.9	14.3	2.1	22.3	10.9
Slovenia	2005	265.0	97.0	13.0	12.2	10.7	1.1	13.4	4.9	2.7	22.4	4.9
Spain	2005	4 784.8	2 494.7	490.5	23.5	16.7	1.4	19.7	7.7	2.6	25.6	10.3
Sweden	2005	983.0	538.0	120.0	21.6	23.0	0.9	22.3	5.8	3.8	33.3	12.2
Switzerland	2005	875.1	575.3	50.8	9.2	8.5	1.1	8.8	3.7	2.4	27.5	5.8
The former Yugoslav Republic of Macedonia	2005	326.5	107.3	67.2	62.1	63.0	1.0	62.6	33.7	1.9	20.7	20.6
Ukraine	2005	7 491.7	3 011.7	448.3	14.4	15.2	0.9	14.9	6.0	2.5	28.0	6.0
United Kingdom	2005	6 726.0	4 430.0	521.0	10.0	13.4	0.7	11.8	3.3	3.6	38.6	7.7
LATIN AMERICA AND THE CARIBBEAN												
Anguilla	2001	1.8	1.1	0.1	17.8	10.0	1.8	13.5	5.2	2.6	36.8	8.3
Antigua and Barbuda	1991	..	6.4	0.8	..	..	..	13.1	4.1	3.2	47.5	..
Argentina	2005	4 083.3	1 859.9	450.1	28.0	21.6	1.3	24.2	7.7	3.1	39.6	11.0
Aruba	1997	..	5.0	1.0	24.5	16.7	1.5	20.4	5.8	3.5	31.1	6.0
Bahamas	2005	..	30.7	6.2	24.1	16.9	1.4	20.2	8.1	2.5	34.3	..

Annex table 8. Youth unemployment indicators (most recent data available)

Region, country	Year	Numbers (in thousands) of:			Youth unemployment rates by sex (percentages)		Ratio of female to male youth unemployment	Total unemployment rates (percentage)		Ratio of youth to adult unemployment rate	Share of unemployed youth in total unemployed (percentage)	Percentage of unemployed youth in youth population
		Youth population	Youth labour force	Unemployed youth	Female	Male		Youth unemployment rate	Adult unemployment rate			
Barbados	2003	36.1	20.6	5.4	28.7	24.1	1.2	26.2	8.5	3.1	33.8	15.0
Belize	2005	..	29.2	5.7	28.9	13.8	2.1	19.5	8.0	2.4	46.8	..
Bolivia	2002	..	911.3	84.0	11.8	7.3	1.6	9.2	4.1	2.2	42.1	11.6
Brazil	2004	34 814.4	22 254.1	4 021.8	23.3	14.2	1.6	18.1	5.9	3.1	49.8	..
British Virgin Islands	1991	1.7	1.7	0.1	7.2	7.6	0.9	7.5	2.7	2.8	40.6	..
Cayman Islands	1997	2.7	2.7	0.3	..	..	..	9.3	3.4	2.7	28.1	..
Chile	2005	2 639.6	819.8	141.9	21.0	15.2	1.4	17.3	5.4	3.2	32.2	5.4
Colombia	2005	10 469.6	4 447.8	660.9	19.4	11.6	1.7	14.9	8.0	1.9	34.0	6.3
Costa Rica	2005	856.7	419.3	63.0	21.5	11.3	1.9	15.0	4.2	3.6	50.3	7.4
Dominica	2001	11.0	4.7	1.2	26.7	25.5	1.0	26.0	7.7	3.4	40.0	11.1
Dominican Republic	2004	..	..	301.8	..	..	..	..	..	..	42.5	..
Ecuador	2005	1 731.5	863.9	134.1	20.6	12.2	1.7	15.5	5.7	2.7	41.7	7.7
El Salvador	2004	1 333.2	626.6	72.2	9.4	12.7	0.7	11.5	5.3	2.2	40.2	5.4
French Guiana	2005	..	..	2.9	..	..	..	..	..	..	18.5	..
Grenada	1998	16.0	9.7	3.0	39.4	25.4	1.6	31.5	10.2	3.1	49.0	19.0
Guadeloupe	2005	..	..	6.3	..	..	..	..	..	..	14.9	..
Guyana	2001	..	61.0	12.2	24.4	17.5	1.4	20.0	5.8	3.4	51.0	..
Haiti	1999	1 553.9	496.5	89.1	21.1	15.1	1.4	17.9	5.0	3.6	42.6	5.7
Honduras	2005	1 562.3	756.9	53.2	11.2	5.2	2.2	7.0	3.0	2.3	50.2	3.4
Jamaica	2005	..	..	51.9	..	..	..	..	..	..	39.8	..
Martinique	2005	..	..	5.5	..	..	..	..	..	..	15.7	..
Mexico	2005	19 553.7	9 145.5	600.5	7.4	6.1	1.2	6.6	2.7	2.4	40.4	3.1
Netherlands Antilles	2000	16.8	5.7	1.5	29.7	25.4	1.2	26.9	12.7	2.1	18.0	9.1
Nicaragua	2003	1 165.1	589.6	73.8	15.8	10.8	1.5	12.5	6.1	2.0	45.7	6.3
Panama	2005	523.0	255.9	57.6	29.6	18.5	1.6	22.5	7.4	3.0	42.1	11.0
Paraguay	2003	..	664.0	101.3	20.5	12.1	1.7	15.3	5.2	2.9	52.3	..
Peru	2005	1 723.6	836.3	174.5	20.7	21.0	1.0	20.9	8.8	2.4	39.9	10.1
Puerto Rico	2005	539.0	215.0	50.0	20.9	24.8	0.8	23.3	9.2	2.5	31.3	9.3
Saint Helena	1998	0.8	0.5	0.1	30.5	32.5	0.9	25.2	16.0	1.6	28.1	16.8
Saint Lucia	2003	..	16.2	6.5	49.2	31.8	1.5	40.0	20.5	2.0	35.6	..
Saint Vincent and the Grenadines	1991	..	12.6	4.6	43.0	32.8	1.3	36.3	12.7	2.9	55.3	8.7
Suriname	1999	47.6	12.2	4.1	58.1	24.1	2.4	33.9	10.4	3.3	35.0	..
Trinidad and Tobago	2005	..	..	21.7	..	..	..	..	..	..	43.7	..
Uruguay	2005	457.8	219.6	64.8	34.9	25.4	1.4	29.5	8.6	3.4	41.8	14.2
Venezuela	2003	4 976.8	2 691.6	752.5	34.8	23.7	1.5	28.0	13.5	2.1	37.3	15.1
NORTH AMERICA												
Canada	2005	4 280.2	2 822.7	350.2	10.6	14.2	0.7	12.4	5.7	2.2	29.9	8.2
United States of America	2005	36 674.0	22 291.0	2 521.0	10.1	12.4	0.8	11.3	4.0	2.8	33.2	6.9
OCEANIA												
Australia	2005	2 842.9	2 025.8	219.1	10.5	11.1	0.9	10.8	3.7	2.9	40.8	7.7
New Zealand	2005	590.9	371.2	34.9	9.8	9.1	1.1	9.4	2.5	3.8	44.0	5.9
New Caledonia	1996	..	29.5	9.9	38.5	29.7	1.3	33.6	19.4	1.7	66.0	..

Source: International Labour Organization, *Key Indicators of the Labour Market*, fifth edition (Geneva: 2007).

Notes:

Two dots (..) indicate that data are not available or are not separately reported.

Data repositories are mainly LABORSTA, an International Labour Office database on labour statistics; and the Organization for Economic Cooperation and Development (OECD). Detailed information on data, including types of surveys, geographic and coverage limitations, reference periods and other remarks, are available from the source publications listed above.

Annex table 9. Youth living in poverty (most recent data available)

Region and subregion	Country	HDI Rank*	Percentage of national population living in poverty			Youth population (thousands)	Total population (thousands)	Estimated number of youth living in poverty	
			Survey year**	Less than US$ 1 per day	Less than US$ 2 per day			Extreme poverty (less than US$ 1 per day) (thousands)	Poverty (less than US$ 2 per day) (thousands)
AFRICA									
Eastern Africa	Burundi	169	1998	54.6	87.6	1 830	8 141	999	1 603
	Comoros	132	..	..	..	171	841	..	..
	Djibouti	148	..	..	..	168	820	..	..
	Eritrea	157	..	..	..	962	4 708	..	..
	Ethiopia	170	1999-2000	23.0	77.8	16 675	81 176	3 835	12 973
	Kenya	152	1997	22.8	58.3	8 078	36 012	1 842	4 709
	Madagascar	143	2001	61.0	85.1	3 856	19 609	2 352	3 281
	Malawi	166	1997-1998	41.7	76.1	2 705	13 452	1 128	2 058
	Mauritius	63	..	..	..	198	1 267	..	..
	Mozambique	168	1996	37.8	78.4	4 245	20 522	1 604	3 328
	Rwanda	158	1999-2000	51.7	83.7	2 236	9 442	1 156	1 871
	Seychelles	47	..	..	..	..	..	..	..
	Tanzania, United Republic of	162	20002001	57.8	89.9	8 624	39 718	4 985	7 753
	Uganda	145	..	..	..	6 262	30 945	..	..
	Zambia	165	2002-2003	75.8	94.1	2 701	12 056	2 047	2 541
	Zimbabwe	151	1995-1996	56.1	83.0	3 370	13 162	1 891	2 797
Middle Africa	Angola	161	..	..	..	3 437	16 867	..	..
	Cameroon	144	2001	17.1	50.6	3 662	16 874	626	1 853
	Central African Republic	172	1993	66.6	84.0	893	4 151	595	750
	Chad	171	..	..	..	2 030	10 303	..	..
	Congo	140	..	..	..	840	4 238	..	..
	Congo, Democratic Republic of	167	..	..	..	12 155	61 174	..	..
	Equatorial Guinea	120	..	..	..	104	527	..	..
	Gabon	124	..	..	..	302	1 429	..	..
	Sao Tome and Principe	127	..	..	..	37	164	..	..
Northern Africa	Algeria	102	1995	2.0	15.1	7 449	33 861	149	1 125
	Egypt	111	1999-2000	3.1	43.9	15 601	76 853	484	6 849
	Libyan Arab Jamahiriya	64	..	..	..	1 268	6 085	..	..
	Morocco	123	1999	2.0	14.3	6 468	32 412	129	925
	Sudan	141	..	..	..	7 541	37 793	..	..
	Tunisia	87	2000	2.0	6.6	2 099	10 319	42	139
Southern Africa	Botswana	131	1993	23.5	50.1	437	1 753	103	219
	Lesotho	149	1995	36.4	56.1	465	1 785	169	261
	Namibia	125	1993	34.9	55.8	467	2 072	163	260
	South Africa	121	2000	10.7	34.1	9 747	47 699	1 043	3 324
	Swaziland	146	..	..	..	282	1 025	..	..

Annex table 9. Youth living in poverty (most recent data available)

Region and subregion	Country	HDI Rank*	Percentage of national population living in poverty			Youth population (thousands)	Total population (thousands)	Estimated number of youth living in poverty	
			Survey year**	Less than US$ 1 per day	Less than US$ 2 per day			Extreme poverty (less than US$ 1 per day) (thousands)	Poverty (less than US$ 2 per day) (thousands)
Western Africa	Benin	163	2003	30.9	73.7	1 839	8 971	568	1 355
	Burkina Faso	174	2003	27.2	71.8	2 917	14 042	793	2 094
	Cape Verde	106	..	..	..	120	530	..	..
	Côte d'Ivoire	164	2002	14.8	48.8	4 141	18 770	613	2 021
	Gambia	155	1998	59.3	82.9	304	1 594	180	252
	Ghana	136	1998-1999	44.8	78.5	4 914	22 995	2 202	3 858
	Guinea	160	..	..	..	1 903	9 808	..	..
	Guinea-Bissau	173	..	..	..	319	1 682	..	..
	Mali	175	1994	72.3	90.6	2 903	14 325	2 099	2 630
	Mauritania	153	2000	25.9	63.1	617	3 247	160	389
	Niger	177	1995	60.6	85.8	2 877	14 907	1 744	2 469
	Nigeria	159	2003	70.8	92.4	28 821	137 243	20 405	26 631
	Senegal	156	1995	22.3	63.0	2 624	12 218	585	1 653
	Sierra Leone	176	1989	..	74.5	1 110	5 802	..	827
	Togo	147	..	..	..	1 343	6 470	..	..
ASIA									
Eastern Asia	China	81	2001	16.6	46.7	221 282	1 331 356	36 733	103 339
	Hong Kong, China SAR	22	..	..	..	891	7 194	..	..
	Japan	7	..	..	..	13 428	128 325	..	..
	Korea, Republic of	26	1998	2.0	..	6 770	48 142	135	..
	Mongolia	116	1998	27.0	74.9	598	2 711	161	448
South-central Asia	Bangladesh	137	2000	36.0	82.8	29 689	147 059	10 688	24 583
	Bhutan	135	..	..	..	483	2 260	..	..
	India	126	1999-2000	34.7	79.9	217 598	1 135 614	75 506	173 861
	Iran, Islamic Republic of	96	1998	2.0	7.3	17 635	71 220	353	1 287
	Kazakhstan	79	2003	2.0	16.0	2 920	14 802	58	467
	Kyrgyzstan	110	2003	2.0	21.4	1 134	5 386	23	243
	Maldives	98	..	..	..	76	346	..	..
	Nepal	138	2003-2004	24.1	68.5	5 749	28 226	1 386	3 938
	Pakistan	134	2002	17.0	73.6	35 532	164 594	6 040	26 151
	Sri Lanka	93	2002	5.6	41.6	3 628	21 078	203	1 509
	Tajikistan	122	2003	7.4	42.8	1 556	6 682	115	666
	Turkmenistan	105	..	..	..	1 092	4 965	..	..
	Uzbekistan	113	..	..	..	6 050	27 371	..	..
South-eastern Asia	Brunei Darussalam	34	..	..	..	69	390	..	..
	Cambodia	129	1997	34.1	77.7	3 495	14 638	1 192	2 715
	Indonesia	108	2002	7.5	52.4	42 020	228 121	3 151	22 018
	Lao People's Democratic Republic	133	2002	27.0	74.1	1 276	6 193	344	945
	Malaysia	61	1997	2.0	9.3	4 749	26 240	95	442
	Myanmar	130	..	..	..	10 127	51 475	..	..
	Philippines	84	2000	15.5	47.5	17 415	85 884	2 699	8 272
	Singapore	25	..	..	..	593	4 434	..	..
	Thailand	74	2002	2.0	25.2	10 807	65 283	216	2 723
	Timor-Leste	142	..	..	..	245	1 068	..	..
	Viet Nam	109	..	..	..	17 971	86 445	..	..

Poverty

Annex table 9. Youth living in poverty (most recent data available)

Region and subregion	Country	HDI Rank*	Percentage of national population living in poverty			Youth population (thousands)	Total population (thousands)	Estimated number of youth living in poverty	
			Survey year**	Less than US$ 1 per day	Less than US$ 2 per day			Extreme poverty (less than US$ 1 per day) (thousands)	Poverty (less than US$ 2 per day) (thousands)
Western Asia	Armenia	80	2003	2.0	31.1	604	2 999	12	188
	Azerbaijan	99	2002	2.0	..	1 788	8 536	36	..
	Bahrain	39	..	..	..	116	751	..	..
	Cyprus	29	..	..	..	132	854	..	..
	Georgia	97	2003	6.5	25.3	733	4 396	48	185
	Israel	23	..	..	..	1 102	6 967	..	..
	Jordan	86	2002-2003	2.0	7.0	1 170	5 966	23	82
	Kuwait	33	..	..	..	429	2 839	..	..
	Lebanon	78	..	..	..	665	3 653	..	..
	Occupied Palestinian Territory	100	..	..	..	776	3 945	..	..
	Oman	56	..	..	..	550	2 668	..	..
	Qatar	46	..	..	..	114	857	..	..
	Saudi Arabia	76	..	..	..	4 878	25 809	..	..
	Syrian Arab Republic	107	..	..	..	4 426	19 988	..	..
	Turkey	92	2003	3.4	18.7	13 444	75 161	457	2 514
	United Arab Emirates	49	..	..	..	821	4 775	..	..
	Yemen	150	1998	15.7	45.2	4 810	22 325	755	2 174
EUROPE									
Eastern Europe	Belarus	67	..	2.0	..	1 594	9 645	32	..
	Bulgaria	54	2003	2.0	6.1	1 011	7 616	20	62
	Czech Republic	30	1996	2.0	..	1 299	10 198	26	..
	Hungary	35	2002	2.0	..	1 258	10 045	25	..
	Republic of Moldova	114	2001	22.0	63.7	782	4 186	172	498
	Poland	37	2002	2.0	..	5 948	38 467	119	..
	Romania	60	2003	2.0	12.9	3 188	21 544	64	411
	Russian Federation	65	2002	2.0	12.1	23 090	141 900	462	2 794
	Slovakia	42	1996	2.0	2.9	819	5 401	16	24
	Ukraine	77	2003	2.0	4.9	7 111	45 509	142	348
Nothern Europe	Denmark	15	..	..	..	621	5 461	..	..
	Estonia	40	2003	2.0	7.5	204	1 321	4	15
	Finland	11	..	..	..	657	5 274	..	..
	Iceland	2	..	..	..	44	300	..	..
	Ireland	4	..	..	..	593	4 267	..	..
	Latvia	45	2003	2.0	4.7	353	2 284	7	17
	Lithuania	41	2003	2.0	7.8	545	3 403	11	42
	Norway	1	..	..	..	584	4 665	..	..
	Sweden	5	..	..	..	1 173	9 095	..	..
	United Kingdom	18	..	..	..	8 019	60 018	..	..
Southern Europe	Albania	73	2002	2.0	11.8	597	3 163	12	70
	Bosnia and Herzegovina	62	..	..	..	536	3 920	..	..
	Croatia	44	2001	2.0	..	580	4 555	12	..
	Greece	24	..	..	..	1 292	11 160	..	..
	Italy	17	..	..	..	5 790	58 173	..	..
	The former Yugoslav Republic of Macedonia	66	2003	2.0	..	321	2 040	6	..
	Malta	32	..	..	..	58	405	..	..

Annex table 9. Youth living in poverty (most recent data available)

Region and subregion	Country	HDI Rank*	Percentage of national population living in poverty			Youth population (thousands)	Total population (thousands)	Estimated number of youth living in poverty	
			Survey year**	Less than US$ 1 per day	Less than US$ 2 per day			Extreme poverty (less than US$ 1 per day) (thousands)	Poverty (less than US$ 2 per day) (thousands)
	Portugal	28	1994	2.0	..	1 229	10 593	25	..
	Slovenia	27	1998	2.0	..	245	1 965	5	..
	Spain	19	..	..	..	4 793	43 604	..	..
Western Europe	Austria	14	..	..	..	978	8 218	..	..
	Belgium	13	..	..	..	1 244	10 453	..	..
	France	16	..	..	..	7 632	60 940	..	..
	Germany	21	..	..	..	9 804	82 729	..	..
	Luxembourg	12	..	..	..	53	477	..	..
	Netherlands	10	..	..	..	1 951	16 429	..	..
	Switzerland	9	..	..	..	877	7 275	..	..
LATIN AMERICA AND THE CARIBBEAN									
Caribbean	Antigua and Barbuda	59	..	..	..	..	..	..	..
	Bahamas	52	..	..	..	58	332	..	..
	Barbados	31	..	..	..	40	271	..	..
	Cuba	50	..	..	..	1 616	11 317	..	..
	Dominica	68	..	..	..	..	..	..	..
	Dominican Republic	94	2003	2.5	11.0	1 860	9 148	46	205
	Grenada	85	..	..	..	..	..	..	..
	Haiti	154	2001	53.9	78.0	2 030	8 773	1 094	1 583
	Jamaica	104	2000	2.0	13.3	519	2 672	10	69
	Saint Kitts and Nevis	51	..	..	..	33	163	..	..
	Saint Lucia	71	..	..	..	25	120	..	..
	Saint Vincent and the Grenadines	88	..	..	..	..	..	..	..
	Trinidad and Tobago	57	1992	12.4	39.0	257	1 313	32	100
Central America	Belize	95	..	..	..	58	280	..	..
	Costa Rica	48	2001	2.2	7.5	876	4 468	19	66
	El Salvador	101	2002	19.0	40.6	1 340	7 116	255	544
	Guatemala	118	2002	13.5	31.9	2 683	13 230	362	856
	Honduras	117	1999	20.7	44.0	1 584	7 521	328	697
	Mexico	53	2002	4.4	20.4	20 597	109 594	906	4 202
	Nicaragua	112	2001	45.1	79.9	1 255	5 715	566	1 003
	Panama	58	2002	6.5	17.1	591	3 343	38	101
South America	Argentina	36	2003	7.0	23.0	6 682	39 531	468	1 537
	Bolivia	115	2002	23.2	42.2	1 870	9 525	434	789
	Brazil	69	2003	7.5	21.2	34 781	191 341	2 609	7 374
	Chile	38	2000	2.0	9.6	2 881	16 635	58	277
	Colombia	70	2003	7.0	17.8	8 553	46 952	599	1 522
	Ecuador	83	1998	15.8	37.2	2 608	13 611	412	970
	Guyana	103	..	2.0	..	137	752	3	..
	Paraguay	91	2002	16.4	33.2	1 315	6 445	216	437
	Peru	82	2002	12.5	31.8	5 534	28 797	692	1 760
	Suriname	89	..	..	..	86	455	..	..
	Uruguay	43	2003	2.0	5.7	523	3 509	10	30
	Venezuela	72	2000	8.3	27.6	5 300	27 684	440	1 463

Annex table 9. Youth living in poverty (most recent data available)

Region and subregion	Country	HDI Rank*	Percentage of national population living in poverty			Youth population (thousands)	Total population (thousands)	Estimated number of youth living in poverty	
			Survey year**	Less than US$ 1 per day	Less than US$ 2 per day			Extreme poverty (less than US$ 1 per day) (thousands)	Poverty (less than US$ 2 per day) (thousands)
NORTHERN AMERICA									
	Canada	6	..	..	..	4 426	32 852	..	..
	United States of America	8	..	..	..	43 599	303 851	..	..
OCEANIA									
	Australia	3	..	..	..	2 868	20 576	..	..
	New Zealand	20	..	..	..	607	4 093	..	..
Melanesia	Fiji	90	..	..	..	162	861	..	..
	Papua New Guinea	139	..	..	..	1 225	6 114	..	..
	Solomon Islands	128	..	..	..	104	502	..	..
	Vanuatu	119	..	..	..	44	219	..	..
Polynesia	Samoa	75	..	..	..	35	187	..	..
	Tonga	55	..	..	..	21	103	..	..

Source: Estimates of youth living in poverty are extrapolations of the United Nations Programme on Youth, based on data drawn from World Bank, World Development Indicators (2006).

Notes: Also see United Nations Development Programme, *Human Development Report 2006* (http://hdr.undp.org/en/). The percentage of the population living below the specified poverty line: • US$ 1 per day—at 1985 international prices (equivalent to $1.08 at 1993 international prices), adjusted for purchasing power parity. •US$ 2 per day—at 1985 international prices (equivalent to $2.15 at 1993 international prices), adjusted for purchasing power parity. Two dots (..) indicate that data are not available or are not separately reported.
* The first Human Development Report (1990) introduced a new way of measuring development by combining indicators of life expectancy, educational attainment and income into a composite Human Development Index, or HDI (see http://hdr.undp.org/en/statistics/indices/hdi/).
** Survey data reflect both expenditure and income data (*World Development Indicators*, 2006, table 2.7, p. 70).
United Nations Population Division, *World Population Prospects 2004*. Population data estimates for 2007.

Annex table 10. Indicators of youth undernutrition and shelter deprivation (most recent data available)

Region, subregion and country	Percentage of underweight youth				Percentage of youth severely underweight				Percentage of youth deprived of shelter by sex and age (years)								
	Survey year*	Females by age (years)			Survey year*	Females by age (years)			Survey year*	Females 15-19	Males 15-19	Females 20-24	Males 20-24	Females 15-24	Males 15-24	All youth 15-24
		15-19	20-24	15-24		15-19	20-24	15-24								
AFRICA																
Eastern Africa																
Comoros	..	..	..	..	..	..	..	..	1996	46.0	42.5	43.6	38.9	44.9	40.9	42.9
Ethiopia	2000	37.2	22.3	30.4	2000	9.2	1.6	5.7	2000	90.0	92.1	91.6	91.8	90.7	91.9	91.3
Kenya	2003	19.9	9.5	15.2	2003	3.5	0.6	2.2	2003	63.3	68.6	54.3	56.5	59.3	63.2	61.3
Madagascar	2004	21.4	17.6	18.9	2004	1.1	1.0	1.1	2004	6.8	7.0	7.7	8.1	7.2	7.2	7.4
Malawi	2000	15.3	6.1	10.9	2000	1.3	0.7	1.0	2000	76.2	74.4	77.2	73.7	76.7	74.1	75.4
Mozambique	2003	13.6	10.5	11.5	2003	0.2	0.5	0.4	2003	81.8	79.7	86.1	83.8	83.9	81.5	82.7
Tanzania, United Republic of	..	..	..	..	..	..	..	..	2003	79.8	78.5	73.1	74.8	76.8	76.8	76.8
Uganda	2001	12.0	6.2	9.2	2001	1.3	0.5	1.0	2001	73.0	77.1	73.2	75.7	73.1	76.4	74.8
Zambia	..	19.5	11.7	15.8	2002	1.9	0.8	1.4	2002	54.5	58.7	56.4	49.9	55.4	54.7	55.0
Zimbabwe	..	..	..	..	..	..	..	..	1999	27.8	29.9	25.9	23.5	27.0	27.1	27.0
Middle Africa																
Angola	..	..	..	..	..	..	..	..	2001	62.2	59.6	62.8	58.2	62.5	59.0	60.8
Cameroon	2004	10.4	6.7	8.8	2004	1.5	1.0	1.3	2004	41.9	44.6	43.4	36.6	42.5	41.0	41.8
Central African Republic	1995	13.6	13.8	13.8	1995	0.6	1.4	1.1	1995	78.7	76.8	80.0	79.5	79.3	78.1	78.7
Chad	..	..	..	..	..	..	..	..	2000	94.6	95.1	95.1	92.2	94.8	93.8	94.3
Congo, Democratic Republic of the	..	..	..	..	..	—	—	—	2000	84.2	84.6	81.3	82.1	82.9	83.5	83.2
Equatorial Guinea	..	..	..	..	..	..	..	..	2000	65.8	63.6	60.8	59.5	63.5	61.8	62.7
Gabon	2000	9.2	9.1	9.1	2000	0.8	0.3	0.5	2000	16.0	19.0	16.1	13.6	16.0	16.5	16.3
Sao Tome and Principe	..	..	..	..	..	..	..	..	2000	21.5	24.3	18.8	18.9	20.3	21.9	21.1
Northern Africa																
Egypt	2003	1.6	0.8	1.0	..	..	..	..	2003	28.2	27.6	23.6	27.6	26.1	27.7	26.9
Morocco	2004	14.6	9.4	12.2	2004	1.0	0.5	0.8	2004	40.1	40.6	37.3	36.3	38.8	38.6	38.7
Sudan	..	..	..	..	..	..	..	..	2000	92.6	92.3	91.3	89.7	92.0	91.1	91.5
Southern Africa																
Lesotho	..	..	..	..	..	..	..	..	2000	55.2	54.9	57.5	56.2	56.2	55.5	55.8
Namibia	2000	18.0	15.0	15.8	..	..	..	..	2000	77.4	76.7	71.6	72.1	74.8	74.6	74.7
South Africa	..	..	..	..	..	..	..	..	1998	17.7	17.5	15.3	14.4	16.6	16.0	16.3
Swaziland	..	..	..	..	..	..	..	..	2000	33.6	31.7	30.7	28.0	32.3	30.1	31.3

Nutrition and Shelter

Annex table 10. Indicators of youth undernutrition and shelter deprivation (most recent data available)

Region, subregion and country	Percentage of underweight youth				Percentage of youth severly underweight				Percentage of youth deprived of shelter by sex and age (years)							
	Survey year*	Females by age (years)			Survey year*	Females by age (years)			Survey year*	Females	Males	Females	Males	Females	Males	All youth
		15-19	20-24	15-24		15-19	20-24	15-24		15-19	15-19	20-24	20-24	15-24	15-24	15-24
Western Africa																
Benin	2001	14.8	10.5	13.0	2001	2.0	0.4	1.3	2001	36.4	36.3	39.3	40.8	37.7	38.3	38.0
Burkina Faso	2003	26.5	15.4	21.4	2003	4.9	1.2	3.2	2003	52.9	59.0	55.3	52.0	54.0	55.9	54.9
Côte d'Ivoire	1999	11.2	6.6	9.2	1999	1.1	0.7	0.9	1999	14.5	14.6	14.0	14.9	14.3	14.7	14.5
Gambia	..	..	..	..	..	..	..	..	2000	54.5	58.0	50.0	51.3	52.4	54.9	53.7
Ghana	2003	14.7	7.1	7.9	2003	1.6	0.8	0.8	2003	9.2	12.9	10.1	9.9	10.0	11.6	11.1
Guinea	..	..	..	..	..	..	..	..	2000	45.8	45.1	49.6	42.4	47.5	43.9	45.6
Guinea-Bissau	..	..	..	..	..	..	..	..	2000	64.8	64.1	64.9	56.5	64.8	60.5	62.7
Mali	2001	20.4	9.9	15.5	2001	2.0	0.6	1.3	2001	69.2	74.1	74.6	66.2	71.6	70.6	71.1
Mauritania	2001	24.5	14.8	20.0	2001	4.9	2.5	3.8	2001	61.1	59.0	59.1	56.1	60.1	57.6	58.9
Niger	1998	21.5	20.4	20.8	1998	1.1	0.6	0.8	1998	80.4	78.4	80.9	76.0	80.6	77.4	78.9
Nigeria	2003	24.1	13.6	19.4	2003	2.7	1.3	2.1	2003	46.7	45.4	50.1	39.4	48.3	42.7	45.4
Senegal	..	..	..	..	..	..	..	..	1999	33.0	36.8	34.0	32.8	33.4	35.0	34.2
Sierra Leone	..	..	..	..	..	..	..	..	2000	74.8	73.3	76.7	70.5	75.7	72.0	73.9
Togo	1998	15.2	13.0	13.6	1998	0.9	0.3	0.5	1998	20.9	25.4	19.8	23.8	20.4	24.7	22.5
ASIA																
Eastern Asia																
China **	2000	26.0	14.0	20.0	2000	4.0	1.0	2.5	1992	5.6	4.5	5.6	4.5	5.6	4.5	5.0
Mongolia	..	..	..	..	..	..	..	..	2000	37.3	36.8	32.6	34.1	35.1	35.5	35.3
South-central Asia																
Bangladesh	2004	48.1	43.8	45.3	2004	5.6	4.6	4.9	2004	82.8	82.8	81.2	81.0	82.0	82.0	82.0
Kazakhstan	1999	13.6	12.5	13.0	1999	1.2	1.4	1.3	1999	0.8	1.3	1.3	1.7	1.0	1.5	1.3
Kyrgyzstan	1997	14.4	6.4	10.8	1997	0.9	0.5	0.7	1997	5.1	5.2	5.8	6.2	5.4	5.7	5.5
Nepal	2001	20.1	21.6	21.1	2001	0.6	1.9	1.5	2001	85.4	85.8	83.6	81.4	84.6	83.9	84.2
Tajikistan	..	..	..	..	..	..	..	..	2000	61.4	61.2	58.9	61.3	60.3	61.2	60.8
Uzbekistan	1996	17.5	10.1	14.1	1996	1.3	0.7	1.0	1996	14.4	16.3	18.4	17.3	16.2	16.8	16.5
South-eastern Asia																
Cambodia	2000	25.3	16.5	22.4	2000	3.6	1.3	2.8	2000	36.4	37.4	42.0	38.4	38.2	37.7	38.0
Indonesia	..	..	..	..	..	..	..	..	2003	13.4	14.2	13.4	12.8	13.5	13.4	13.4
Lao People's Democratic Republic	..	..	..	..	..	..	..	..	2000	36.0	32.4	37.5	37.4	36.7	34.7	35.7
Myanmar	..	..	..	..	..	..	..	..	2000	67.4	67.6	65.9	64.1	66.7	65.9	66.3
Philippines	..	..	..	..	..	..	..	..	2003	10.7	12.4	9.4	11.5	10.1	12.0	11.0
Viet Nam	..	..	..	..	..	..	..	..	2002	26.4	24.5	26.5	29.0	26.5	26.6	26.6
Western Asia																
Armenia	2000	6.3	6.1	6.2	2000	0.4	0.4	0.4	2000	1.0	1.4	1.3	0.9	1.1	1.2	1.1
Azerbaijan	..	..	..	..	..	..	..	..	2000	32.1	31.9	34.4	32.6	33.2	32.2	32.7
Iraq	..	..	..	..	..	..	..	..	2000	27.6	28.6	22.1	24.3	25.0	26.6	25.8
Jordan	2002	4.8	4.5	4.5	..	..	..	..	..	..	..	..	..	..	..	..
Turkey	1998	6.3	3.6	4.0	1998	0.9	..	0.1	1998	8.3	8.4	6.7	8.1	7.5	8.2	7.9
Yemen	1997	29.3	27.9	28.2	..	..	..	..	..	..	..	..	..	..	..	..
EUROPE ***																
Eastern Europe																
Bulgaria	..	..	..	19.4	..	..	..	..	..	..	..	..	..	..	..	..
Czech Republic	..	..	..	13.0	..	..	..	..	..	..	..	..	..	..	..	..
Hungary	..	..	..	15.4	..	..	..	..	..	..	..	..	..	..	..	..
Poland	..	..	..	16.9	..	..	..	..	..	..	..	..	..	..	..	..

Annex table 10. Indicators of youth undernutrition and shelter deprivation (most recent data available)

Region, subregion and country	Percentage of underweight youth				Percentage of youth severely underweight				Percentage of youth deprived of shelter by sex and age (years)							
	Survey year*	Females by age (years)			Survey year*	Females by age (years)			Survey year*	Females 15-19	Males 15-19	Females 20-24	Males 20-24	Females 15-24	Males 15-24	All youth 15-24
		15-19	20-24	15-24		15-19	20-24	15-24								
Republic of Moldova	..	..	..	..	..	..	..	..	2000	12.4	12.5	14.5	13.0	13.3	12.8	13.0
Romania	..	..	..	15.7	..	..	..	..	..	..	..	..	..	..	..	..
Russian Federation ****	..	..	..	..	..	..	..	..	2004	4.1	4.4	3.7	2.2	3.8	3.4	3.6
Slovakia	..	..	..	19.0	..	..	..	..	..	..	..	..	..	..	..	..
Northern Europe																
Denmark	..	..	..	9.4	..	..	..	..	..	..	..	..	..	..	..	..
Estonia	..	..	..	14.9	..	..	..	..	..	..	..	..	..	..	..	..
Finland	..	..	..	11.7	..	..	..	..	..	..	..	..	..	..	..	..
Iceland	..	..	..	6.9	..	..	..	..	..	..	..	..	..	..	..	..
Ireland	..	..	..	3.7	..	..	..	..	..	..	..	..	..	..	..	..
Latvia	..	..	..	17.9	..	..	..	..	..	..	..	..	..	..	..	..
Lithuania	..	..	..	8.5	..	..	..	..	..	..	..	..	..	..	..	..
Norway	..	..	..	32.6	..	..	..	..	..	..	..	..	..	..	..	..
Sweden	..	..	..	9.9	..	..	..	..	..	..	..	..	..	..	..	..
United Kingdom	..	..	..	16.8	..	..	..	..	..	..	..	..	..	..	..	..
Southern Europe																
Albania	..	..	..	..	..	..	..	..	2000	40.5	39.6	37.5	36.0	39.1	38.0	38.6
Bosnia and Herzegovina	..	..	..	..	..	..	..	..	..	..	..	..	..	..	..	..
Greece	..	..	..	9.2	..	..	..	..	..	..	..	..	..	..	..	..
Italy	..	..	..	18.3	..	..	..	..	..	..	..	..	..	..	..	..
Malta	..	..	..	10.5	..	..	..	..	..	..	..	..	..	..	..	..
Portugal	..	..	..	10.0	..	..	..	..	..	..	..	..	..	..	..	..
Slovenia	..	..	..	9.9	..	..	..	..	..	..	..	..	..	..	..	..
Spain	..	..	..	14.2	..	..	..	..	..	..	..	..	..	..	..	..
Western Europe																
Austria	..	..	..	12.7	..	..	..	..	..	..	..	..	..	..	..	..
Belgium	..	..	..	14.7	..	..	..	..	..	..	..	..	..	..	..	..
France	..	..	..	19.3	..	..	..	..	..	..	..	..	..	..	..	..
Germany	..	..	..	3.5	..	..	..	..	..	..	..	..	..	..	..	..
Netherlands	..	..	..	13.4	..	..	..	..	..	..	..	..	..	..	..	..
Switzerland	..	..	..	17.2	..	..	..	..	..	..	..	..	..	..	..	..
LATIN AMERICA AND THE CARIBBEAN																
Caribbean																
Dominican Republic	2002	10.7	6.7	7.8	..	..	..	..	2002	11.3	12.5	12.2	14.1	11.7	13.3	12.5
Haiti	2000	18.7	9.0	14.4	2000	2.2	0.8	1.6	2000	36.7	43.0	40.0	39.4	38.2	41.5	39.8
Central America																
Guatemala	1999	1.8	1.5	1.6	1999	0.5	0.1	0.2	1999	35.2	46.0	34.4	35.9	34.9	41.6	38.2
Nicaragua	2001	6.6	4.2	5.5	2001	0.6	0.5	0.5	2001	64.4	67.2	58.5	63.0	61.7	65.3	63.5
South America																
Bolivia	2003	4.1	2.2	3.2	2003	0.3	0.0	0.2	2003	27.5	32.4	25.4	25.6	26.5	29.2	27.9
Brazil	1996	8.1	7.3	7.5	1996	0.3	0.3	0.3	1996	7.7	9.6	6.5	8.7	7.1	9.2	8.2
Colombia	2005	13.8	7.5	10.8	2005	1.1	0.7	0.9	2005	7.7	11.2	6.1	8.0	6.9	9.7	8.3
Guyana	..	..	..	..	..	..	..	..	2000	35.3	37.2	35.5	32.1	35.3	34.8	35.1
Peru	2003	2.0	1.1	1.3	..	..	..	..	2003	46.8	52.8	42.6	48.2	44.7	50.6	47.7
Suriname	..	..	..	..	..	..	..	..	2000	13.0	10.8	12.7	6.8	12.9	9.1	11.0
Venezuela	..	..	..	..	..	..	..	..	2000	47.1	44.1	47.4	43.9	47.3	44.0	45.6

Source: Calculated by Townsend Centre for International Poverty Research, University of Bristol.

Notes:
Two dots (..) indicate that data are not available or are not separately reported. An dash (—) indicates that the amount is nil or negligible.
* Data are taken from demographic health surveys (DHS) or Multiple Indicator Cluster Surveys (MICS) for the latest available year (range: 1995-2004).
** China, excluding Hong Kong (SAR) and Macao (SAR). Data sources: China Health and Nutrition Survey (CHNS) and National Statistical Society of China (NSSC).
*** Europe: data are taken from the New Cronos and European Community Household Panel survey (ECHP).
**** Russian Federation: data are taken from Russian Longitudinal Monitoring Surveys (RLMS).

Sanitation and water

Annex table 11. Youth access to sanitation and water (most recent data available)

Region, subregion and country	Percentage of youth deprived of sanitation by age (years) and sex								Percentage of youth deprived of water by age (years) and sex							
	Survey year*	15-19 years		20-24 years		15-24 years		All youth 15-24 years	Survey year*	15-19 years		20-24 years		15-24 years		All youth 15-24 years
		Females	Males	Females	Males	Females	Males	Both sexes		Females	Males	Females	Males	Females	Males	Both sexes
AFRICA																
Eastern Africa																
Comoros	1996	0.0	0.1	0.3	0.1	0.1	0.1	0.1	1996	11.9	9.8	11.8	11.9	10.4	11.9	11.3
Ethiopia	2000	75.3	79.0	77.0	80.5	76.1	79.7	77.9	2000	85.3	85.4	86.0	86.6	85.6	85.9	85.8
Kenya	2003	13.7	17.9	11.9	12.8	12.9	15.6	14.3	2003	64.1	69.4	53.9	54.8	59.5	62.8	61.2
Madagascar	2004	58.4	57.0	57.4	56.9	57.9	57.0	57.4	2004	78.1	77.0	77.6	77.7	77.8	77.3	77.6
Malawi	2000	14.4	12.8	15.2	12.3	14.8	12.6	13.7	2000	66.9	66.6	66.4	64.5	66.6	65.6	66.1
Mozambique	2003	53.5	52.3	62.1	57.1	57.6	54.4	56.0	2003	51.7	46.6	61.1	49.4	56.1	47.9	52.1
Tanzania, United Republic of	2003	12.4	8.8	9.7	9.3	11.2	9.1	10.1	2003	68.5	68.5	61.2	60.9	65.2	65.0	65.1
Uganda	2001	12.9	11.1	13.2	13.8	13.1	12.3	12.7	2001	80.3	82.6	77.4	79.0	79.0	81.0	80.0
Zambia	2002	23.3	23.0	26.5	22.1	24.7	22.6	23.7	2002	55.1	56.4	52.4	52.2	53.9	54.5	54.2
Zimbabwe	1999	24.3	27.4	21.6	19.0	23.2	23.7	23.4	1999	40.2	45.2	32.0	28.5	36.5	37.8	37.2
Middle Africa																
Angola	2001	37.9	34.6	41.3	38.2	39.5	36.2	37.9	2001	36.7	34.8	36.7	34.1	36.7	34.4	35.6
Cameroon	2004	4.4	5.6	6.1	4.7	5.2	5.2	5.2	2004	45.2	47.7	45.3	42.8	45.2	45.4	45.3
Central African Republic	1995	22.9	23.8	25.0	23.8	23.9	23.8	23.9	1995	50.6	48.4	50.6	47.2	50.6	47.9	49.2
Chad	2000	73.1	70.2	73.1	65.4	73.1	68.0	70.6	2000	49.9	53.5	52.1	53.5	50.9	53.5	52.2
Democratic Republic of the Congo	2000	90.4	91.1	87.3	88.5	89.0	89.9	89.5	2000	75.6	76.1	71.0	74.1	73.5	75.2	74.3
Equatorial Guinea	2000	7.9	8.2	9.9	9.3	8.8	8.7	8.7	2000	57.2	59.6	60.1	55.8	58.5	57.9	58.2
Gabon	2000	1.8	1.7	2.0	1.6	1.9	1.6	1.8	2000	23.5	26.9	24.7	22.2	24.1	24.7	24.4
Sao Tome and Principe	2000	68.3	68.9	69.0	70.1	68.6	69.4	69.0	2000	46.4	44.5	42.7	46.0	44.7	45.2	45.0
Northern Africa																
Egypt	2003	1.1	1.6	0.9	1.2	1.0	1.4	1.2	2003	1.7	1.9	1.3	1.5	1.5	1.7	1.6
Morocco	2004	16.6	18.2	15.8	15.8	16.3	17.1	16.7	2004	25.4	25.9	24.4	23.2	24.9	24.6	24.8
Sudan	2000	31.4	28.5	29.5	24.3	30.5	26.5	28.5	2000	23.5	22.6	22.5	19.5	23.0	21.1	22.1
Southern Africa																
Lesotho	2000	75.8	77.4	74.6	77.6	75.3	77.5	76.3	2000	46.4	47.0	44.6	46.8	45.6	46.9	46.2
Namibia	2000	60.9	57.0	50.7	53.6	56.2	55.4	55.8	2000	34.7	33.5	27.9	26.9	31.5	30.4	31.0
South Africa	1998	17.0	18.7	16.3	15.0	16.7	16.9	16.8	1998	24.4	24.6	19.9	18.4	22.2	21.7	21.9
Swaziland	2000	62.9	68.3	64.2	66.5	63.4	67.6	65.4	2000	56.6	64.4	52.6	55.7	54.9	60.8	57.7
Western Africa																
Benin	2001	57.6	59.6	64.0	58.5	60.4	59.1	59.7	2001	40.9	43.1	45.4	44.2	42.8	43.6	43.2
Burkina Faso	2003	61.7	68.5	61.7	59.5	61.7	64.5	63.1	2003	55.4	57.2	57.2	53.9	56.2	55.7	56.0
Côte d'Ivoire	1999	24.5	28.9	26.8	27.7	25.6	28.3	27.0	1999	18.0	18.5	18.4	13.4	18.2	16.3	17.2
Gambia	2000	9.6	12.0	9.6	7.9	9.6	10.1	9.9	2000	41.8	41.9	37.2	41.3	39.7	41.7	40.7
Ghana	2003	20.8	23.7	20.4	25.9	20.4	24.7	23.3	2003	42.9	44.7	40.7	39.7	40.9	42.4	41.9
Guinea	2000	29.5	28.2	31.4	28.1	30.3	28.2	29.2	2000	36.4	37.0	37.5	33.6	36.9	35.5	36.2
Guinea-Bissau	2000	33.4	34.4	32.8	31.0	33.1	32.8	32.9	2000	51.7	53.6	51.3	49.4	51.5	51.6	51.6
Mali	2001	17.3	17.3	19.7	16.1	18.4	16.8	17.6	2001	56.4	60.8	60.5	55.2	58.2	58.3	58.3
Mauritania	2001	48.9	45.5	43.1	39.0	46.2	42.5	44.3	2001	53.8	53.9	51.7	48.5	52.8	51.3	52.1
Niger	1998	75.5	74.9	77.0	70.5	76.2	72.9	74.5	1998	56.0	54.3	57.2	50.7	56.6	52.6	54.5
Nigeria	2003	22.9	24.3	23.5	23.3	23.1	23.8	23.5	2003	68.1	69.0	68.5	68.3	68.3	68.7	68.5
Senegal	1999	27.3	29.6	26.9	26.9	27.1	28.4	27.8	1999	20.9	20.3	20.8	16.7	20.9	18.7	19.8
Sierra Leone	2000	23.6	23.6	25.3	22.3	24.4	23.0	23.7	2000	65.1	61.6	62.7	63.1	64.0	62.2	63.1
Togo	1998	97.2	96.7	97.6	97.3	97.4	97.0	97.2	1998	38.5	44.1	39.4	41.2	38.9	42.8	40.9

Annex table 11. Youth access to sanitation and water (most recent data available)

Region, subregion and country	Percentage of youth deprived of sanitation by age (years) and sex								Percentage of youth deprived of water by age (years) and sex							
	Survey year*	15-19 years		20-24 years		15-24 years		All youth 15-24 years	Survey year*	15-19 years		20-24 years		15-24 years		All youth 15-24 years
		Females	Males	Females	Males	Females	Males	Both sexes		Females	Males	Females	Males	Females	Males	Both sexes
ASIA																
Eastern Asia																
China **	1992	7.7	6.9	7.7	6.8	7.7	6.9	7.3	1992	34.0	34.2	32.3	32.5	33.1	33.3	33.2
Mongolia	2000	24.8	23.9	26.3	26.0	25.5	24.9	25.2	2000	63.8	62.6	65.1	63.1	64.4	62.8	63.6
South-central Asia																
Bangladesh	2004	38.2	35.6	36.7	36.3	37.6	35.9	36.7	2004	3.5	3.3	3.9	3.1	3.7	3.2	3.4
Kazakhstan	1999	0.5	—	0.5	0.1	0.5	0.1	0.3	1999	45.3	48.7	45.3	43.7	45.3	46.3	45.8
Kyrgyzstan	1997	—	—	0.1	0.1	0.1	0.1	0.1	1997	34.4	35.6	30.6	34.9	32.7	35.3	34.0
Nepal	2001	65.0	67.5	65.1	63.8	65.1	65.8	65.5	2001	29.1	24.5	26.4	23.6	27.8	24.1	25.9
Tajikistan	2000	8.9	10.1	8.8	8.6	8.8	9.4	9.1	2000	52.9	57.8	53.8	54.8	53.3	56.4	54.9
Uzbekistan	1996	—	—	—	—	—	—	—	1996	14.5	14.8	12.8	16.3	13.8	15.5	14.6
South-eastern Asia																
Cambodia	2000	71.4	75.8	74.1	76.2	72.3	76.0	74.1	2000	64.3	66.5	67.1	66.4	65.2	66.4	65.8
Indonesia	2003	21.0	22.8	21.3	20.6	21.2	21.7	21.5	2003	36.9	37.9	36.5	36.7	36.7	37.3	37.0
Lao People's Democratic Republic	2000	61.0	60.8	63.8	61.6	62.3	61.2	61.7	2000	53.3	48.7	50.3	52.1	51.9	50.3	51.1
Myanmar	2000	80.3	79.9	79.5	80.4	79.9	80.1	80.0	2000	68.3	68.1	67.2	68.4	67.8	68.3	68.0
Philippines	2003	17.0	21.5	15.7	16.9	16.4	19.4	17.9	2003	20.0	21.2	20.3	19.2	20.1	20.3	20.2
Viet Nam	2002	18.0	19.1	15.5	18.9	16.8	19.0	17.9	2002	15.5	16.3	17.1	17.1	16.3	16.7	16.5
Western Asia																
Armenia	2000	—	0.1	—	—	—	—	—	2000	10.5	12.5	9.3	10.0	10.0	11.3	10.6
Azerbaijan	2000	19.7	19.5	18.0	18.4	18.9	19.0	19.0	2000	36.0	37.8	34.5	39.6	35.3	38.6	36.9
Iraq	2000	6.7	7.2	5.9	5.8	6.3	6.5	6.4	2000	17.5	18.1	16.5	16.1	17.0	17.1	17.1
Turkey	1998	36.9	36.2	30.2	33.1	33.7	34.7	34.2	1998	36.6	31.8	34.7	34.5	35.7	33.1	34.4
EUROPE																
Eastern Europe																
Republic of Moldova	2000	1.1	0.8	0.9	1.3	1.0	1.0	1.0	2000	15.3	15.7	13.4	16.5	14.4	16.1	15.3
Russian Federation ***	2004	—	—	—	—	—	—	—	2004	1.6	3.3	1.5	1.5	1.5	2.4	2.0
Southern Europe																
Albania	2000	9.2	9.9	9.1	9.2	9.1	9.6	9.3	2000	16.5	15.4	14.8	14.0	15.8	14.8	15.3
Bosnia and Herzegovina	2000	4.6	5.2	5.3	6.1	4.9	5.7	5.3	2000	5.4	5.4	5.0	5.0	5.2	5.2	5.2
LATIN AMERICA AND THE CARIBBEAN																
Caribbean																
Dominican Republic	2002	3.9	4.3	4.6	5.7	4.3	5.0	4.6	2002	62.0	57.0	66.5	59.4	64.1	58.1	61.0
Haiti	2000	45.1	55.4	49.4	50.3	47.1	53.2	50.2	2000	35.9	46.1	35.3	37.7	35.6	42.4	39.1
Central America																
Guatemala	1999	11.3	14.0	12.8	11.5	12.0	12.9	12.4	1999	25.2	22.8	26.1	25.4	25.6	23.9	24.8
Nicaragua	2001	12.4	14.1	15.3	15.2	13.7	14.6	14.1	2001	14.5	16.8	13.3	15.8	14.0	16.4	15.2
South America																
Bolivia	2003	27.9	30.6	25.0	25.8	26.6	28.4	27.5	2003	10.2	11.9	9.7	11.1	9.9	11.5	10.7
Brazil	1996	10.6	12.8	9.4	11.6	10.0	12.2	11.2	1996	2.9	2.1	3.0	2.1	3.0	2.1	2.5
Colombia	2005	6.8	9.0	6.0	6.9	6.5	8.0	7.2	2005	10.7	13.6	10.3	12.0	10.5	12.9	11.7
Guyana	2000	1.5	1.6	1.1	1.3	1.3	1.5	1.4	2000	14.8	18.9	21.6	19.3	18.2	19.1	18.7
Peru	2003	13.0	15.3	9.6	13.4	11.4	14.4	12.9	2003	18.7	20.6	17.0	20.3	17.9	20.4	19.2
Suriname	2000	13.0	5.9	13.7	4.1	13.3	5.1	9.2	2000	13.8	8.2	14.7	5.1	14.2	6.8	10.5
Venezuela	2000	5.5	6.7	7.4	4.9	6.4	5.8	6.1	2000	9.4	10.0	11.8	12.5	10.5	11.2	10.9

Source: Calculated by Townsend Centre for International Poverty Research, University of Bristol.

Notes: An em dash (—) indicates that the amount is nil or negligible.

* Data are taken from demographic health surveys (DHS) or Multiple Indicator Cluster Surveys (MICS) for the latest available year (range: 1992-2004).

** China, excluding Hong Kong and Macao (male data in parentheses); data sources are China Health and Nutrition Survey (CHNS) and National Statistical Society of China (NSSC).

*** Russian Federation: data is from Russian Longitudinal Monitoring Surveys (RLMS).

Annex table 12. Leading causes of death among youth aged 15-24 years (most recent data available)

Region and country	Year	Leading cause of death	Second leading cause of death	Third leading cause of death	Number of deaths for leading cause of death	Total number of deaths	Deaths from leading cause as a proportion of total deaths (percentage)
AFRICA							
Egypt	2000	Event of undetermined intent	Heart failure and complications and ill-defined descriptions of heart disease	Land transport accidents	1,675	11,977	14
Mauritius*	2004	Land transport accidents	Intentional self-harm (suicide)	Chronic lower respiratory diseases	36	126	29
South Africa	2004	Event of undetermined intent	Tuberculosis	Influenza and pneumonia	7,704	34,194	23
ASIA							
Bahrain	2000	Land transport accidents	Event of undetermined intent	Malignant neoplasms of lymphoid, haematopoietic and related tissue	10	71	14
Brunei Darussalam	2000	Transport accidents	Accidental drowning and submersion	..	12	46	26
Georgia	2001	Influenza and pneumonia	Chronic lower respiratory diseases	Assault (homicide)	72	391	18
Israel	2003	Land transport accidents	Assault (homicide)	Intentional self-harm (suicide)	105	550	19
Japan	2004	Intentional self-harm (suicide)	Land transport accidents	Malignant neoplasms of lymphoid, haematopoietic and related tissue	1,812	5,169	35
Kazakhstan	2004	Intentional self-harm (suicide)	Transport accidents	Assault (homicide)	912	4,687	19
Kuwait	2002	Land transport accidents	Malignant neoplasms of lymphoid, haematopoietic and related tissue	Epilepticus and status epilepticus/**congenital malformations, deformations and chromosomal abnormalities	97	211	46
Korea, Republic of	2004	Land transport accidents	Intentional self-harm (suicide)	Malignant neoplasms of lymphoid, haematopoietic and related tissue	707	2,787	25
Singapore*	2003	Land transport accidents	Intentional self-harm (suicide)	Event of undetermined intent	55	257	21
Thailand	2002	Land transport accidents	Event of undetermined intent	Intentional self-harm (suicide)	3,856	16,613	23
EUROPE							
Austria	2004	Land transport accidents	Intentional self-harm (suicide)	Mental and behavioural disorders due to psychoactive substance use	195	609	32
Belarus	2003	Transport accidents	Intentional self-harm (suicide)	Accidental drowning and submersion	383	1,740	22
Bulgaria*	2004	Land transport accidents	Intentional self-harm (suicide)	Heart failure and complications and ill-defined descriptions of heart disease	142	666	21
Croatia	2004	Land transport accidents	Intentional self-harm (suicide)	Accidental poisoning	142	327	43
Czech Republic	2004	Land transport accidents	Intentional self-harm (suicide)	Event of undetermined intent	259	750	35
Denmark	2001	Land transport accidents	Intentional self-harm (suicide)	Accidental poisoning	94	250	38
Estonia	2004	Accidental poisoning	Intentional self-harm (suicide)	Land transport accidents	54	213	25
Finland	2004	Intentional self-harm (suicide)	Land transport accidents	Accidental poisoning	141	403	35
France	2003	Land transport accidents	Intentional self-harm (suicide)	Malignant neoplasms of lymphoid, haematopoietic and related tissue	1,445	4,022	36
Germany	2004	Land transport accidents	Intentional self-harm (suicide)	Event of undetermined intent	1,511	4,071	37
Greece*	2004	Land transport accidents	Accidental poisoning	Accidental drowning and submersion	407	824	49
Hungary	2003	Land transport accidents	Intentional self-harm (suicide)	Malignant neoplasms of lymphoid, haematopoietic and related tissue	189	656	29
Iceland	2004	Intentional self-harm (suicide)	Land transport accidents		7	22	32
Ireland*	2004	Intentional self-harm (suicide)	Land transport accidents	Accidental drowning and submersion	92	299	31
Italy*	2002	Land transport accidents	Intentional self-harm (suicide)	Malignant neoplasms of lymphoid, haematopoietic and related tissue	1,432	3,077	47
Latvia	2004	Land transport accidents	Intentional self-harm (suicide)	Event of undetermined intent	99	336	29
Lithuania	2004	Land transport accidents	Intentional self-harm (suicide)	Assault (homicide)	155	536	29
Luxembourg	2004	Land transport accidents	Malignant neoplasm of brain	Intentional self-harm (suicide)	11	30	37
Malta	2004	Land transport accidents	Intentional self-harm (suicide)	Congenital malformations, deformations and chromosomal abnormalities	5	27	19

Annex table 12. Leading causes of death among youth aged 15-24 years (most recent data available)

Region and country	Year	Leading cause of death	Second leading cause of death	Third leading cause of death	Number of deaths for leading cause of death	Total number of deaths	Deaths from leading cause as a proportion of total deaths (percentage)
Netherlands	2004	Land transport accidents	Intentional self-harm (suicide)	Malignant neoplasms of lymphoid, haematopoietic and related tissue	189	641	29
Norway	2004	Intentional self-harm (suicide)	Land transport accidents	Accidental poisoning	78	319	24
Poland	2004	Land transport accidents	Intentional self-harm (suicide)	Event of undetermined intent	1,047	3,658	29
Portugal	2003	Land transport accidents	Intentional self-harm (suicide)	Malignant neoplasms of lymphoid, haematopoietic and related tissue	349	870	40
Republic of Moldova	2004	Land transport accidents	Intentional self-harm (suicide)	Accidental drowning and submersion	118	524	23
Romania	2004	Land transport accidents	Intentional self-harm (suicide)	Accidental drowning and submersion	420	2,075	20
Russian Federation	2004	Transport accidents	Intentional self-harm (suicide)	Assault	8,062	44,203	18
Serbia and Montenegro (former)	2002	Intentional self-harm (suicide)	Land transport accidents	Event of undetermined intent	88	607	14
Slovakia	2002	Land transport accidents	Intentional self-harm (suicide)	Event of undetermined intent	164	509	32
Slovenia	2004	Land transport accidents	Intentional self-harm (suicide)	Event of undetermined intent	58	168	35
Spain	2004	Land transport accidents	Intentional self-harm (suicide)	Malignant neoplasms of lymphoid, haematopoietic and related tissue	974	2,447	40
Sweden	2002	Land transport accidents	Intentional self-harm (suicide)	Event of undetermined intent	117	448	26
Switzerland	2004	Land transport accidents	Intentional self-harm (suicide)	Mental and behavioural disorders due to psychoactive substance use/**accidental falls	109	384	28
The former Yugoslav Republic of Macedonia*	2003	Land transport accidents	Intentional self-harm (suicide)	Assault (homicide)	23	171	13
Ukraine*	2004	Transport accidents	Intentional self-harm (suicide)	Other violence	1,620	8,320	19
United Kingdom	2004	Land transport accidents	Intentional self-harm (suicide)	Event of undetermined intent	873	3,511	25
LATIN AMERICA AND THE CARIBBEAN							
Argentina	2003	Assault (homicide)	Intentional self-harm (suicide)	Land transport accidents	831	5,526	15
Bahamas	2000	Assault (homicide)	Land transport accidents	Human immunodeficiency virus (HIV) disease	14	55	25
Barbados	2001	Assault (homicide)	Heart failure and complications and ill-defined descriptions of heart disease	Land transport accidents	5	25	20
Belize	2001	Land transport accidents	Assault (homicide)	Intentional self-harm (suicide)	16	77	21
Brazil	2002	Assault (homicide)	Land transport accidents	Event of undetermined intent	19,206	48,142	40
Chile	2003	Land transport accidents	Intentional self-harm (suicide)	Assault (homicide)	320	1,615	20
Costa Rica	2004	Land transport accidents	Intentional self-harm (suicide)	Assault (homicide)	117	518	23
Cuba	2004	Land transport accidents	Assault (homicide)	Intentional self-harm (suicide)	172	850	20
Ecuador	2002	Assault (homicide)	Land transport accidents	Intentional self-harm (suicide)	583	3,249	18
El Salvador	2003	Assault (homicide)	Land transport accidents	Intentional self-harm (suicide)	754	1,952	39
Guatemala*	2003	Assault (homicide)	Event of undetermined intent	Influenza and pneumonia	1,312	4,724	28
Mexico	2003	Land transport accidents	Assault (homicide)	Intentional self-harm (suicide)	3,235	16,717	19
Panama	2003	Assault (homicide)	Land transport accidents	Intentional self-harm (suicide)	122	568	21

Deaths

Annex table 12. Leading causes of death among youth aged 15-24 years (most recent data available)

Region and country	Year	Leading cause of death	Second leading cause of death	Third leading cause of death	Number of deaths for leading cause of death	Total number of deaths	Deaths from leading cause as a proportion of total deaths (percentage)
Paraguay	2000	Assault (homicide)	Land transport accidents	Pregnancy, childbirth and the puerperium/**intentional self-harm (suicide)	203	836	24
Saint Lucia	2002	Assault (homicide)	Land transport accidents	Intentional self-harm (suicide)	8	33	24
Saint Vincent and the Grenadines	2002	Accidental drowning and submersion	Assault (homicide)	Human immunodeficiency virus (HIV) disease	5	24	21
Trinidad and Tobago	2000	Human immunodeficiency virus (HIV) disease	Intentional self-harm (suicide)	Assault (homicide)	43	275	16
Uruguay	2001	Land transport accidents	Intentional self-harm (suicide)	Accidental drowning and submersion	69	397	17
Venezuela	2002	Assault (homicide)	Event of undetermined intent	Land transport accidents	3,242	9,348	35
NORTH AMERICA							
Canada	2003	Land transport accidents	Intentional self-harm (suicide)	Assault (homicide)	711	2,299	31
United States of America	2002	Land transport accidents	Assault (homicide)	Intentional self-harm (suicide)	11,618	33,046	35
OCEANIA							
Australia	2003	Land transport accidents	Intentional self-harm (suicide)	Accidental poisoning	438	1,435	31
New Zealand	2003	Land transport accidents	Intentional self-harm (suicide)	Assault (homicide)	140	408	34

Source: World Health Organization, WHO Mortality Database (as of 4 December 2006); these data are as reported by countries to WHO.

Notes:
Two dots (..) indicate that data are not available or are not separately reported.
Population data are from the United Nations Population Division (2004 Revision estimates).
The number of deaths and population are in units.
Countries with fewer than 20 deaths among those aged 15-24 years in the table have been excluded.
* Country data for all causes of death are ICD Code 9; all others are ICD Code 10. (ICD = International Classification of Diseases. Countries use either the 9th or the 10th revision for coding causes of death.)
** Where there are similar numbers of deaths, the ranking is shared.

Annex table 13. Premarital sexual behaviour and condom use among youth (most recent data available)

A = Young people who have had premarital sex in the past year (percentage); B = Young people using a condom during premarital sex (percentage); C = Young people using a condom at last higher-risk sex (percentage). Values grouped by Sex and age in years (15-19, 20-24, 16-24; Males / Females).

Region, subregion and country	Notes	Year*	A 15-19 M	A 15-19 F	A 20-24 M	A 20-24 F	A 16-24 M	A 16-24 F	B 15-19 M	B 15-19 F	B 20-24 M	B 20-24 F	B 16-24 M	B 16-24 F	C 15-19 M	C 15-19 F	C 20-24 M	C 20-24 F	C 16-24 M	C 16-24 F
AFRICA																				
Sub-Saharan Africa																				
Benin	12,18,23,28,35	1996	..	29	72	59	..	36	..	7	26	12	..	9	..	8	24	12	..	9
Benin		2001	40	35	74	69	53	44	35	17	37	21	36	19	34	18	35	20	34	19
Botswana		1998	..	59	..	89	..	72	..	..	..	..	..	..	..	..	..	..	..	..
Botswana		2001	..	..	..	..	39	42	..	..	..	..	89	76	..	..	..	..	..	..
Burkina Faso		1992/93	..	16	..	46	..	18	..	..	..	..	..	..	..	..	..	..	..	..
Burkina Faso	35,42	1998/99	23	20	53	56	34	24	45	41	64	52	55	44	45	39	63	48	55	41
Burkina Faso		2003	22	21	54	54	32	26	61	47	71	72	66	55	62	46	71	68	67	54
Burundi	3	1987	..	1	..	5	..	2	..	..	..	..	..	..	..	..	..	..	..	..
Cameroon	3	1991	..	39	..	78	..	48	..	..	..	..	..	..	..	..	..	..	..	..
Cameroon	35,42	1998	41	42	81	79	58	52	31	16	33	18	32	17	30	16	32	17	31	16
Cameroon		2004	31	26	69	60	45	34	54	50	59	53	57	51	56	47	58	45	57	46
Central African Republic		1994/95	45	32	85	73	58	41	..	..	..	..	..	..	..	..	..	..	..	..
Côte d'Ivoire	5,20,26	1994	..	56	..	79	..	62	..	20	..	20	..	20	..	..	..	..	..	..
Côte d'Ivoire	35,42	1998	51	48	76	79	61	56	..	..	89**	..	81**	52**	53	21	89**	58	81**	25
Eritrea		1995	2	—	29	3	10	1	..	..	..	..	..	..	..	..	..	..	..	..
Eritrea		2002	..	2	..	2	..	2	..	..	..	..	..	..	..	..	..	..	..	..
Ethiopia	36,44	2000	10	2	26	5	16	2	28	25	32	22	30	24	28	22	32	14	30	17
Ghana		1988	..	31	..	69	..	40	..	..	..	..	..	..	..	..	..	..	..	..
Ghana		1993	29	44	73	66	46	49	..	..	..	..	..	..	..	..	..	..	..	..
Ghana		1998	15	21	41	58	24	31	26**	21	49	23	40	22	28	..	..	..	..	..
Ghana		2003	14	23	45	45	24	30	47	35	54	35	52	35	46	34	55	32	52	33
Guinea	35,42	1999	43	22	66	51	52	27	27	17	38	25	33	20	27	15	37	20	32	17
Kenya	3	1989	..	25	..	58	..	33	..	..	..	..	..	..	..	..	..	..	..	..
Kenya		1993	..	28	86	51	86	35	..	..	..	..	..	..	..	..	..	..	..	..
Kenya	35,42	1998	46	26	75	51	56	32	38	15	49	16	43	15	38	14	48	14	43	14
Kenya	36,44	2003	29	18	59	31	41	21	41	25	52	30	47	27	41	23	51	28	47	25
Liberia		1986	..	70	..	91	..	75	..	..	..	..	..	..	..	..	..	..	..	..
Madagascar		1992	..	33	..	54	..	39	..	..	..	..	..	..	..	..	..	..	..	..
Madagascar		1997	..	31	..	58	..	38	..	3	..	3	..	3	..	..	..	..	..	..
Malawi		2000	42	24	62	41	49	27	28	32	45	34	36	32	29	31	47	33	38	32
Mali		1987	..	3	..	..	..	5	..	..	..	..	..	..	..	..	..	..	..	..
Mali	42	1995/96	26	30	60	69	37	37	26	14	35	13	31	13	27	14	34	16	31	14
Mali		2001	23	24	59	51	36	29	22	14	34	17	29	15	23	14	35	16	31	14
Mozambique		1997	53	38	81	69	61	43	12	4	15	11	13	6	30	14	35	16	33	16
Mozambique		2003	61	48	88	77	67	54	31	33	44	37	35	35	30	30	38	27	33	29
Namibia		1992	45	35	77	64	59	46	..	..	..	..	..	..	..	..	..	..	..	..
Namibia	36,44	2000	..	35	..	61	59	46	62	54	77	47	70	50	63	52	74	45	69	48
Niger	3	1992	..	4	..	19	..	6	..	..	..	..	..	..	..	..	..	..	..	..
Nigeria		1990	..	25	..	59	..	34	..	..	..	..	..	..	..	..	..	..	..	..
Nigeria		1999	20	19	51	50	31	28	27	19	46	23	38	21	33	22	53	26	46	24
Nigeria		2003	17	23	43	49	29	32	33	23	54	27	47	25	49	28	61	18	55	23
Rwanda	3	1992	6	3	16	7	9	4	..	..	..	..	..	..	..	..	..	..	..	..
Rwanda	35,42	2000	..	7	..	23	9	12	49	30	61	20	55	25	..	..	..	..	..	..
Senegal		1992/93	..	7	..	15	..	9	..	..	..	..	..	..	..	..	..	..	..	..
Senegal		1997	..	7	..	..	..	..	..	..	..	..	..	..	..	..	..	..	..	..
South Africa		1998	..	37	..	75	..	53	..	21	..	20	..	20	..	..	..	..	..	..

Annex table 13. Premarital sexual behaviour and condom use among youth (most recent data available)

Region, subregion and country	Notes	Year*	A. Young people who have had premarital sex in the past year (percentage) Sex and age in years						B. Young people using a condom during premarital sex (percentage) Sex and age in years						C. Young people using a condom at last higher-risk sex (percentage) Sex and age in years					
			16-19		20-24		16-24		16-19		20-24		16-24		16-19		20-24		16-24	
			Males	Females	Males	Females	Males	Females	Males	Females	Males	Females	Males	Females	Males	Females	Males	Females	Males	Females
Tanzania, United Republic of		1991/92	58	29	83	54	65	35	..	..	..	..	..	..	23	17	37	20	31	18
Tanzania, United Republic of	34,42	1996	32	23	66	49	44	29	19	14	29	15	25	14	26	19	36	24	31	18
Tanzania, United Republic of	36,44	1999	49	32	75	64	57	39	25	18	39	21	31	19	39	40	51	37	46	39
Tanzania, United Republic of		2004	33	23	63	51	43	29	39	38	54	35	46	37	39	40	51	37	46	39
Togo		1988	..	48	..	68	..	53	..	..	..	..	..	..	..	..	..	..	..	..
Togo	35,42	1998	33	45	68	76	46	53	39	24	44	19	42	22	39	24	43	18	41	22
Uganda		1988/89	..	30	..	57	..	35	..	..	..	..	..	..	..	..	..	..	..	..
Uganda	34,42	1995	23	17	53	43	33	22	27	25	60	30	44	26	28	20	50	31	42	25
Uganda		2000/01	22	21	52	54	31	27	51	54	65	43	58	50	52	50	71	37	62	44
Uganda		2004/05	23	19	48	46	30	24	50	57	59	49	54	54	50	56	59	49	55	53
Zambia		1992	..	38	..	63	..	42	..	..	..	..	..	..	..	..	..	..	..	..
Zambia	35,42	1996	51	33	68	48	57	36	30	18	48	29	38	21	30	18	47	23	39	20
Zambia	7,14	1998	41	34	..	..	36	31	..	..	..	..	..	..	..	..	..	..	..	..
Zambia	32,36,40,44	2000	43	28	66	41	51	31	33	30	51	38	41	36	36	41	45	35	41	38
Zambia		2001/02	..	..	..	..	33	31	..	..	..	..	41	32	32	30	51	38	42	33
Zambia		2003	..	..	..	..	33	27	..	..	..	..	39	35	..	..	..	..	..	..
Zimbabwe		1988	..	13	36	36	..	18	..	..	..	..	..	..	..	..	..	..	..	..
Zimbabwe	6,21,27,31,38	1994	24	8	66	28	38	13	50	28	65	34	59	31	48	26	69	51	61	42
Zimbabwe	36,44	1999	22	10	57	31	34	15	60	37	77	40	69	39	59	37	75	45	69	42
ASIA																				
West Asia																				
Armenia	36,44	2000	13	—	51	—	27	—	47**	—	41	—	43	—	49**	..	41	..	44	..
Central Asia																				
Kazakhstan		1995	..	8	70	21	..	11	..	..	..	..	..	..	..	..	..	..	..	..
Kazakhstan	36,44	1999	27	9	70	21	42	12	73	39	62	31	66	35	73	36	60	28	65	32
Kyrgyz Republic		1997	..	1	..	1	..	1	..	..	..	..	..	..	..	..	..	..	..	..
Uzbekistan		1996	..	—	..	—	..	—	..	..	..	..	..	..	..	..	..	..	..	..
Uzbekistan	4	2002	7	—	23	2	13	1	53**	..	43	..	46	..	56*	..	48	..	50	..
South & Southeast Asia																				
Cambodia		2000	..	—	..	—	..	—	..	..	..	..	..	..	..	..	..	..	..	..
Nepal	1,36,44	2001	..	..	..	:	..	:	..	..	..	..	..	..	..	..	..	..	52**	..
Philippines		1993	:	—	:	1	:	1	:	:	:	:	:	:	:	:	:	:	:	:
Viet Nam			2	—	5	—	3	—	..	..	68	..	68	..	..	..	68	..	68	..

Annex table 13. Premarital sexual behaviour and condom use among youth (most recent data available)

Region, subregion and country	Notes	Year*	A. Young people who have had premarital sex in the past year (percentage) Sex and age in years						B. Young people using a condom during premarital sex (percentage) Sex and age in years						C. Young people using a condom at last higher-risk sex (percentage) Sex and age in years					
			15-19		20-24		16-24		15-19		20-24		15-24		16-19		20-24		16-24	
			Males	Females	Males	Females	Males	Females	Males	Females	Males	Females	Males	Females	Males	Females	Males	Females	Males	Females
LATIN AMERICA AND THE CARIBBEAN																				
Bolivia		1989	..	7	..	15	..	9	..	..	..	..	..	..	..	..	..	..	..	..
Bolivia		1998	33	6	74	17	47	9	40	13	38	20	39	17	..	..	..	..	..	..
Bolivia	36,44	2003	33	12	70	28	45	16	37	23	37	19	37	21	37	21	36	20	37	20
Brazil		1986	..	5	..	15	..	8	..	..	..	..	..	..	..	..	..	..	..	..
Brazil	2	1991	..	6	..	15	..	9	..	..	..	..	..	..	..	..	..	..	..	..
Brazil		1996	54	17	83	37	65	23	61	35	59	32	60	33	60	34	59	31	59	32
Colombia		1986	..	5	..	14	..	8	..	..	..	..	..	..	..	..	..	..	..	..
Colombia		1990	..	7	..	20	..	12	..	..	..	..	..	..	..	.*	..	..	..	..
Colombia		1995	..	13	..	31	..	19	..	20	..	22	..	21	..	..	..	..	..	..
Colombia		2000	..	23	..	49	..	32	..	33	..	31	..	32	..	..	..	..	..	..
Dominican Republic		1991	..	4	..	6	..	5	..	..	..	..	..	..	..	..	..	..	..	..
Dominican Republic	35,42	1996	38	4	76	16	52	8	46	14	49	15	48	15	45	11	50	12	48	12
Dominican Republic		2002	38	9	74	25	52	13	50	32	55	29	53	31	51	29	53	30	52	29
Guatemala		1987	..	2	..	5	..	2	..	..	..	..	..	..	..	..	..	..	..	..
Haiti		1994	40	13	71	28	52	17	..	..	..	..	..	..	..	..	..	..	..	..
Haiti		2000	39	14	65	37	47	21	31	25	31	28	31	26	33	20	27	18	30	19
Honduras		1996	..	3	..	10	..	5	..	..	..	..	..	..	..	..	..	..	..	..
Paraguay		1990	..	13	..	37	..	20	..	..	..	..	..	..	..	..	..	..	..	..
Peru		1991/92	..	7	..	16	..	10	..	..	..	..	..	..	..	..	..	..	..	..
Peru		2000	..	8	..	22	..	13	..	16	..	23	..	20	..	..	..	..	..	..
Trinidad and Tobago		1987	..	1	..	1	..	1	..	..	..	..	..	..	..	..	..	..	..	..

Source: MEASURE DHS (2007) (accessed at http://www.measuredhs.org on 23 March 2007).

Indicator information:

A. Young people who have had premarital sex in the past year
Definition: the percentage of young never-married people (aged 15-24 years) who have had sex in the past 12 months of all young single people surveyed.
Numerator: the number of young never-married respondents aged 15-24 years who report having had any sex in the past 12 months.
Denominator: total number of never-married respondents aged 15-24 years.

B. Young people using a condom during premarital sex
Definition: the percentage of young never-married people (aged 15-24 years) who used a condom at last sex, of all young, single, sexually active people surveyed.
Numerator: the number of never-married respondents aged 15-24 years who report having used a condom the last time they had sex in the past 12 months.
Denominator: total number of never-married respondents aged 15-24 years who report having had sex in the past 12 months.

C. Young people using a condom at last higher-risk sex
Definition: the percentage of young people (aged 15-24 years) who used a condom at last sex with a non-marital, non-cohabiting partner, of those who have had sex with a non-marital, non-cohabiting partner in the past 12 months.
Numerator: the number of respondents aged 15-24 years who report having used a condom the last time they had sex with a non-marital, non-cohabiting partner in the past 12 months.
Denominator: total number of respondents aged 15-24 years who report having had sex with a non-marital, non-cohabiting partner in the past 12 months.

In certain cases, definitions of samples, numerators and denominators vary. Please see MEASURE DHS (2007) at http://www.measuredhs.org for full details.

Notes:
Two dots (..) indicate that data are not available or are not separately reported. A dash (—) indicates that the amount is nil or negligible.
* Year(s) as indicated in each respective survey.
** Figures marked with an asterisk are based on small denominators (typically 25-49 unweighted cases). Figures with denominators of fewer than 25 cases are not displayed.

Reproductive health and HIV/AIDS

Annex table 14. Precocious sexual behaviour and condom use at first sex among youth (most recent data available)

Region, subregion and country	Notes	Year	A. Percentage of youth having sex before the age of 15 years						B. Percentage of youth using a condom at first sex					
			15-19		20-24		15-24		15-19		20-24		15-24	
			Males	Females	Males	Females	Males	Females	Males	Females	Males	Females	Males	Females
AFRICA														
Sub-Saharan Africa														
Burkina Faso		2003	5	7	2	7	4	7	..	..	..	..	..	..
Cameroon		2004	11	18	11	22	11	20	31	24	25	14	27	18
Côte d'Ivoire		1998	14	22	18	24	16	23	..	..	..	..	..	..
Ethiopia		2000	5	13	3	19	4	16	..	..	..	..	..	..
Ghana		2003	4	7	4	8	4	7	34	28	39	19	37	22
Kenya		1993	..	15	28	18	..	16	..	..	..	..	..	..
Kenya		1998	32	15	34	17	32	16	..	..	..	..	..	..
Kenya		2003	..	..	..	..	..	..	10	12	17	12	14	12
Mali		2001	11	26	11	30	11	28	..	..	..	..	..	..
Mozambique		1997	24	29	13	32	19	30	..	..	..	..	..	..
Mozambique		2003	31	28	18	28	26	28	8	13	8	5	8	8
Namibia		2000	31	10	23	8	27	9	..	..	..	..	..	..
Nigeria		1990	..	24	..	28	..	26	..	..	..	..	..	..
Nigeria		1999	8	16	11	21	9	18	..	..	..	..	..	..
Nigeria		2003	8	20	5	21	7	21	11	7	20	6	17	6
Rwanda		2000	9	3	7	4	8	3	..	..	..	..	..	..
Tanzania, United Republic of		1999	24	14	14	16	20	15	..	..	..	..	..	..
Tanzania, United Republic of		2004	13	11	5	14	9	12	18	20	21	10	20	14
Uganda		2000/01	16	14	8	21	12	17	..	..	..	..	..	..
Uganda		2004/05	16	12	11	17	14	14	31	42	34	22	33	29
Zambia		1996	39	22	32	22	36	22	..	..	..	..	..	..
Zambia		2001/02	27	17	24	18	26	18	..	..	..	..	..	..
LATIN AMERICA AND THE CARIBBEAN		2003												
Bolivia	1	2003	15	6	21	7	18	6	18	..	13	..	15	..
Brazil		1991	..	..	..	..	..	..	..	6	..	2	..	3
Brazil		1996	..	..	..	..	..	..	33	19	19	12	25	14
Ecuador		1999	..	..	..	..	..	..	..	3	..	3	..	3
Haiti		1994	20	8	14	9	17	9	..	2	..	2	..	3
Honduras		1996	27	..	24	..	26	..	..	2	..	2	..	2

Source: MEASURE DHS (2007) (accessed at http://www.measuredhs.org on 23 March 2007).

Notes:

Two dots (..) indicate that data are not available or are not separately reported. An em dash (—) indicates that an amount is nil or negligible.

1. Survey was only of the north-east region of Brazil, and the sample included husbands (instead of all men).

Indicator information:

A. Percentage of youth having sex before the age of 15 years
Definition: percentage of young people aged 15-24 years who have had sex before the age of 15.
Numerator: young people aged 15-24 years who report their age at first sex as under 15 years.
Denominator: all young people aged 15-24 years.

B. Percentage of youth using a condom at first sex
Definition: percentage of young people aged 15-24 years who used a condom the first time they ever had sex, of those who have ever had sex.
Numerator: the number of respondents aged 15-24 years who report having used a condom the first time they ever had sex.
Denominator: total number of respondents aged 15-24 years who report that they have ever had sex.